Eye Diseases - Recent Advances, New Perspectives and Therapeutic Options

Edited by Salvatore Di Lauro, Sara Crespo Millas and David Galarreta Mira

Published in London, United Kingdom

Eye Diseases - Recent Advances, New Perspectives and Therapeutic Options
http://dx.doi.org/10.5772/intechopen.100984
Edited by Salvatore Di Lauro, Sara Crespo Millas and David Galarreta Mira

Contributors
María del Rosario Sánchez Valerio, Nazario Bautista-Elivar, Ricardo Cruz-Castillo, Ilaria Piano, Claudia Gargini, Francesca Corsi, Khadija Abdulaziz Lawan, Abdulhadi Sale Kumurya, Stephanie M. Llop, Erick Rivera-Grana, Mohamed Al-Abri, Ahmed Al-Hinai, Nawal Al-Fadhil, Alada Joel James, Jordana Sandes, Giulia Regattieri, Gabriela Cecilio Ventura Bariani Belem, Maria Cristina Curatolo, Maria Grazia Mazzone, Santa Viola, Carmela Giovanna Spoto, Luca Rosario La Rosa, Andrea Sudano Roccaro, Cristina Zappulla, Manuela Santonocito, Claudine Civiale, May Griffith, Kamal Malholtra, Ejaz Ansari, Cristian de los Santos, Lidia Cocho, Josê María Herreras, Salvatore Di Lauro, Sara Crespo Millas, David Galarreta Mira, Maria Isabel López Gálvez

First published in London, United Kingdom, 2023 by IntechOpen
IntechOpen is the global imprint of INTECHOPEN LIMITED, registered in England and Wales, registration number: 11086078, 5 Princes Gate Court, London, SW7 2QJ, United Kingdom

British Library Cataloguing-in-Publication Data
A catalogue record for this book is available from the British Library

Additional hard and PDF copies can be obtained from orders@intechopen.com

Eye Diseases - Recent Advances, New Perspectives and Therapeutic Options
Edited by Salvatore Di Lauro, Sara Crespo Millas and David Galarreta Mira
p. cm.
Print ISBN 978-1-80356-416-6
Online ISBN 978-1-80356-417-3
eBook (PDF) ISBN 978-1-80356-418-0

For EU product safety concerns:
IN TECH d.o.o., Prolaz Marije Krucifikse Kozulić 3, 51000 Rijeka, Croatia,
info@intechopen.com or visit our website at intechopen.com.

Meet the editors

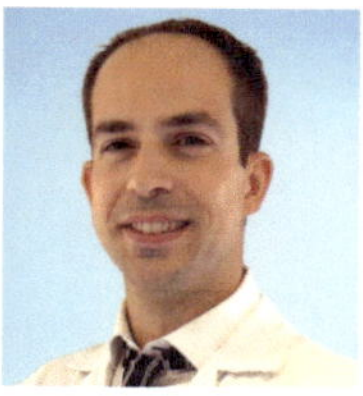

Salvatore Di Lauro graduated in medicine and surgery from the University of Naples "Federico II" (Italy) in 2009. He obtained a Master's degree in vitreo-retina from the University of Valladolid (Spain), becoming a specialist in ophthalmology. He is a Fellow of the European Board of Ophthalmology and has been an Honorific Collaborator of the University of Valladolid. He is an active researcher in retinal and ocular surface diseases, participating as investigator and study coordinator in numerous clinical trials, and has published several papers and book chapters. He is part of the REPRISE (database of expert reviewers created by the Italian Ministry of Education, Universities and Research).

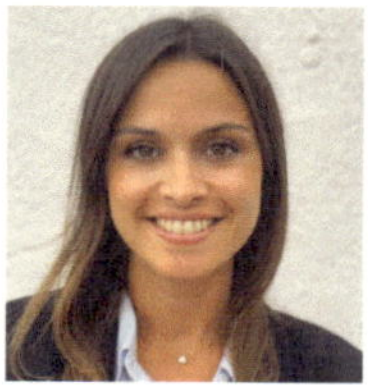

Sara Crespo Millas graduated in medicine and surgery from the Autonomous University of Madrid (Spain), receiving a Master's degree in vitreo-retina from the University of Valladolid (Spain), and the title of specialist in ophthalmology. She is a researcher in retinal and ocular surface diseases, participating as an investigator in various clinical trials, and has presented at several recent international congresses.

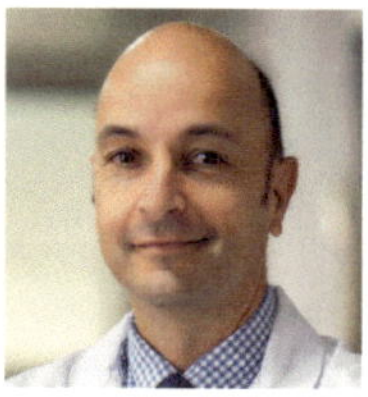

David Galarreta Mira graduated in medicine and surgery from the University of Navarra (Spain) and obtained his Ph.D. in medicine and surgery from the University of Valladolid (Spain). He is an associate researcher at the Recognized Research Group (GIR) of Optical Diagnostic Techniques (TOD) at the University of Valladolid, an associate researcher in the Results-Oriented Cooperative Research Networks in Health (RICORS), and has been the principal investigator for many clinical trials and competitive projects. He is the author of multiple publications and book chapters.

Contents

Preface

Ophthalmology is continuously evolving, with new imaging techniques, diagnostic tools and therapeutic options. The reader will find in this book a combination of review chapters from international experts and original research chapters, including recent innovations in ophthalmology.

The chapters in Section 1 are written by authors working on the ground with direct experience with diagnostic and therapeutic challenges. They discuss infectious diseases associated with ophthalmic surgery and diseases from developing countries that are often forgotten.

Section 2 discusses uveitis and immune-mediated diseases, a challenging and constantly growing area with new diagnostic and therapeutic options.

Section 3 reviews biomaterials for corneal regeneration, elucidating recent advances in this rapidly growing and important field.

Finally, Section 4 looks at fascinating advances in retinal imaging, such as optic coherence tomography angiography, which are changing our clinical practice and understanding of retinal diseases.

Our special thanks go to Prof. Ejaz Ansari and Prof. May Griffith for their scientific contributions, and to Marica Novakovic for her excellent work during the preparation of this book.

Salvatore Di Lauro MD, FEBO
Hospital Clínico Universitario de Valladolid (HCUV),
Ophthalmology Department,
Valladolid, Spain

Instituto Oftalmológico Recoletas (IOR),
Vitreo- Retinal Department,
Valladolid, Spain

Sara Crespo Millas MD
Hospital Clínico Universitario de Valladolid (HCUV),
Ophthalmology Department,
Valladolid, Spain

David Galarreta Mira Ph.D., MD
Hospital Clínico Universitario de Valladolid (HCUV),
Ophthalmology Department,
Valladolid, Spain

Instituto Oftalmológico Recoletas (IOR),
Ocular Surface Department,
Valladolid, Spain

Section 1

Infectious Diseases

Chapter 1

Infectious Endophthalmitis: Ongoing Challenges and New Prospectives

Mohamed Al-Abri, Ahmed Al-Hinai and Nawal Al-Fadhil

Abstract

Endophthalmitis is a rare but potentially sight and organ-threatening ocular emergency characterized by marked intraocular inflammation. It can be categorized into two broad categories of exogenous and endogenous types. Exogenous endophthalmitis is caused by inoculation of the globe by either bacterial or fungal microorganisms from an external environment and most commonly occurs as a complication of intraocular surgeries or procedures and open globe injuries. Blurred vision and pain are the main symptoms, and gram-positive coagulase-negative organisms are the main etiology of exogenous endophthalmitis. Endogenous endophthalmitis is caused by the hematogenous spread of microorganisms from distant sites of the body into the globe. Both categories lead to subsequent intraocular inflammation and potentially severe visual and anatomical devastating consequences. In addition, they have different risk factors and causative microorganisms, and thus, require somehow different diagnostic and treatment approaches. In this review chapter, further review of infectious endophthalmitis in terms of risk factors, causative pathogens, clinical presentations, prognosis, prevention, and the latest therapeutic recommendations are discussed.

Keywords: endophthalmitis, exogenous, endogenous, causes, treatment, prognosis

1. Introduction

Endophthalmitis in general is classified into infectious and non-infectious categories. Furthermore, infectious endophthalmitis is subclassified into exogenous and endogenous (**Box 1**) [1–5].

Although the term endophthalmitis refers to an infectious or non-infectious inflammation, its use often refers to an infectious origin. Exogenous endophthalmitis is caused by inoculation of the eye by either bacterial or fungal microorganisms from an external environment and most commonly occurs as a complication of ocular surgery, traumatic open globe injuries, or intravitreal injections [2]. Acute postoperative endophthalmitis occurs within 6 weeks of the intraocular surgery or procedure [3].

The incidence of endophthalmitis after various intraocular procedures is low, and it is illustrated in **Table 1** [6–15].

Endophthalmitis
- Infectious
  - ○ Exogenous
    - • Postoperative
      - • Acute
      - • Delayed onset
      - • Filtering bleb-associated
    - • Post-intraocular Injections
    - • Traumatic
  - ○ Endogenous
- Non-infectious
  - ○ Toxic Anterior Segment Syndrome (TASS)
  - ○ Lens-induced
  - ○ Others

Box 1.
Classification of Endophthalmitis.

Procedure	Incidence of endophthalmitis
Cataract extraction	0.053% to 0.145%
Pars Plana Vitrectomy	0.03% to 0.05%
Glaucoma filtering surgery	0.06% to 1.32%
Penetrating Keratoplasty	0.11% to 0.16%
Intravitreal injections	0.04% to 0.08%

Table 1.
Different intraocular procedures and incidence of endophthalmitis.

Pathogen	Percentage (%)	Pathogen	Percentage (%)
Gram-positive bacteria	75–85%	**Gram-negative bacteria**	10–15%
Staphylococcus epidermidis	43%	*Pseudomonas*	8%
Staphylococcus spp.	57%	*Proteus*	5%
Staphylococcus aureus	15%	*Hemophilus influenzae*	Less than 1% (higher in late-onset bleb-associated)
Propionibacterium acnes	Rare	*Klebsiella*	Less than 1%
Bacillus cereus	1%	*Coliform* spp.	Less than 1%
Fungi	Rare		
Candida parapsilosis			
Aspergillus			
Cephalosporium spp.			

Table 2.
Microorganisms causing infectious endophthalmitis.

Causative microorganisms of infectious endophthalmitis in general are listed and summarized in **Table 2** [15]. Intraocular inflammation caused by viruses, protozoa, or helminths is usually named uveitis.

2. Acute postoperative infectious endophthalmitis

The onset of acute postoperative infectious endophthalmitis (APIE) onset is within 6 weeks from the intraocular procedure [3]. It has a typical presentation of severe ocular pain and reduction in vision. In addition; eyelid edema is observed in around one-third of the patients. The conjunctiva is congested and corneal edema is commonly present. Intraocular inflammatory signs (cells, fibrin, and hypopyon) are the main findings and these involve both anterior chamber (AC) and the vitreous cavity. The red reflex is usually absent in the affected eye. Hypopyon and fibrinous reaction in the AC are typical features of APIE. B-scan ultrasound, usually, reveals vitreous hyperechoic opacities due to vitritis (**Figure 1**).

The APIE can be also subclassified into early (within 7 days after surgery) or late (8 days to 6 weeks after surgery) [16]. The early type is usually caused by gram-negative bacteria and usually has worse visual acuity at presentation and carries a poor visual prognosis. However, the late type is usually caused by gram-positive bacteria (frequently coagulase-negative staphylococci) and the presenting visual acuity is usually better than the early type with better visual prognosis.

Early diagnosis and prompt intervention of APIE are crucial. The guidelines from Endophthalmitis Vitrectomy Study (EVS) are usually adopted to treat patients with APIE based on the visual acuity on presentation. If the affected eye has a visual acuity of hand motion or better than a tapping-injection procedure is recommended. Pars plana vitrectomy with vitreous specimen collection and intravitreal injection of antibiotics, is recommended for an eye with visual acuity of light perception or worse. According to EVS, tapping of the vitreous yields more positive microbial results than taping from the anterior chamber. Intravitreal injection of antibiotics should cover both gram-positive and gram-negative bacteria. The most common intravitreal antibiotics being used are vancomycin (1 gm/0.1 ml) and ceftazidime (2.25 mg/0.1 ml).

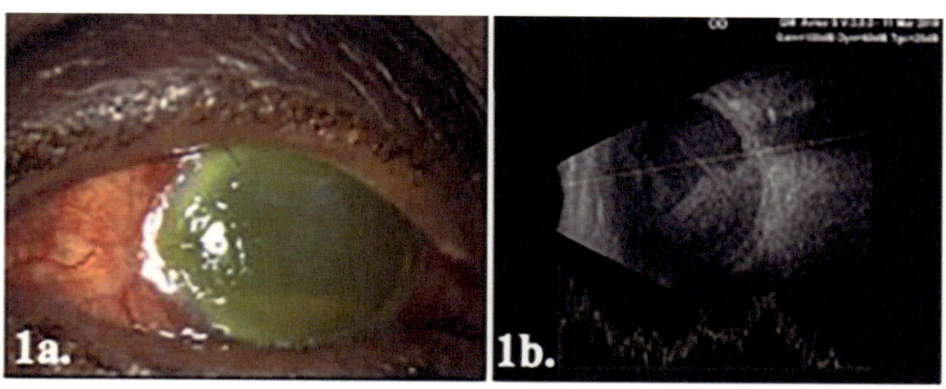

Figure 1.
Acute postoperative (phaco +PCIOL) endophthalmitis secondary to Serratia marcescens. Anterior segment photo of the right eye shows diffuse lid edema, diffuse and severe conjunctival chemosis, diffuse corneal cloudiness, organized hypopyon, iris details not visualized (1a) and B-scan shows diffuse vitreous hyperechoic opacities and attached retina (1b).

Amikacin (0.4 mg/0.1 ml) can be used as an alternative for ceftazidime. The visual prognosis for an eye with APIE is promising after early and appropriate intervention. After 9–12 months of follow-up of treated eyes; 53% of eyes had visual acuity of 6/12 or better and only 11% had worse than 6/240 [3].

3. Delayed-onset postoperative infectious endophthalmitis

Delayed-onset postoperative infectious endophthalmitis occurs beyond 6 weeks after the intraocular procedure [3]. It is a synonym that is usually used to describe chronic postoperative endophthalmitis (CPE) [17]. This type of endophthalmitis has a diagnostic and therapeutic dilemma and requires a high index of suspension because other causes may mimic its presentation. Hence, patients with CPE are frequently treated with corticosteroids due to the masquerading presentation of autoimmune intraocular inflammation. CPE was first described in the 1980s and the microorganisms that are responsible for CPE are somewhat different from that of APIE. They are usually low virulent and indolent. Specific groups of bacteria and fungi are considered to be causative pathogens for CPE (**Table 3**) [17–21].

It was observed that CPE has a lower incidence rate than APIE. Its incidence is around 0.017% after cataract surgery [20]. Some studies reported a ratio of acute to chronic postoperative endophthalmitis between 5:1 and 2:1 [17].

Propionibacterium acne, which is a gram-positive, non-spore-forming anaerobic bacillus bacteria, and found usually in skin and hair follicles; is considered to be the most common causative pathogen for CPE. Around two-thirds of the CPE, cases are found to have Propionibacterium acne [21].

The clinical features of CPE are less aggressive than that of APIE. It occurs 6 weeks to months after the intraocular procedure. Usually, the affected eye shows a persistent or recurrent low-grade indolent inflammation [22, 23]. The inflammation is often granulomatous with large keratic precipitates. The ocular pain is usually not severe, but reduced vision is common in almost all patients. Hypopyon is not a frequent

Bacteria	**Fungi**
Propionibacterium acnes	Aspergillus species
Staphylococcus species	*Candida species*
Corynebacterium	*Curvularia lunata*
Nocardia	*Fonsecaea pedrosoi*
Cephalosporium and Acremonium	*Paecilomyces species*
Paecilomyces	*Acremonium strictum*
Ochrobactrum anthropic	
Hafnia alvei	
Sphingomona spaucimobilis	
Mycobacterium chlonae	
Pseudomonas stutzeri	
Achromobacter	

Table 3.
Microorganisms that are associated with CPE.

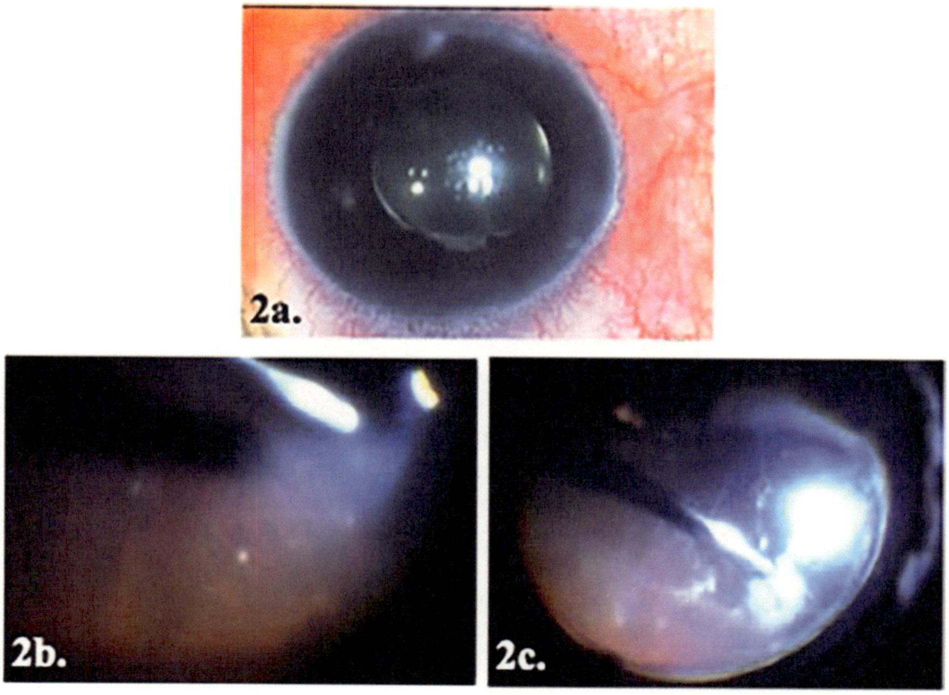

Figure 2.
Delayed-onset endophthalmitis due to P. acne. Anterior segment photo shows clear cornea and plaques on the posterior capsule (2a) and intraoperatively photos show moderately inflamed vitreous (2b & 2c) (Courtesy of Dr. Hemant Trehan).

finding, but microhypopyon may present. Other associated clinical features include conjunctival congestion and photophobia. An important feature in CPE is the presence of white plaques in the capsule. These plaques are associated with a different variety of microorganisms that causes CPE and not only P. acne (**Figure 2**) [20].

Management of CPE is somewhat challenging due to the ambiguous presentation. Many patients with CPE are treated initially with steroids and which may result in a partial response. However; the indolent inflammation persists and recurs after tapering down or discontinuation of the steroids. Furthermore, patients with fungal etiology might get worsening signs if steroid treatment is commenced. There is no standard treatment protocol known for CPE like the one which is known for APIE (i.e., EVS recommendations). However, in real-life practice, treatment may include intravitreal injection of antibiotics alone as an initial treatment or with pars plana vitrectomy (PPV) along with partial or total capsulotomy and removal or exchange of the intraocular lens (IOL) is performed [17]. In addition, sending the IOL with the capsule to a microbiology lab is recommended in the management plan of CPE. The use of empiric intravitreal antibiotics is recommended when treating chronic endophthalmitis. Patients with highly suspected or culture-proven fungal endophthalmitis to be monitored and treated with anti-fungal therapy, such as intraocular amphotericin (5–10 μg in 0.1 ml).

The outcome after treating CPE depends on the causative pathogen. In general, visual acuity of 20/40 or better can be achieved in 29–50% after treatment. Eyes with CPE caused by P. acne or other gram-positive bacteria has a better outcome [17]. However, CPE caused by fungus carries poor visual outcome [20].

4. Bleb-associated postoperative infectious endophthalmitis

Endophthalmitis is a sight-threatening rare complication of glaucoma surgery. Mostly delayed in onset. The rates of endophthalmitis associated with glaucoma filtering surgeries vary with surgical technique and use of antimetabolite agents. A study based on 5-year, retrospective data showed a 0.55% risk of blebitis and 0.45–1.3% risk of endophthalmitis after glaucoma filtering surgery [21]. The tube versus trabeculectomy study (TVT) reported endophthalmitis developed in 1 of 107 in the tube group and 5 of 105 in the trabeculectomy group over five years [22].

Early bleb-associated postoperative endophthalmitis is rare with a reported incidence of 0.1% [22]. Majority of bleb-associated postoperative endophthalmitis occurs months to years after the original procedure.

There are multiple reported risk factors under this entity. Among these are; cystic bleb, which may create direct access of pathogens to the eye either by the high permeability of the cystic wall or by the relatively frequent coexistence of a conjunctival leak [23]. Use of antimetabolites, such as mitomycin C and 5-fluorouracil, changes the thickness, cellularity, and vascularity of the overlying conjunctiva, which increases the risk of developing endophthalmitis. Furthermore, the use of these agents weakens the barrier against the migration of bacteria across the bleb wall. Patients with recurrent or persistent bleb leak are more at risk of developing endophthalmitis [24]. Hence, screening for bleb leakage following each visit is recommended among patients with trabeculectomy surgery. Finally, an inferiorly located bleb is more likely to lead to endophthalmitis than a superiorly located one probably due more to exposure of the bleb to the bacteria-rich tear film [23].

Patients with bleb-associated postoperative endophthalmitis may present with a drop in vision, redness, and eye discharges. It is often preceded by the accelerated prodromal syndrome of brow ache, ocular pain, and headache, which progress rapidly over a short period of few hours [3].

Clinically, the visual acuity is significantly reduced and anterior segment evaluation may reveal discoloration or mucopurulent discharge within the bleb described as a "white on red" appearance against conjunctival erythema. The anterior chamber may show the cellular reaction of cells, flare, and/or hypopyon. Seidel test may identify early bleb leak. Posterior segment evaluation may show vitreous cells and filaments, however, if dense vitritis, fundus view might be obscured, and hence, the B-scan ultrasonography is indicated to confirm vitreous involvement and rule out complications, such as retinal detachment.

True bleb-associated postoperative endophthalmitis must be differentiated from blebitis. In blebitis, there is a chalky white bleb surrounded by conjunctival injection and might be associated with a bleb leak and mild anterior chamber cellular reaction without significant vitritis. The diagnosis is based on a clinical exam and confirmed by standard adequate vitreous or aqueous sample for culture and sensitivity.

The array of organisms associated with bleb-related endophthalmitis differs from those associated with cataract surgery. Bleb-related endophthalmitis is mostly preceded by bleb infection, therefore, clinicians must be more aggressive in the treatment of blebitis. This includes oral and hourly topical fourth-generation antibiotics and daily monitoring for signs of progression, which includes assessment of the bleb, anterior chamber, and anterior vitreous face until a positive response to therapy is observed [25].

Intravitreal antibiotics, the combination of vancomycin (for gram-positive coverage) and ceftazidime (for gram-negative coverage) commonly administered during vitreous tap & inject. Intravitreal amphotericin B and voriconazole are considered if a fungal infection is suspected and/or confirmed. The use of corticosteroids is controversial since their effect on the visual outcome is not yet known [26].

Following the endophthalmitis vitrectomy study (EVS) guidelines; patients presented with hand motion or better vision may be treated with tap and inject; on the other hand, patients with light perception or worse should be considered for immediate pars plana vitrectomy (PPV) and intravitreal antibiotics. However; the population EVS study did not include patients with post-glaucoma surgery endophthalmitis. Therefore, it might be fair to consider early vitrectomy in patients with more virulent organisms, and it has been shown that vitrectomy in such cases may produce more favorable outcomes [24, 26].

Although bleb-associated endophthalmitis carries a poor visual prognosis; early recognition and treatment are necessary for optimizing the outcome of filtering surgery. Therefore, it is important to inspect the bleb or tube at each visit for any evidence of leak or erosion and if endophthalmitis is suspected, immediate aggressive and appropriate treatment is initiated.

5. Endophthalmitis Post Pars Plana Vitrectomy (PPV)

Endophthalmitis post-PPV is relatively rare. The incidence has decreased from 0.3–0.14% to 0.0180.076% with improvement in VR instrumentations and techniques [27].

There are several reported predisposing factors under this entity; insufficient wound closure, hypotony from a sclerotomy leak, and vitreous incarceration at a sclerotomy site, are some risk factors as it allows migration of microorganisms into the vitreous cavity from the ocular surface [28–30].

Patients may present with symptoms and signs similar to endophthalmitis following cataract surgery in particular hypopyon and dense vitritis (**Figure 3**).

Vitreous samples should be obtained if endophthalmitis is suspected. A combination of broad-spectrum intravitreal antibiotics is injected intravitreally.

Multiple studies have reported several bacteria under such entity which include coagulase-negative staphylococci, Pseudomonas species, Propionibacterium, enterococci, and Bacillus species. However, coagulase-negative staphylococci are the most common organism [31].

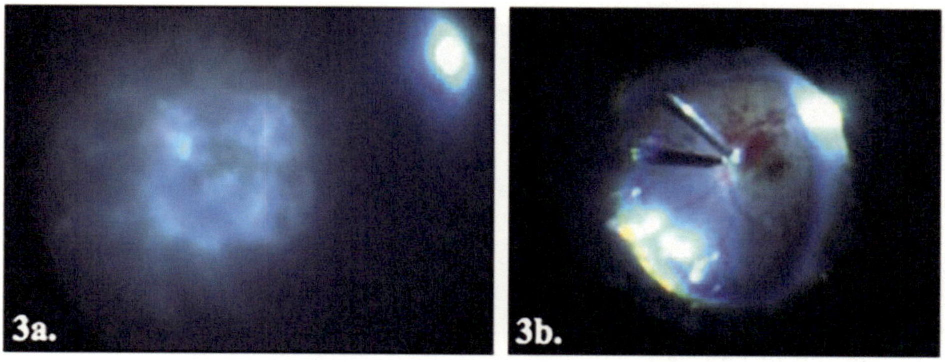

Figure 3.
Intraoperative photos of post PPV endophthalmitis. Intraoperatively photos showing dense vitritis suggestive of aggressive inflammation (3a) and clear vitreous after silicone oil removal (3b). (Courtesy of Dr. Hemant Trehan).

EVS did not enroll patients with post-PPV endophthalmitis, therefore, the results do not directly apply to the management of such entity. Nevertheless, certain principles apply.

On average, about 70% of all samples across studies have shown positive microbiology cultures. In a large multicenter study, Cohen et al. reported16 culture-positive cases out of 18 cases (89%) of endophthalmitis post-vitrectomy [32].

Despite treatment, the visual outcome varies. As described by Park et al., a significant proportion of cases have poor visual outcomes, with vision ranging from 20/200 to no light perception [33]. However, some cases achieved 20/40 vision [34, 35].

6. Endophthalmitis post-intravitreal injections

The use of intravitreal agents (e.g., Anti-VEGF and steroids) to treat various retinal diseases has increased significantly since the 1990s.

The incidence rate of infectious endophthalmitis after intravitreal injection is low when compared to other post-surgical infectious endophthalmitis, it varies between 0.038% and 0.053% [36].

The most commonly causative pathogens are Streptococcus or Staphylococcus species suggesting the commensal flora of the ocular adnexa and oropharynx as the source. Published reports confirmed that Streptococcus is significantly more frequent after intravitreal injection than after other intraocular surgeries [37, 38].

The use of post-injection antibiotics does not decrease the frequency of subsequent endophthalmitis; however, it may possibly cause drug-resistant bacteria in the nasopharynx [39].

Post-intravitreal infectious endophthalmitis should be differentiated from sterile endophthalmitis, a well-recognized condition that can occur after intravitreal injections. In the latter patients present with painless reduction in vision, no or minimum redness, anterior chamber cells, fibrin, and/or hypopyon. In the MARINA trial, there was a 1% rate of serious inflammation in patients who received intravitreal injection with ranibizumab [40].

In contrary, the presentation post-intravitreal infectious endophthalmitis is more aggressive similar to the presentation seen after other intraocular procedures; this may include significant painful loss of vision, marked anterior chamber cells, fibrinous reaction, hypopyon, and/or vitritis [41].

The outcome is variable. In a large series of post-intravitreal infectious endophthalmitis; most of the eyes that developed (15 of 23) returned to baseline vision within 3 months after treatment and there was no significant difference in the rate of endophthalmitis between the types of anti-VEGF injected [42].

7. Endophthalmitis post-penetrating keratoplasty

Endophthalmitis following penetrating keratoplasty (PK) occurs at a slightly higher rate compared to other intraocular procedures. The incidence ranges from 0.2% to 0.4% [43, 44].

Risk factors include; large circumferential incision, wound dehiscence, suture abscess, and contaminated donor tissue [44]. In addition, chronic use of topical steroids which are known to decrease immune defense may increase the risk of endophthalmitis.

Symptoms are similar to other types of postoperative endophthalmitis. The causative agents are predominantly gram-positive bacteria (Streptococcus and Staphylococcus). On the other hand, gram-negative bacteria account for nearly 20% of cases.

The outcomes can be devastating with severe visual loss in 50% of cases and often a requirement of repeat keratoplasty [45].

Overall, the frequency of endophthalmitis in modern corneal transplant surgery is expected to decrease significantly with the advancement in lamellar keratoplasty. In a study conducted by Heinzelmann et al., it was apparent that the outcome of lamellar endothelial keratoplasty and Descemet membrane endothelial keratoplasty is superior to PK without serious complications, such as exogenous endophthalmitis [46].

8. Post-traumatic infectious endophthalmitis

Post-traumatic endophthalmitis is an uncommon yet devastating complication of open globe injuries. It has a poorer outcome compared to postoperative endophthalmitis due to concomitant ocular tissue damage, presence of more virulent pathogens, and possibly due delay in diagnosis and treatment.

The reported incidence of infectious endophthalmitis following open globe injuries ranges from 3.1% to 11.9% of open globe injuries in the absence of an intraocular foreign body (IOFB) [47–52]. The incidence increases from 3.8% to 48.1%, in the presence of an IOFB, with higher infection rates with retained IOFBs contaminated with organic matter from a rural setting [53–57].

The following factors are associated with an increased risk of post-traumatic endophthalmitis: intraocular foreign bodies (IOFB) [58–62], violation of the lens capsule [58, 60–62], contamination of the wound [59, 61] and delayed primary repair [58, 61, 63]. Interestingly, the existence of hyphema or iris prolapse was associated with lower rates of endophthalmitis [64].

Recognizing symptoms of post-traumatic endophthalmitis might be challenging due to the presence of injury-induced inflammation and the disruption of ocular structures [65]. Pain and decreased visual acuity often occur with ocular injury with or without infection. Presence of worsening symptoms of photophobia, tearing and pain are suggestive of infectious endophthalmitis. Pain from ocular injury can be distinguished from that of endophthalmitis if it is progressive and out of proportion to the degree of injury [66–70]. Inflammatory signs are almost similar to other types of endophthalmitis (i.e., eyelid edema, chemosis, corneal edema, hypopyon, variable degree of vitritis, etc.), however, purulent discharge from the site of injury is a feature of post-traumatic endophthalmitis. Inflammation that progresses slowly following primary repair may be indicative of fungal endophthalmitis [67, 69].

The broad spectrum of pathogens causing post-traumatic endophthalmitis, with gram-positive cocci the most frequently identified causative organism, followed by Bacillus species, fungi, and mixed infections. In a large cohort of post-traumatic endophthalmitis cases, Long et al. have reported that 38.1% of cases of post-traumatic endophthalmitis were culture-positive, and 3.2% showed mixed infections (gram-negative bacilli and fungi). Culture proven pathogens included gram-positive cocci (41.9%), gram-negative bacilli (29.1%), gram-positive bacilli (12.3%), and fungi (16.8%). In the same reported series, the coagulase-negative staphylococcal (CNS) species S. epidermidis (21.8%) and S. saprophyticus (12.0%) were the predominant pathogens, followed by Bacillus subtilis (8.7%), Pseudomonas aeruginosa (7.8%),

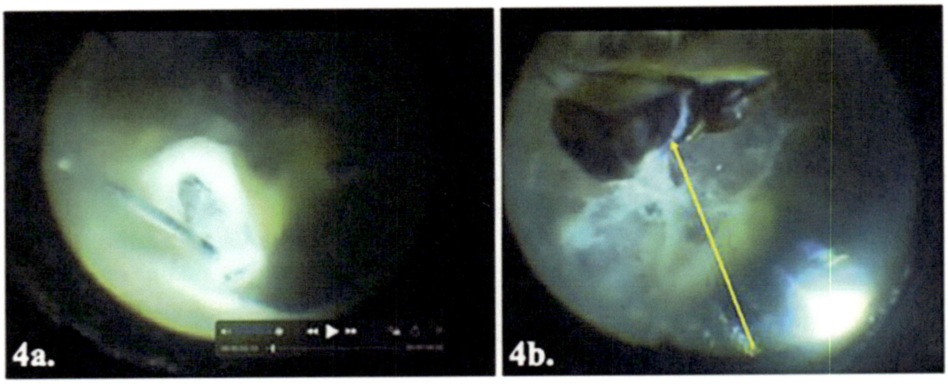

Figure 4.
Post-traumatic endophthalmitis with IOFB. Intraoperatively photos showing densely infiltrated vitreous suggest aggressive organism (4a) and large IOFB being removed with suture snare (yellow arrow) (4b). (Courtesy of Dr. Hemant Trehan).

and Escherichia coli (6.4%). Delayed repair over 24 hours and metallic injury were significantly associated with a positive culture of CNS. The most frequent fungal species were Aspergillus (33%), followed by yeast-like fungi (30%) [51]. In another cohort of post-traumatic endophthalmitis; Clostridium perfringens were isolated in 16.6% of culture-positive cases [71].

To reduce the risk of post-traumatic endophthalmitis, it is widely accepted common practice to immediate initiation of empirical prophylactic systemic antibiotics (either intravenous or oral administration) at initial presentation for all open globe injuries and an injection of intravitreal antibiotics at the time of primary repair for high-risk patients [72–75].

In a meta-analysis report, it has been noted that the incidence of endophthalmitis post open globe injuries has reduced significantly when intravitreal/intracameral antibiotics were used intraoperatively without additional benefit on the final visual outcome [76].

The threshold for vitrectomy in cases of post-traumatic endophthalmitis is low. Vitrectomy should be performed if there is no response to intravitreal antibiotics within 24 hours or if associated with complications like retinal detachment or intraocular foreign body (**Figure 4**).

In general, the visual prognosis of post-traumatic endophthalmitis is worse than that of post-operative endophthalmitis [77, 78]. The virulence of the microorganisms in post-traumatic endophthalmitis, for example, Bacillus cereus carries a very high risk of progressing to a final visual acuity of NLP [79]. A delay in diagnosis and initiation of appropriate therapy is an important risk factor that contributes to poor visual prognosis. Moreover, the presence of an afferent pupillary defect, perforating injury, expelled lens, corneoscleral wound (vs corneal wound), and retinal detachment at the time of ocular injury is associated with a poor visual prognosis even in the absence of endophthalmitis [80].

9. Endogenous endophthalmitis

Endogenous endophthalmitis (EE), also called metastatic endophthalmitis, occurs as a result of the hematogenous spread of microorganisms from the body to the eye. The microorganism primarily spreads through the posterior segment vessels. The right eye is more commonly affected due to dominant and direct blood flow from the right carotid artery, however, approximately 25% of cases have a bilateral presentation [81].

The reported incidence of EE is 2 to 8% [82, 83]. However, it has been reported that the causative pathogens have geographical variations. They can be fungal or bacterial, with fungal pathogens being the commonest [82]. According to reported cases from Asia, fungal EE accounts for nearly 11.1 to 17.54% of total cases [84]. In bacterial EE, gram-positive streptococcus and staphylococcus are the most common pathogens. Gram-negative bacterial EE, however, is more common in Asian countries [85]. Among fungal species, *Candida albicans* account for many cases being the most common yeast, and among the molds, *Aspergillus flavus* is the commonest [86].

The risk factors for EE are primarily systemic conditions or medications which reduce immunity. Among these are diabetes mellitus, malignancies, asplenia, cardiac or renal transplant, and severe infections (e.g., pneumonia, urinary tract infection, vertebral osteomyelitis, liver abscess, and acquired immune deficiency syndrome), chronic alcoholism, intravenous catheters, and drug abuse and long-term use of steroids or other immunosuppressants [87–90].

The patients with the aforementioned risk factors and associated with ophthalmic symptoms require a thorough ophthalmic assessment to rule out EE. Such symptoms vary from eye pain, redness, photophobia, blurred vision, floaters, and flashes. The clinical signs are similar to other types of endophthalmitis, however, in EE the vitreous involvement, for example, vitreous haze, vitreous cells and floaters as well as subretinal membranes and exudates are the most important associated findings to look for [91, 92]. Aspergillus flavus is known to cause yellow/white exudates in the vitreous, which vary from focal to diffuse. The hallmark feature of Candida EE is the presence of fluffy cotton wool-like white retinal exudates or colonies along with vitritis (**Figure 5**) [92].

The management of EE should be focused on systemic evaluation and management of underlying causes. In addition to clinical evaluation, a B scan ultrasound may delineate choroidal abscess, which appears as a dome-shaped elevation on B scan similar to choroidal detachment [93].

Blood cultures and urine cultures are important adjuvant diagnostic modality in the diagnosis of possible systemic infection. It was reported that blood culture has shown a higher culture positivity than the vitreous sample, probably due to the

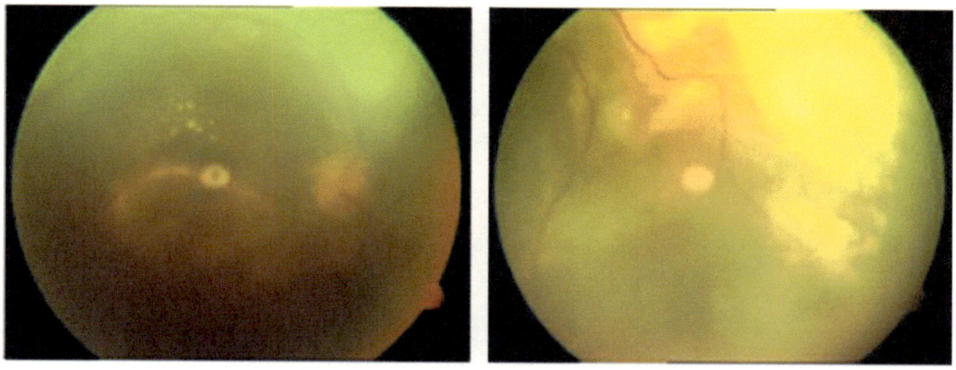

Figure 5.
Bilateral endogenous Nocardia endophthalmitis. Note the subretinal infiltrates and vitirtis. (Courtesy of Dr. Hemant Trehan).

sample volume obtained. Moreover, culture at extraocular sites has yielded a 21–100% positivity rate as per previous reports [94].

Medical management includes topical and systemic antibiotics or antifungals, intravitreal antibiotics or antifungals, and pars plana vitrectomy (PPV). PPV is recommended for non-resolving vision-threatening EE cases. PPV serves both diagnostic and therapeutic purposes. Sato et al. suggested early vitrectomy in Candida EE cases [95]. Yoon et al. suggested early PPV in Klebsiella endophthalmitis, which may result in better visual effects [96]. The collaboration of the treating ophthalmologist or vitreoretinal surgeon, microbiologists, pathologists, and the critical care physician plays a vital role in determining the patient's final systemic and ocular outcome [82].

Prognosis of EE similar to other endophthalmitis depends on the duration of the condition, the extent of the ocular structures involved, the virulence of the causative agents, and the timing of initiation of treatment as well as the response to the treatment. Reported studies have shown that yeasts have a better prognosis, followed by bacteria followed by molds, which have the worst prognosis.

10. Conclusion

Endophthalmitis is a devastating ophthalmic emergency that may lead to total loss of vision and possibly the eye if it is not recognized and managed promptly. In addition to eye caregivers, patients undergoing intraocular surgeries must be counseled about this rare condition as well as the potential further sequala that might occur with or without treatment are critical. With the advancements in VR instrumentations and techniques, the threshold of diagnostic and therapeutic PPV and appropriate intravitreal antibiotics and/or antifungals in the management of endophthalmitis is very low. Finally, frontline health care providers must be aware and critical if they encounter patients with suspicious of endophthalmitis as early recognition, prompt referral, and timely treatment are very crucial aspects for better visual prognosis.

Acknowledgements

We would like to thank Dr. Hemant Trehan, sr. consultant VR surgeon, Al Nahdha hospital, Ministry of Health, Muscat, Sultanate of Oman, for sharing clinical photos.

Author details

Mohamed Al-Abri*, Ahmed Al-Hinai and Nawal Al-Fadhil
Department of Ophthalmology, Sultan Qaboos University Hospital, Muscat, Sultanate of Oman

*Address all correspondence to: msalabri@squ.edu.om

References

[1] Mamalis N. Endophthalmitis. Journal of Cataract and Refractive Surgery. 2002;**28**:729-730

[2] Smith SR, Kroll AJ, Lou PL, Ryan EA. Endogenous bacterial and fungal endophthalmitis. International Ophthalmology Clinics. 2007;**47**:173-183

[3] Results of the Endophthalmitis Vitrectomy Study. A Randomized Trial of immediate vitrectomy and of intravenous antibiotics for the treatment of postoperative bacterial endophthalmitis. Archives of Ophthalmology. 1995;**113**(12):1479-1496

[4] Vaziri K, Schwartz SG, Kishor K, Flynn HW Jr. Endophthalmitis: State of the art. Clinical Ophthalmology. 2015;**9**:95-08

[5] Kresloff MS, Castellarin AA, Zarbin MA. Endophthalmitis. Survey Ophthalmology. 1998;**43**(3):193-224

[6] Kattan HM, Flynn HW Jr, Pflugfelder SC, Robertson C, Forster RK. Nosocomial endophthalmitis survey: Current incidence of infection after intraocular surgery. Ophthalmology. 1991;**98**(2):227-238

[7] Shi S-L, Yu X-N, Cui Y-L, Zheng S-F, Shentu X-C. Incidence of endophthalmitis after phacoemulsification cataract surgery: A Meta-analysis. International Journal of Ophthalmology. 2022;**15**(2):327-335

[8] Simonett JM, Choi RY, Flaxel CJ. Filtering-associated endophthalmitis after trabeculectomy or tube-shunt implant. Ophthalmology Retina. 2021;**5**(3):279-284

[9] Shah CP, Garg SJ, Vander JF, Brown GC, Kaiser RS, Haller JA. Outcomes and risk factors associated with endophthalmitis after intravitreal injection of anti-vascular endothelial growth factor agents. Ophthalmology. 2011 Oct;**118**(10):2028-2034

[10] Taban M, Behrens A, Newcomb RL, Nobe MY, Saedi G, Sweet PM, et al. Acute endophthalmitis following cataract surgery: A systematic review of the literature. Archives of Ophthalmology. 2005 May;**123**(5):613-620

[11] Bhende M, Raman R, Jain M, Shah PK, Sharma T, Gopal L, et al. Incidence, microbiology, and outcomes of endophthalmitis after 111,876 pars plana vitrectomies at a single, tertiary eye care hospital. PLoS One. 2018;**13**(1):e0191173

[12] Creuzot-Garcher C, Benzenine E, Mariet A-S, de Lazzer A, Chiquet C, Bron AM, et al. Incidence of Acute Postoperative Endophthalmitis after Cataract Surgery. A Nationwide Study in France from 2005 to 2014. Ophthalmology. 2016;**123**:1414-1420

[13] Chen JY, Jones MN, Srinivasan S, Neal TJ, John Armitage W, Kaye SB, et al. Endophthalmitis after penetrating keratoplasty. Ophthalmology. 2015;**122**:25-30

[14] Torres-Costa S, Ramos D, Brandão E, Carneiro Â, Rosas V, Rocha-Sousa A, et al. Incidence of endophthalmitis after intravitreal injection with and without topical antibiotic prophylaxis. European Journal of Ophthalmology. 2021;**31**(2):600-606

[15] Sunaric-Mégevand G, Pournaras CJ. Current approach to postoperative endophthalmitis. The British Journal of Ophthalmology. 1997;**81**(11):1006-1015

[16] Quinn CD, Flynn HW, Scott IU, Smiddy WE. Acute–onset endophthalmitis following cataract surgery: Association between time of diagnosis, causative organism, and final visual acuity outcome. Investigative Ophthalmology and Visual Science. 2004;**45**(13):522

[17] Maalouf F, Abdulaal M, Hamam RN. Chronic postoperative endophthalmitis: A review of clinical characteristics,microbiology, treatment strategies, and outcomes. International Journal of Inflammation. 2012;**2012**:6

[18] Meisler DM, Zakov ZN, Bruner WE, Hall GS, McMahon JT, Zachary AA, et al. Endophthalmitis associated with sequestered intraocular Propionibacterium acnes. American Journal of Ophthalmology. 1987;**104**(4):428-429

[19] Roussel TJ, Culbertson WW, Jaffe NS. Chronic postoperative endophthalmitis associated with Propionibacterium acnes. Archives of Ophthalmology. 1987;**105**(9):1199-1201

[20] Al-Mezaine HS, Al-Assiri A, Al-Rajhi AA. Incidence, clinical features, causative organisms, and visual outcomes of delayed-onset pseudophakic endophthalmitis. European Journal of Ophthalmology. 2009;**19**(5):804-811

[21] Kishor K, Vaziri K, Moshfeghi D, Schwartz S, Maharaj A, Moshfeghi A, et al. Incidence of bleb-associated endophthalmitis in the United States. Clinical Ophthalmology. 2015;**2015**:317

[22] Gedde S, Herndon L, Brandt J, Budenz D, Feuer W, Schiffman J. Postoperative complications in the tube versus trabeculectomy (TVT) Study during five years of follow-up. American Journal Of Ophthalmology. 2012;**153**(5):804

[23] Lehmann OJ, Bunce C, Matheson MM, Maurino V, Khaw PT, Wormald R, et al. Risk factors for development of post-trabeculectomy endophthalmitis. British Journal of Ophthalmology. 2000;**84**(12):1349-1353

[24] Busbee B, Recchia F, Kaiser R, Nagra P, Rosenblatt B, Pearlman R. Bleb-associated endophthalmitis. Ophthalmology. 2004;**111**(8):1495-1503

[25] Al-Turki TA, Al-Shahwan S, Al-Mezaine HS, Kangave D, Abu El-Asrar AM. Microbiology and visual outcome of bleb-associated endophthalmitis. Ocular Immunology and Inflammation. 2010;**18**(2):121-126

[26] Lemley C, Han D. Endophthalmitis. Retina. 2007;**27**(6):662-680

[27] Patel K, Rahman R. Incidence of post-operative endophthalmitis following 23-gauge transconjunctival sutureless vitrectomy in the United Kingdom: A survey. Eye. 2011;**25**(7):956-956

[28] Acar N, Kapran Z, Unver Y, Altan T, Ozdogan S. Early postoperative hypotony after 25-gauge sutureless vitrectomy with straight incisions. Retina. 2008;**28**:545-552

[29] Chen D, Lian Y, Cui L, Lu F, Ke Z, Song Z. Sutureless vitrectomy incision architecture in the immediate post-operative period evaluated in vivo using optical coherence tomography. Ophthalmology. 2010;**117**:2003-2009

[30] Gupta OP, Maguire JI, Eagle RC Jr, et al. The competency of pars plana vitrectomy incisions: A comparative histologic and spectrophotometric analysis. American Journal of Ophthalmology. 2009;**147**:243-250

[31] Oshima Y, Kadonosono K, Yamaji H, Inoue M, Yoshida M, Kimura H, et al.

Multicenter survey with a systematic overview of acute-onset endophthalmitis after transconjunctival microincision vitrectomy surgery. American Journal of Ophthalmology. 2010;**150**:716-725

[32] Cohen SM, Flynn HW Jr, Murray TG, Smiddy WE. Endophthalmitis after pars plana vitrectomy. The post vitrectomy endophthalmitis study group. Ophthalmology. 1995;**102**:702-712

[33] Park J, Ramasamy B, Ling R, Prasad S. Endophthalmitis following vitrectomy. Eye. 2011;**26**(3):482-482

[34] Bacon A, Davison C, Patel B, Frazer D, Ficker L, Dart J. Infective endophthalmitis following vitreoretinal surgery. Eye. 1993;**7**(4):529-534

[35] Scott I, Flynn H, Acar N, Dev S, Shaikh S, Mittra R, et al. Incidence of endophthalmitis after 20-gauge vs 23-gauge vs 25-gauge pars plana vitrectomy. Graefe's Archive for Clinical and Experimental Ophthalmology. 2011;**249**(3):377-380

[36] Levison A, Mendes T, Bhisitkul R. Postprocedural endophthalmitis: A review. Expert Review of Ophthalmology. 2013;**8**(1):45-62

[37] Irigoyen C, Ziahosseini K, Morphis G, Stappler T, Heimann H. Endophthalmitis following intravitreal injections. Graefe's Archive for Clinical and Experimental Ophthalmology. 2011;**250**(4):499-505

[38] Shah C, Garg S, Vander J, Brown G, Kaiser R, Haller J. Outcomes and risk factors associated with endophthalmitis after intravitreal injection of anti-vascular endothelial growth factor agents. Ophthalmology. 2011;**118**(10):2028-2034

[39] Kim SJ, Toma HS. Ophthalmic antibiotics and antimicrobial resistance a randomized, controlled study of patients undergoing intravitreal injections. Ophthalmology. 2011;**118**:1358-1353

[40] Rosenfeld PJ, Brown DM, Heier JS, et al. Ranibizumab for neovascular age-related macular degeneration. New England Journal of Medicine. 2006;**355**:1419-1431

[41] Roth DB, Modi KK, Scott IU, Flynn JR. Update on the Use of Intraocular Steroids for Posterior-Segment Diseases. 2013. Available from: https://www.retinalphysician.com/issues/2013/september-2013/update-on-the-use-of-intraocular-steroids-for-post

[42] Taban M, Behrens A, Newcomb RL, Nobe MY, McDonnell PJ. Incidence of acute endophthalmitis following penetrating keratoplasty: A systematic review. Archives of Ophthalmology. 2005;**123**(5):605-609

[43] Kitazawa K, Wakimasu K, Yoneda K, Iliakis B, Sotozono C, Kinoshita S. A case of fungal keratitis and endophthalmitis post penetrating keratoplasty resulting from fungal contamination of the donor cornea. American Journal of Ophthalmology Case Reports. 2017;**5**:103-106

[44] Bor E, Kremer I. Endophthalmitis and wound dehiscence following late removal of penetrating keratoplasty sutures. Ophthalmic Surgery, Lasers & Imaging. 2011;**42**(3):234-240

[45] Heinzelmann S, Böhringer D, Eberwein P, et al. Outcomes of Descemet membrane endothelial keratoplasty, Descemet stripping automated endothelial keratoplasty and penetrating keratoplasty from a single centre study. Graefes Archivrs for Clinical and Experimental Ophthalmology. 2016;**254**:515-522

[46] Fox GM, Joondeph BC, Flynn HW Jr, Pflugfelder SC, Roussel TJ. Delayed-onset

pseudophakic endophthalmitis. American Journal of Ophthalmology. 1991;**111**(2):163-173

[47] Hashemian H, Mirshahi R, Khodaparast M, Jabbarvand M. Post-cataract surgery endophthalmitis: Brief literature review. Journal of Current Ophthalmoogy. 2016;**28**(3):101-105

[48] Dave VP, Pathengay A, Sharma S, Govindhari V, Karolia R, Pappuru RR, et al. Clinical presentations and comparative outcomes of primary versus deferred intraocular lens explantation in delayed-onset endophthalmitis. Indian Journal of Ophthalmology. Jul 2019;**67**(7):1101-1104

[49] Barr CC. Prognostic factors in corneoscleral lacerations. Archives of Ophthalmology. 1983;**101**(6):919-924

[50] Essex RW, Yi Q, Charles PG, et al. Post-traumatic endophthalmitis. Ophthalmology. 2004;**111**(11):2015-2022

[51] Rubsamen PE, Cousins SW, Martinez JA. Impact of cultures on management decisions following surgical repair of penetrating ocular trauma. Ophthalmic Surgery and Lasers. 1997;**28**(1):43-49

[52] Sabaci G, Bayer A, Mutlu FM, et al. Endophthalmitis after deadly-weapon-related open-globe injuries: Risk factors, value of prophylactic antibiotics, and visual outcomes. American Journal of Ophthalmology. 2002;**133**(1):62-69

[53] Verbraeken H, Rysselaere M. Post-traumatic endophthalmitis. European Journal of Ophthalmology. 1994;**4**(1):1-5

[54] Zhang Y, Zhang MN, Jiang CH, Yao Y, Zhang K. Endophthalmitis following open globe injury. The British Journal of Ophthalmology. 2010;**94**(1):111-114

[55] Busbee BG. Advances in knowledge and treatment: An update on endophthalmitis. Current Opinion in Ophthalmology. 2004;**15**(3):232-237

[56] Campochiaro PA, Green WR. Toxicity of intravitreous ceftazidime in primate retina. Archives of Ophthalmology. 1992;**110**(11):1625-1629

[57] Cardillo JA, Stout JT, LaBree L, et al. Post-traumatic proliferative vitreoretinopathy. The epidemiologic profile, onset, risk factors, and visual outcome. Ophthalmology. 1997;**104**(7):1166-1173

[58] Cavallo JD, Ramisse F, Girardet M, et al. Antibiotic susceptibilities of 96 isolates of Bacillus anthracis isolated in France between 1994 and 2000. Antimicrobial Agents and Chemotherapy. 2002;**46**(7):2307-2309

[59] Cebulla CM, Flynn HW Jr. Endophthalmitis after open globe injuries. American Journal of Ophthalmology. 2009;**147**(4):567-568

[60] Mansouri M, Faghihi H, Hajizadeh F, et al. Epidemiology of open-globe injuries in Iran: Analysis of 2,340 cases in 5 years (report no. 1). Retina. 2009;**29**:1141-1149

[61] Jonas JB, Knorr HL, Budde WM. Prognostic factors in ocular injuries caused by intraocular or retrobulbar foreign bodies. Ophthalmology. 2000;**106**:823-828

[62] Ariyasu RG, Kumar S, Labrec LD, et al. Microorganisms cultured from the anterior chamber of ruptured globes at the time of repair. American Journal of Ophthalmology. 1995;**119**:181-188

[63] Duch-Samper AM, Menezo JL, Hurtado-Sarrio M. Endophthalmitis following penetrating eye injuries.

Acta Ophthalmologica Scandinavica. 1997;**75**:104-106

[64] Mieler WF, Ellis MK, Williams DF, Han DP. Retained intraocular foreign bodies and endophthalmitis. Ophthalmology. 1990;**97**:1532-1538

[65] William DF, Mieler WF, Abrams GW, Lewis H. Results and prognostic factors in penetrating ocular injuries with retained intraocular foreign bodies. Ophthalmology. 1988;**95**:911-916

[66] Aghihi H, Hajizadeh F, Esfahani MR, Rasoulinejad SA, Lashay A, Mirshahi A, et al. Posttraumatic endophthalmitis. Retina. 2012;**32**:146-151

[67] Parrish CM, O'Day DM. Traumatic endophthalmitis. International Ophthalmology Clinics. 1987;**27**(2):112-119

[68] Danis RP. Endophthalmitis. Ophthalmology Clinics of North America. 2002;**15**(2):243-248

[69] Peyman GA, Carroll CP, Raichand M. Prevention and management of traumatic endophthalmitis. Ophthalmology. 1980;**87**(4):320-324

[70] Reynolds DS, Flynn HW Jr. Endophthalmitis after penetrating ocular trauma. Current Opinion in Ophthalmology. 1997;**8**(3):32-38

[71] Long et al. Causative organisms of post-traumatic endophthalmitis: A 20-year retrospective study. BMC Ophthalmology. 2014;**14**:34

[72] Abu AM, Amro SA, Mosallam AA, Obeidan S. Post-traumatic endophthalmitis: Causative organisms and visual outcome. European Journal of Ophthalmology. 1999;**9**(1):21-31

[73] Narang S, Gupta V, Gupta A, Dogra MR, Pandav SS, Das S. Role of prophylactic intravitreal antibiotics in open globe injuries. Indian Journal of Ophthalmology. 2003;**51**(1):39-44

[74] Tabatabaei SA, Soleimani M, Behrooz MJ, Sheibani K. Systemic oral antibiotics as a prophylactic measure to prevent endophthalmitis in patients with open globe injuries in comparison with intravenous antibiotics. Retina. 2016;**36**(2):360-365

[75] Du Toit N, Mustak S, Cook C. Randomised controlled trial of prophylactic antibiotic treatment for the prevention of endophthalmitis after open globe injury at Groote Schuur Hospital. The British Journal of Ophthalmology. 2017;**101**(7):862-867

[76] Abouammoh MA, Al-Mousa A, Gogandi M, Al-Mezaine H, Osman E, Alsharidah AM, et al. Prophylactic intravitreal antibiotics reduce the risk of post-traumatic endophthalmitis after repair of open globe injuries. Acta Ophthalmologica. 2018;**96**(3):e361-e365

[77] Thevi T, Abas AL. Role of intravitreal/intracameral antibiotics to prevent traumatic endophthalmitis - Meta-analysis. Indian Journal of Ophthalmology. 2017;**65**(10):920-925

[78] Bohigian GM, Olk RJ. Factors associated with a poor visual result in endophthalmitis. American Journal of Ophthalmology. 1986;**101**(3):332-341

[79] Nobe JR, Gomez DS, Liggett P, et al. Post-traumatic and postoperative endophthalmitis: A comparison of visual outcomes. The British Journal of Ophthalmology. 1987;**71**(8):614-617

[80] Lieb DF, Scott IU, Flynn HW Jr, et al. Open globe injurie with positive intraocular cultures: Factors influencing final visual acuity outcomes. Ophthalmology. 2003;**110**(8):1560-1566

[81] Greenwald MJ, Wohl LG, Sell CH. Metastatic bacterial endophthalmitis: A contemporary reappraisal. Survey of Ophthalmology. 1986;**31**(2):81-101

[82] Schiedler V, Scott IU, Flynn HW, Davis JL, Benz MS, Miller D. Culture-proven endogenous endophthalmitis: Clinical features and visual acuity outcomes. American Journal of Ophthalmology. 2004;**137**(4):725-731

[83] Novosad BD, Callegan MC. Severe bacterial endophthalmitis: Towards improving clinical outcomes. Expert Review in Ophthalmology. 2010;**5**(5):689-698

[84] Sharma S, Padhi TR, Basu S, Kar S, Roy A, Das T. Endophthalmitis patients seen in a tertiary eye care centre in Odisha: A clinico-microbiological analysis. The Indian Journal of Medical Research. 2014;**139**(1):91-98

[85] Jackson TL, Paraskevopoulos T, Georgalas I. Systematic review of 342 cases of endogenous bacterial endophthalmitis. Survey of Ophthalmology. 2014;**59**(6):627-635

[86] Sridhar J, Flynn HW, Kuriyan AE, Miller D, Albini T. Endogenous fungal endophthalmitis: Risk factors, clinical features, and treatment outcomes in mold and yeast infections. Journal of Ophthalmic Inflammatory Infection. 2013;**3**(1):60

[87] Durand ML. Endophthalmitis. Clinical Microbiology and Infection. 2013;**19**(3):227-234

[88] Lamaris GA, Esmaeli B, Chamilos G, Desai A, Chemaly RF, Raad II, et al. Fungal endophthalmitis in a tertiary care cancer center: A review of 23 cases. European Journal of Clinical Microbiology & Infectious Diseases. 2008;**27**(5):343-347

[89] Keyashian K, Malani PN. Endophthalmitis associated with intravenous drug use. Southern Medical Journal. 2007;**100**(12):1219-1220

[90] Cheng HH, Ding Y, Wu M, Tang CC, Zhang RJ, Lin XF, et al. Endogenous aspergillus endophthalmitis after kidney transplantation. International Journal of Ophthalmology. 2011;**4**(5):567-571

[91] Agarwal M, Biswas J, Mathur U, Sijwali MS, Singh AK. Aspergillus iris granuloma in a young male: A case report with review of literature. Indian Journal of Ophthalmology. 2007;**55**(1):73-74

[92] Oude Lashof AM, Rothova A, Sobel JD, Ruhnke M, Pappas PG, Viscoli C, et al. Ocular manifestations of candidemia. Clinical Infectious Diseases. 2011;**53**(3):262-268

[93] Rodrigues IA, Jackson TL. A high-definition view of endogenous fungal endophthalmitis. The Lancet Infectious Diseases. 2014;**14**(4):358

[94] Wu ZH, Chan RP, Luk FO, Liu DT, Chan CK, Lam DS, et al. Review of clinical features, microbiological spectrum, and treatment outcomes of endogenous endophthalmitis over an 8-year period. Journal of Ophthalmology. 2012;**2012**:265078

[95] Sato Y, Miyasaka S, Shimada H. Prognosis of endogenous fungal endophthalmitis and utility of Ishibashi's classification. Japanese Journal of Ophthalmology. 2001;**45**(2):181-186

[96] Yoon YH, Lee SU, Sohn JH, Lee SE. Result of early vitrectomy for endogenous Klebsiella pneumoniae endophthalmitis. Retina. 2003;**23**(3):366-370

Chapter 2

Post-Operative Infections Following Glaucoma Drainage Surgery

Ejaz Ansari

Abstract

Glaucoma drainage surgery is performed commonly throughout the world for the surgical treatment of glaucoma. Typically, a guarded fistula is fashioned leading to a drainage bleb that represents subconjunctival collection and egress of aqueous humour from the eye. Bleb related infections (BRI) include blebitis and bleb related endophthalmitis (BRE). Although rare, BRI can be blinding, and appropriate vigilance is needed to ensure prompt diagnosis and treatment to save sight. Pre-operatively, blepharoconjunctivitis must be treated as well as any potential sources of infection. Clinicians must examine thoroughly to exclude bleb leaks and conjunctival erosions post-operatively. Patients must be educated about seeking care immediately if ocular redness, pain, discharge, or decreased vision develops. If BRI is diagnosed, sampling of ocular tissues is necessary for culture and sensitivity, followed by administration of broad-spectrum antibiotics. The interval from onset of symptoms to treatment, initial visual acuity, clarity of cornea at presentation, type of infecting organism, and presence or absence of diabetes mellitus are associated with final visual outcome particularly for BRE.

Keywords: glaucoma drainage surgery, blebitis, endophthalmitis, micro-organisms, antibiotics, vitrectomy

1. Introduction

Trabeculectomy with antimetabolites is the most commonly performed glaucoma surgery worldwide [1], being indicated for cases of progressive optic neuropathy despite maximum medical therapy. Other forms of drainage surgery include glaucoma drainage device (GDD) implantation, XEN45 gel stent, microshunt implantation and non-penetrating glaucoma surgery such as deep sclerectomy (DS).

Bleb-related infections (BRI), although rare can be very aggressive with poor prognosis and variable response to antimicrobial therapy. BRI includes blebitis and endophthalmitis, which may represent a continuum of infection. Early onset BRI occurs within 1 month of surgery and late onset BRI is defined as occurring after 1 month.

IntechOpen

Several studies have addressed the possible risk factors associated with BRI and new surgical techniques have been developed to improve safety. In this chapter, we will discuss the risk factors for BRI following trabeculectomy, the pathogens involved, the treatment protocol and antimicrobial agents that are typically used in treatment.

2. Incidence

The incidence of BRI is difficult to determine because of variable modes and times of presentation. Long-term studies are useful in ascertaining the lifetime risk of BRI, which is important to discuss with patients as part of the informed consent process.

In the Collaborative Initial Glaucoma Treatment Study, the 5-year risk of blebitis and bleb related endophthalmitis (BRE) was 1.5% and 1.1%, respectively [2]. In the Tube Versus Trabeculectomy Study, [3] the 5-year incidence of BRI following trabeculectomy was 4.8% (n = 105). A 20-year study (n = 460) reported cumulative probabilities of blebitis and BRE of 2% and 5%, respectively [4].

In the trabeculectomy versus tube trial, at 5 years, blebitis and endophthalmitis occurred in 1% and 4.8% of cases in the tube and trabeculectomy groups, respectively, but this was not statistically significant [3]. In a large case series of GDD implantations, exposed implants were more likely to be associated with infection than the group generally (16% v 1%), and exposed inferior GDD had a higher rate of infection compared to superior y placed GDD (47% v 8%) [5]. Multiple studies have shown a higher rate of endophthalmitis in patients younger than 18 years of age [6]. Removal of GDD in the clinical setting of BRI is controversial but recommended by the author once the infection has been treated.

The reported rate of BRI after various nonpenetrating surgeries has been 0–1.6% [7–10]. Cases of BRI in this setting usually occur after laser goniopuncture [10]. In a large case series (n = 199) with relatively short follow-up there was 1 case of late onset endophthalmitis following XEN 45 gel stent implantation [11]. Apart from this, there have been a few case reports of BRE following XEN 45 implantation [12–15]. In the author's experience, after 5 years of follow up of 90 eyes implanted with XEN45 gel stent, there were no cases of BRI (unpublished data). One case of BRE has been reported following bleb needling in an eye implanted with microshunt [16].

3. Symptoms and signs of bleb related infection

BRI can lead to severe and permanent loss of vision if not detected and treated in a timely and directed manner. Early on there may be mild signs similar to viral or bacterial conjunctivitis, leading to a delay in seeking medical attention. Cases typically present with a painful red eye, often associated with discharge, eyelid swelling, photophobia, and reduced vision. There may be a prodromal history of headache, conjunctivitis, blepharitis, and coryza [17].

The findings include a milky bleb appearance due to a mucopurulent infiltrate. There is usually swelling and hyperaemia of the conjunctiva with upper eyelid oedema. These findings are known as a "white on red" appearance (**Figure 1**). The anterior chamber may be shallow if there is a bleb leak. Later on, an anterior chamber inflammatory reaction occurs, and anterior vitritis.

Generally, BRE and blebitis present similarly, but the symptoms and signs in BRE are more fulminant with greater reduction in vision and a more accelerated course.

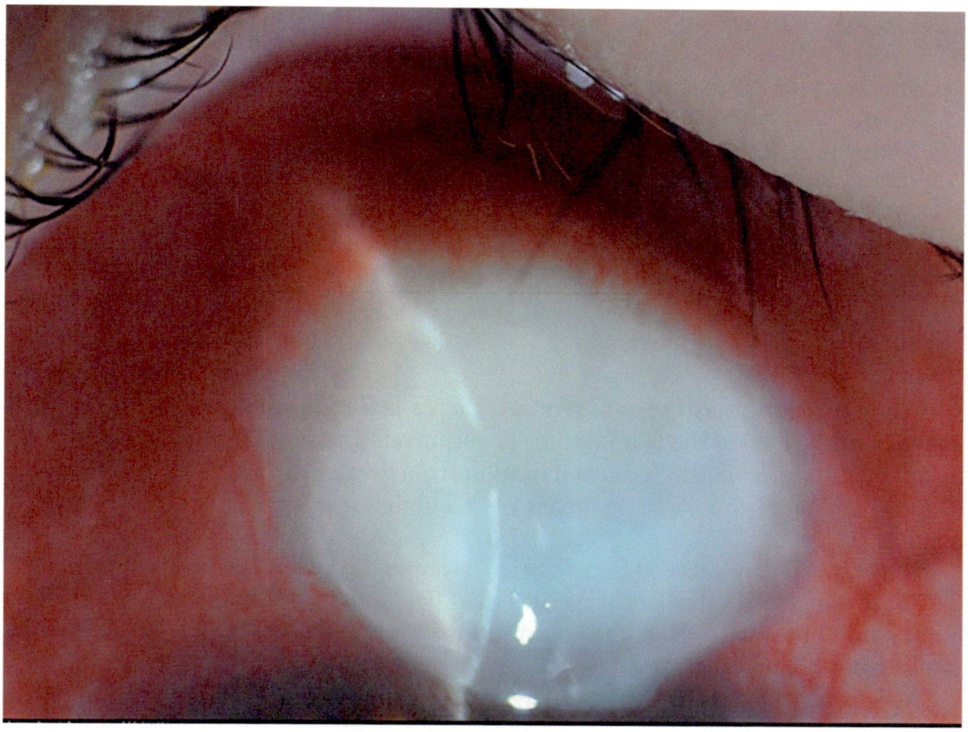

Figure 1.
"White on red" appearance of bleb related infection (notice adjacent blepharitis).

In the author's experience, blebitis can progress to BRE very rapidly, so that if suspected, there must be a low threshold to admit the patient immediately for appropriate targeted treatment (vide infra).

4. Risk factors

Risk factors for BRI can be broadly classified under ocular and systemic conditions.

4.1 Ocular risk factors

- Bleb leak, inferior or nasal bleb, high bleb
- Intraoperative and post-operative MMC/5-FU
- Conjunctivitis
- Blepharitis
- Nasolacrimal duct obstruction
- Lens status
- Trabeculectomy alone compared to combined procedure

4.2 Systemic risk factors

- Upper respiratory tract infection
- Diabetes mellitus
- Age
- Season
- Gender

Blebs located inferiorly are at increased risk of infection since there is greater exposure of the bleb to the tear lake with concentrated bacteria, less protection from the upper lid and more mechanical irritation from greater exposure [18]. The risk of infection in an inferiorly located bleb is x4–x 8 higher in eyes treated with antimetabolites [19].

Fornix-based conjunctival flap trabeculectomies are associated with reduced risk of BRI compared to limbal based conjunctival flap peritomy (hazard ratio 3.39) [20]. In one study, the incidence of late-onset BRI decreased from 5.7% to 1.2% following a change from limbal based to fornix based peritomy [21].

The use of antimetabolite agents, e.g., 5-Fluorouracil (5-FU) and Mitomycin C (MMC) has led to an increase in cases of BRI. The incidence before the use of antimetabolites was 0.2–1.5% [22–24]. This has increased to 2–13.0% in 5-FU treated eyes [25–27] and 1.5%–14% of MMC treated eyes [28–31].

Thin, cystic blebs associated with MMC, and 5-FU use are more prone to infection than blebs with a thick wall [32–35]. They are also associated with late bleb leak (leakage after 4 weeks), another risk factor for BRI [36–38].

In one study, the rate of BRI was 7.9% and 1.7% for blebs with and without leakage, respectively (202). The presence of bleb leak was associated with a 4.7-fold increase in the risk of BRI [38]. Bleb leak must therefore be addressed in an urgent manner by the glaucoma team.

Blepharoconjunctivitis is associated with microbial colonisation of the ocular surface, which is a risk factor for BRI [39–43].

An important practice pearl is to examine the ocular adnexa pre-operatively and to prepare the ocular surface in case of pre-existing blepharoconjunctivitis or nasolacrimal duct obstruction. Furthermore, post-operatively, all patients with an active bleb should be examined for blepharitis.

In patients with a filtering bleb and blepharoconjunctivitis, a short course of topical antibiotic (e.g., fucithalmic, tobramycin, bacitracin, or erythromycin) plus eyelid hygiene is recommended with prompt discontinuation of antibiotic upon resolution. However, the eyelid hygiene must be continued indefinitely. Rosacea blepharitis responds well to topical azithromycin or oral doxycycline [44]. For chronic blepharitis, 0.01% hypochlorous acid, which is a natural product, is an antimicrobial agent that can be used repetitively and long-term without resistance developing [45].

Aphakia and pseudophakia are associated with higher odds of BRI (6.3 v 2.85) [46]. Absence of an intact posterior capsule may enhance microbial penetration into the vitreous cavity [47].

A slightly lower rate of BRI was found in cases of combined trabeculectomy+ cataract surgery (1.4%) compared to trabeculectomy alone (1.5%) at 2.5 years post-operatively. The lower rate of thin-walled blebs after a combined operation could explain this observation [39].

Diabetes mellitus (DM) is associated with higher positive conjunctival culture rate than in patients without DM. The severity of diabetic retinopathy is correlated to culture positivity (98). In some studies, 18% of cases of BRI had DM [29, 35, 37, 40–42, 48].

Younger age was found to be a risk factor for infection [49, 50], and severe bleb leak was associated with younger adults (<55 years) (99). In some studies, a high rate of BRI was found in children [51] including 8% chance of late onset endophthalmitis [52].

The association with gender is not clearly proven. Seasonal variation in temperature and humidity may influence the conjunctival flora and therefore, the rate of BRI [53].

5. Microbiology of bleb related infection

The most common pathogens in blebitis are Staphylococcus aureus and Staphylococcus epidermidis [47, 54, 55]. The microbes most commonly associated with blebitis are less virulent than those in BRE, are part of normal lid/lacrimal flora, and produce no exotoxins; therefore, with successful treatment, visual prognosis is good. In a retrospective study, visual acuity was at least 20/25 in all successfully treated patients [17].

The microbes most commonly associated with early BRE include Staphylococcus epidermidis. Late onset BRE is associated with greater percentage of Streptococcus species 31%, and Gram-negatives such as Haemophilus influenzae 23%, Enterococcus 7%, Pseudomonas 7%, and fewer Staphylococcus species 7–22% [39, 48, 56].

When initiating antibiotic therapy for BRI, it is important to consider antibiotic resistance, which is particularly high in staphylococci; nearly half being resistant to methicillin with a high probability of concurrent resistance among methicillin resistant Staphylococcus aureus to other commonly used antibiotic classes [57]. In such cases it is useful to know that vancomycin is active against all gram-positive organisms, including all the methicillin-resistant staphylococci [57, 58].

6. Diagnostic investigations

Sampling of the intraocular fluid for Gram stain and culture is recommended before treatment is initiated. However, empiric treatment should begin promptly while the specimen is being analysed. Working closely with the microbiology department is mandatory in managing these cases.

Intraocular fluid samples should be sent for Gram and Giemsa staining, culture, and sensitivity. Gram stain is positive in approximately 45% of endophthalmitis cases [59]. Vitreous sampling has a higher positive culture rate than aqueous humour, with vitrectomy samples being more culture positive than vitreous tap [60].

Polymerase chain reaction (PCR) is useful in culture negative cases. It is effective in detecting fastidious bacteria, provides a result in a few minutes and is more sensitive than cultures [61, 62]. However multiple samples have to be sent for each micro-organism that the clinician suspects. Biome representational in silico karyotyping (BRiSK) is a new technique for detection of any DNA-based life form and can detect micro-organisms in PCR negative samples [63]. However, its role in BRI is not established.

Although the majority of glaucoma specialists recommend conjunctival sampling, it must be appreciated that conjunctival culture results in BRI do not generally match the culture results from anterior chamber and vitreous humour samples [32, 39, 64]. Care must be taken not to tear the conjunctiva over the bleb area when taking samples.

7. Treatment modalities

The most effective treatment for BRI consists of a combination of fortified aminoglycoside or ceftazidime with vancomycin, i.e., a broad-spectrum antibiotic combination. Moxifloxacin tends to be the most popular fluoroquinolone of choice due to its higher intraocular penetration and activity against gram-negative bacteria, gram-positive cocci, and atypical pathogens [65–67]. Topical aminoglycosides may be efficacious in BRI caused by fluoroquinolone-resistant Staphylococcus species [68].

Pre-operative 5% povidone iodine instillation in the conjunctival sac is recommended in the prophylaxis of endophthalmitis for cataract surgery, and the author recommends the same for glaucoma drainage surgery. It has also been used in the treatment regimen for BRI. Povidone iodine is an antiseptic agent which is clinically effective against a broad range of bacteria and fungi. In a British survey, 28% of glaucoma surgeons used povidone iodine in the conjunctival sac to treat BRI [64]. Just one drop of 5% povidone iodine acts rapidly within 2 minutes to reduce the positive swab rate of the ocular surface from 75% to 28% in eyes without active infection [69].

For BRE, a broad-spectrum combination of intravitreal antibiotics that cover gram-positive and gram-negative bacteria can be started empirically before culture results are available [70], e.g., vancomycin and ceftazidime. The author recommends amikacin instead of ceftazidime for beta lactam sensitive patients with cephalosporin cross reactivity.

Practice point: before performing vitreous tap and intravitreal injections in BRI cases, a retinal examination must be performed to exclude retinal detachment or choroidal detachment (which can be associated with bleb leaks and hypotony). If the view is not clear, ultrasound biomicroscopy must be performed to exclude the same.

Vitreous sampling and intravitreal injection in the presence of choroidal detachment could lead to catastrophic choroidal haemorrhage.

The short duration of action of intravitreal antibiotics does limit their efficacy, but generally If there is no improvement after 36–48 h, another intravitreal antibiotic injection can be given in line with culture and sensitivity results, or pars plana vitrectomy (PPV) can be performed [71]. The author's advice is to have a low threshold for PPV in BRE since the infecting organisms tend to be more virulent and the disease course more fulminant than in post-cataract surgery endophthalmitis.

Other modes of administration of antibiotics include the subconjunctival and oral routes. However, subconjunctival antibiotics do not achieve therapeutic levels in the vitreous [72]. A combination of topical and oral antibiotics achieves higher levels in the vitreous than topical therapy alone, but there is no consensus on the use of oral therapy.

Although, antibiotics are the mainstay of treatment for BRI, consideration should also be given to treating concurrent intraocular inflammation. Therefore, topical cycloplegics should be used to prevent and release posterior synechiae. Topical steroids should be considered once it is confirmed that the antibiotic treatment is being administered according to sensitivities of cultured organisms and that the treatment is working.

In one study, most of the glaucoma surgeons started topical corticosteroids 24–72 h after the initiation of topical antibiotics [64]. The role of intravitreal steroid therapy lacks evidence but can be considered depending on the response to antimicrobials and the amount of ocular inflammation. Subconjunctival dexamethasone is a reasonable alternative to intravitreal corticosteroids. Steroids are effective in treating inflammation associated with bacterial exotoxins [73] but are contraindicated in fungal disease.

For fungal infections, e.g., severe candida endophthalmitis, a combination of oral amphotericin-B and flucytosine is advised. Fluconazole and oral voriconazole are alternatives that cover a range of fungal species [74, 75]. Usually, a period of 4–6 weeks of treatment is required.

The role of vitrectomy in the setting of endophthalmitis after glaucoma surgery is a matter of debate. The Endophthalmitis Vitrectomy Study (EVS) [60] did not include BRI cases, therefore, strictly speaking, its recommendations cannot be extrapolated to this population. Typically, BRE for example occurs a lot later than the acute setting of post-cataract surgery endophthalmitis. Furthermore, the more virulent organisms found in BRE, would warrant earlier consideration of vitrectomy compared to patients with endophthalmitis following cataract surgery, but evidence-based data to drive this clinical decision are lacking [48, 56]. In cases of fungal BRE, PPV can be sight saving in severe cases [76]. Intravitreal antifungal agents are commonly used in cases of fungal BRE, but evidence for their value is lacking [75]. Intravitreal amphotericin B, voriconazole, and caspofungin are examples of antifungal agents used in BRE [77].

8. Treatment protocol

There is no universally agreed upon regimen, however, the following is the author's preferred practice with reference to what has been discussed in this chapter:

General considerations:

- For all cases of BRI- blebitis and BRE- admit the patient for frequent topical antibiotic therapy and close observation and examination.

- Take ocular samples for culture and sensitivity straight away but start empirical treatment whilst awaiting culture results.

- Blebitis can convert to BRE very quickly, so have a low threshold for pursuing a more aggressive treatment approach if no improvement in the clinical picture is seen in the first 48–72 h (vide infra).

- Examine the patient twice daily during the acute phase of BRI.

- In cases of BRE, fully inform the patient and relatives that there is a high chance of losing vision despite treatment and a low chance of losing the eye.

Specific details:

- If no vitreal involvement, start aggressive broad-spectrum topical antibiotic treatment. Options include fortified antibiotics such as vancomycin (25–50 mg/mL) and cefazolin (50 mg/mL) or fortified tobramycin (14 mg/mL) alternating q30min for 48 h after a loading dose (every 5 min for three doses); or 4th generation fluoroquinolone with same posology.

- Topical cycloplegics, e.g., g Atropine bd can be started straight away; topical steroid, e.g., Prednisolone 1% or Dexamethasone 0.1% qid can be used 48–72 h after initiation of topical antibiotics.

- Taper fortifides after 48 h to regular strength based on improvement.

- If there is vitreal involvement, perform a vitreous tap following all necessary precautions (vide supra) and inject intravitreal antibiotics, e.g., vancomycin + ceftazidime/ amikacin.

- In the absence of fungal infection, consider adjunctive intravitreal dexamethasone (0.4 mg/0.1 mL) which may modify the inflammatory response and consequent damage to retina and other ocular structures.

- If there is improvement in the clinical picture, start tapering the topical antibiotics (vide supra).

- If there is no improvement, refer to retinal surgeons for urgent vitrectomy + intravitreal antibiotics.

9. Visual outcome

In most cases of Infection arising from gram-negative pathogens and streptococci, there is a worse visual prognosis, with only 45–46% achieving best visual acuity (BVA) ≥20/400. In contrast, 89% of eyes achieve BVA ≥20/400 following Infections associated with coagulase-negative staphylococci [78].

Better visual outcomes after BRE are associated with the following:

shorter interval from onset of symptoms to treatment, better initial visual acuity, clear cornea at presentation, isolation of less virulent organisms, and absence of diabetes mellitus [34, 79].

10. Conclusions

- Bleb related infections are uncommon but can lead to blindness in a short space of time.

- Early diagnosis and treatment are crucial to provide the best chance to save sight.

- Patients must be informed of the signs of infection or impending infection- redness, pain, discharge, reduction of vision- and to report to the emergency department immediately if any of these symptoms are experienced.

- Surgeons must play an active role in clinics to look for blepharitis, epiphora or conjunctivitis in the presence of a bleb, and these conditions explained and treated.
- Blebs must be examined at each clinic visit for leakage by Seidel testing, and leaks managed appropriately to prevent further complications.
- Thin, avascular, or sweating blebs, even if not leaking, must be assessed more frequently and the patient informed (vide supra) of the possibility of infection. In such cases it is reasonable to discuss the option of bleb revision.
- Although no clear guidelines have been developed regarding management of BRE, early aggressive treatment is associated with better visual prognosis.

Conflict of interest

"The author declares no conflict of interest."

Author details

Ejaz Ansari[1,2]

1 Eye Ear and Mouth Unit, Maidstone and Tunbridge Wells NHS Trust, Kent, UK

2 Institute of Medical Sciences, Canterbury Christ Church University, Kent, UK

*Address all correspondence to: e.ansari@nhs.net

References

[1] Wang X, Khan R, Coleman A. Device-modified trabeculectomy for glaucoma. Cochrane Database of Systematic Reviews. 2015;**12**:Cd010472

[2] Zahid S, Musch DC, Niziol LM, Lichter PR. Risk of endophthalmitis and other long-term complications of trabeculectomy in the Collaborative Initial GlaucomaTreatment Study (CIGTS). American Journal of Ophthalmology. 2013;**155**(4):674-680, 680.e1

[3] Gedde SJ, Herndon LW, Brandt JD, et al. Postoperative complications in the Tube Versus Trabeculectomy (TVT) study during five years of follow-up. American Journal of Ophthalmology. 2012;**153**(5):804-814.e1

[4] Olayanju JA, Hassan MB, Hodge DO, Khanna CL. Trabeculectomy-related complications in Olmsted County, Minnesota, 1985 through 2010. JAMA Ophthalmology. 2015;**133**(5):574-580

[5] Levinson JD, Giangiacomo AL, Beck AD, et al. Glaucoma drainage devices: Risk of exposure and infection. American Journal of Ophthalmology. 2015;**160**(3):516-521.e2

[6] Wentzloff JN, Grosskreutz CL, Pasquale LR, Walton DS, Chen TC. Endophthalmitis after glaucoma drainage implant surgery. International Ophthalmology Clinics. 2007;**47**(2): 109-115. DOI: 10.1097/IIO.0b013e3180 37766a

[7] Anand N, Arora S, Clowes M. Mitomycin C augmented glaucoma surgery: Evolution of filtering bleb avascularity, transconjunctival oozing, and leaks. The British Journal of Ophthalmology. 2006;**90**(2):175-180

[8] Detry-Morel M, Detry MB. Five-year experience with non-penetrating deep sclerectomy. Bulletin de la Société Belge d'Ophtalmologie. 2006;**299**:83-94

[9] Grieshaber MC, Peckar C, Pienaar A, et al. Long-term results of up to 12 years of over 700 cases of viscocanalostomy for open-angle glaucoma. Acta Ophthalmologica. 2015;**93**(4):362-367

[10] Roy S, Mermoud A. Deep nonpenetrating sclerectomy: Technical aspects. Journal Français d'Ophtalmologie. 2006;**29**(10):1160-1166

[11] Heidinger A, Schwab C, Lindner E, Riedl R, Mossböck G. A retrospective study of 199 Xen45 stent implantations from 2014 to 2016. Journal of Glaucoma. 2019;**28**(1):75-79. DOI: 10.1097/IJG.0000000000001122

[12] Karri B, Gupta C, Mathews D. Endophthalmitis following XEN stent exposure. Journal of Glaucoma. 2018;**27**(10):931-933. DOI: 10.1097/IJG.0000000000001012

[13] de Las B-S, Matas R, Such-Irusta L, Alfonso-Muñoz EA, et al. Late-onset Endophthalmitis after XEN45® Implantation: A retrospective case series and literature review. Journal of Current Glaucoma Practice. 2021;**15**(3):153-160. DOI: 10.5005/jp-journals-10078-1316

[14] Ng AW, Yip VC, Ang BC, Yip LW, Lim BA. Culture-positive exogenous endophthalmitis related to XEN45 gel stent implantation. American Journal of Ophthalmology Case Reports. 2022;**25**:101291, ISSN 2451-9936. DOI: 10.1016/j.ajoc.2022.101291

[15] Kerr NM, Wang J, Sandhu A, Harasymowycz PJ, Barton K. Ab interno

gel implant-associated Bleb-related Infection. American Journal of Ophthalmology. 2018;**189**:96-101. DOI: 10.1016/j.ajo.2018.02.014. Epub 2018. Feb 28

[16] Brambati M, Bettin P, Ramoni A, Battista M, Bandello F. A case of endophthalmitis following needling procedure after PRESERFLO® Micro Shunt implantation. European Journal of Ophthalmology. 2022;**32**(3):NP83-NP86. DOI: 10.1177/11206721211019548. Epub 2021 May 20

[17] Poulsen EJ, Allingham RR. Characteristics and risk factors of infections after glaucoma filtering surgery. Journal of Glaucoma. 2000;**9**(6):438-443

[18] Caronia RM, Liebmann JM, Friedman R, et al. Trabeculectomy at the inferior limbus. Archives of Ophthalmology. 1996;**114**(4):387-391

[19] Yamamoto T. Bleb-related infection: Clinical features and management. Taiwan Journal of Ophthalmology. 2012;**2**(1):2-5

[20] Solus JF, Jampel HD, Tracey PA, et al. Comparison of limbusbased and fornix-based trabeculectomy: Success, bleb related complications, and bleb morphology. Ophthalmology. 2012;**119**(4):703-711

[21] Rai P, Kotecha A, Kaltsos K, et al. Changing trends in the incidence of bleb-related infection in trabeculectomy. The British Journal of Ophthalmology. 2012;**96**(7):971-975

[22] Freedman J, Gupta M, Bunke A. Endophthalmitis after trabeculectomy. Archives of Ophthalmology. 1978;**96**(6):1017-1018

[23] Katz LJ, Cantor LB, Spaeth GL. Complications of surgery in glaucoma. Early and late bacterial endophthalmitis following glaucoma filtering surgery. Ophthalmology. 1985;**92**(7):959-963

[24] Solomon A, Ticho U, Frucht-Pery J. Late-onset, blebassociated endophthalmitis following glaucoma filtering surgery with or without antifibrotic agents. Journal of Ocular Pharmacology and Therapeutics. 1999;**15**(4):283-293

[25] Five-year follow-up of the fluorouracil filtering surgery study. The fluorouracil filtering surgery study group. American Journal of Ophthalmology. 1996;**121**(4):349-366

[26] Ticho U, Ophir A. Late complications after glaucoma filteringsurgery with adjunctive 5-fluorouracil. American Journal of Ophthalmology. 1993;**115**(4):506-510

[27] Uchida S, Suzuki Y, Araie M, et al. Long-term follow-up of initial 5-fluorouracil trabeculectomy in primary open-angle glaucoma in Japanese patients. Journal of Glaucoma. 2001;**10**(6):458-465

[28] Greenfield DS, Liebmann JM, Jee J, Ritch R. Late-onset bleb leaks after glaucoma filtering surgery. Archives of Ophthalmology. 1998;**116**(4):443-447

[29] Mochizuki K, Jikihara S, Ando Y, et al. Incidence of delayed onset infection after trabeculectomy with adjunctive mitomycin C or 5-fluorouracil treatment. The British Journal of Ophthalmology. 1997;**81**(10):877-883

[30] Sharan S, Trope GE, Chipman M, Buys YM. Late-onset bleb infections: Prevalence and risk factors. Canadian Journal of Ophthalmology. 2009;**44**(3):279-283

[31] Shigeeda T, Tomidokoro A, Chen YN, et al. Long-term follow-up of initial

trabeculectomy with mitomycin C for primary open-angle glaucoma in Japanese patients. Journal of Glaucoma. 2006;**15**(3):195-199

[32] Greenfield DS. Bleb-related ocular infection. Journal of Glaucoma. 1998;7(2):132-136

[33] Wallin O, Al-Ahramy AM, Lundstrom M, Montan P. Endophthalmitis and severe blebitis following trabeculectomy. Epidemiology and risk factors; A single centre retrospective study. Acta Ophthalmologica. 2014;**92**(5):426-431

[34] Wolner B, Liebmann JM, Sassani JW, et al. Late bleb-related endophthalmitis after trabeculectomy with adjunctive 5-fluorouracil. Ophthalmology. 1991;**98**(7):1053-1060

[35] Yamamoto T, Kuwayama Y, Kano K, et al. Clinical features of bleb-related infection: A 5-year survey in Japan. Acta Ophthalmologica. 2013;**91**(7):619-624

[36] Higginbotham EJ, Stevens RK, Musch DC, et al. Bleb-related endophthalmitis after trabeculectomy with mitomycin C. Ophthalmology. 1996;**103**(4):650-656

[37] Lehmann OJ, Bunce C, Matheson MM, et al. Risk factors for development of post-trabeculectomy endophthalmitis. The British Journal of Ophthalmology. 2000;**84**(12):1349-1353

[38] Waheed S, Ritterband DC, Greenfield DS, et al. New patterns of infecting organisms in late bleb-related endophthalmitis: A ten year review. Eye (London, England). 1998;**12**(Pt 6): 910-915

[39] Greenfield DS, Suner IJ, Miller MP, et al. Endophthalmitis after filtering surgery with mitomycin. Archives of Ophthalmology. 1996;**114**(8):943-949

[40] Kim EA, Law SK, Coleman AL, et al. Long-term bleb-related infections after trabeculectomy: Incidence, risk factors, and influence of bleb revision. American Journal of Ophthalmology. 2015;**159**(6):1082-1091

[41] Leng T, Miller D, Flynn HW Jr, et al. Delayed-onset bleb associated endophthalmitis (1996-2008): Causative organisms and visual acuity outcomes. Retina. 2011;**31**(2):344-352

[42] Ramakrishnan R, Bharathi MJ, Maheshwari D, et al. Etiology and epidemiological analysis of glaucoma-filtering bleb infections in a tertiary eye care hospital in South India. Indian Journal of Ophthalmology. 2011;**59**(6):445-453

[43] Waheed S, Ritterband DC, Greenfield DS, et al. Bleb-related ocular infection in children after trabeculectomy with mitomycin C. Ophthalmology. 1997;**104**(12): 2117-2120

[44] De Paiva CS, Corrales RM, Villarreal AL, et al. Corticosteroid and doxycycline suppress MMP-9 and inflammatory cytokine expression, MAPK activation in the corneal epithelium in experimental dry eye. Experimental Eye Research. 2006;**83**(3):526-535

[45] Li Z, Wang H, Liang M. Hypochlorous acid can be the novel option for the meibomian gland dysfunction dry eye through ultrasonic atomization. Disease Markers. 2022;**2022**:Article ID 8631038, 12 p. DOI: 10.1155/2022/8631038

[46] Yamamoto T, Kuwayama Y, Nomura E, et al. Changes in visual acuity and intra-ocular pressure following bleb related infection: The Japan Glaucoma Society Survey of Bleb-related Infection

Report 2. Acta Ophthalmologica. 2013;**91**(6):e420-e426

[47] Ciulla TA, Beck AD, Topping TM, Baker AS. Blebitis, early endophthalmitis, and late endophthalmitis after glaucoma filtering surgery. Ophthalmology. 1997;**104**(6):986-995

[48] Song A, Scott IU, Flynn HW Jr, Budenz DL. Delayed-onset bleb-associated endophthalmitis: Clinical features and visual acuity outcomes. Ophthalmology. 2002;**109**(5):985-991

[49] Jampel HD, Musch DC, Gillespie BW, et al. Perioperative complications of trabeculectomy in the Collaborative Initial Glaucoma Treatment Study (CIGTS). American Journal of Ophthalmology. 2005;**140**(1):16-22

[50] Karolina C, Baril C, Bourret-Massicotte D, et al. Risk factors for a severe bleb leak following trabeculectomy: A retrospective case-control study. Journal of Glaucoma. 2015;**24**(7):493-497

[51] Mandelbaum S, Forster RK. Endophthalmitis associated with filtering blebs. International Ophthalmology Clinics. 1987;**27**(2):107-111

[52] Beck AD, Wilson WR, Lynch MG, et al. Trabeculectomy with adjunctive mitomycin C in pediatric glaucoma. American Journal of Ophthalmology. 1998;**126**(5):648-657

[53] Takahashi N, Sawada A, Mochizuki K, et al. Fluctuation of bacteria on bleb surface after trabeculectomy with adjunctive mitomycin C. Journal of Glaucoma. 2016;**25**:433-439

[54] Ayyala RS, Bellows RA, Thomas JV, Hutchinson TB. Bleb infections: Clinically different courses of blebitis and endophthalmitis. Ophthalmic Surgery and Lasers. 1997;**28**:452-460

[55] Waheed S, Ritterband DC, Greenfield DS, et al. Recurrent bleb infections. The British Journal of Ophthalmology. 1998;**82**:926-929

[56] Busbee BG, Recchia FM, Kaiser R, et al. Bleb-associated endophthalmitis: Clinical characteristics and visual outcomes. Ophthalmology. 2004;**118**(8):1495-1503, discussion 1503

[57] Asbell PA, Sanfilippo CM, Pillar CM, et al. Antibiotic resistance among ocular pathogens in the United States: Five-year results from the Antibiotic Resistance Monitoring in Ocular Microorganisms (ARMOR) surveillance study. JAMA Ophthalmology. 2015;**133**:1445-1454

[58] Han DP, Wisniewski SR, Wilson LA, et al. Spectrum and susceptibilities of microbiologic isolates in the endophthalmitis vitrectomy study. American Journal of Ophthalmology. 1996;**122**(1):1-17

[59] Durand ML. Endophthalmitis. Clinical Microbiology and Infection. 2013;**19**(3):227-234

[60] Results of the Endophthalmitis Vitrectomy Study. A randomized trial of immediate vitrectomy and of intravenous antibiotics for the treatment of postoperative bacterial endophthalmitis. Endophthalmitis vitrectomy study group. Archives of Ophthalmology. 1995;**113**(12):1479-1496

[61] Hong BK, Lee CS, Van Gelder RN, Garg SJ. Emerging techniques for pathogen discovery in endophthalmitis. Current Opinion in Ophthalmology. 2015;**26**(3):221-225

[62] Joseph CR, Lalitha P, Sivaraman KR, et al. Real-time polymerase chain

reaction in the diagnosis of acute postoperative endophthalmitis. American Journal of Ophthalmology. 2012;**153**(6):1031-1037.e2

[63] Lee AY, Akileswaran L, Tibbetts MD, et al. Identification of torque teno virus in culture-negative endophthalmitis by representational deep DNA sequencing. Ophthalmology. 2015;**122**(3):524-530

[64] Chiam PJ, Arashvand K, Shaikh A, James B. Management of blebitis in the United Kingdom: A survey. The British Journal of Ophthalmology. 2012;**96**(1):38-41

[65] Caeiro JP, Iannini PB. Moxifloxacin (Avelox): A novel fluoroquinolone with a broad spectrum of activity. Expert Review of Anti-Infective Therapy. 2003;**1**(3):363-370

[66] McCulley JP, Caudle D, Aronowicz JD, Shine WE. Fourth generation fluoroquinolone penetration into the aqueous humor in humans. Ophthalmology. 2006;**113**(6):955-959

[67] Robertson SM, Curtis MA, Schlech BA, et al. Ocular pharmacokinetics of moxifloxacin after topical treatment of animals and humans. Survey of Ophthalmology. 2005;**50**(Suppl1):S32-S45

[68] Kim SJ, Toma HS. Antimicrobial resistance and ophthalmic antibiotics: 1-year results of a longitudinal controlled study of patients undergoing intravitreal injections. Archives of Ophthalmology. 2011;**129**(9):1180-1188

[69] Boes DA, Lindquist TD, Fritsche TR, Kalina RE. Effects of povidone-iodine chemical preparation and saline irrigation on the perilimbal flora. Ophthalmology. 1992;**99**(10):1569-1574

[70] Yam JC, Kwok AK. Update of the management of postoperative endophthalmitis. Hong Kong Medical Journal. 2004;**10**(5):337-343

[71] Yamamoto T, Kuwayama Y. Interim clinical outcomes in the collaborative bleb-related infection incidence and treatment study. Ophthalmology. 2011;**118**(3):453-458

[72] Hawkins AS, Deutsch TA. Infectious endophthalmitis. Current Infectious Disease Reports. 1999;**1**(2):172-177

[73] Jacobs DJ, Pathengay A, Flynn HW Jr, et al. Intravitreal dexamethasone in the management of delayed-onset bleb associated endophthalmitis. International Journal of Inflammation. 2012;**2012**:503912

[74] Espinel-Ingroff A, Boyle K, Sheehan DJ. In vitro antifungal activities of voriconazole and reference agents as determined by NCCLS methods: Review of the literature. Mycopathologia. 2001;**150**(3):101-115

[75] Pappas PG, Kauffman CA, Andes D, et al. Clinical practice guidelines for the management of candidiasis: 2009 update by the Infectious Diseases Society of America. Clinical Infectious Diseases. 2009;**48**(5):503-535

[76] Essman TF, Flynn HW Jr, Smiddy WE, et al. Treatment outcomes in a 10-year study of endogenous fungal endophthalmitis. Ophthalmic Surgery and Lasers. 1997;**28**(3):185-194

[77] Lemley CA, Han DP. Endophthalmitis: A review of current evaluation and management. Retina. 2007;**27**(6):662-680. DOI: 10.1097/IAE.0b013e3180323f96. Erratum in: Retina. 2007 Sep;27(7): table of contents. Dosage error in article text

[78] Jacobs DJ, Leng T, Flynn HW Jr, et al. Delayed-onset bleb associated endophthalmitis: Presentation and outcome by culture result. Clinical Ophthalmology. 2011;**5**:739-744

[79] Al-Turki TA, Al-Shahwan S, Al-Mezaine HS, et al. Microbiology and visual outcome of bleb-associated endophthalmitis. Ocular Immunology and Inflammation. 2010;**18**(2):121-126

Chapter 3

Potency of Netilmicin against Staphylococci Compared to Other Ophthalmic Antibiotics

Andrea Sudano Roccaro, Carmela Giovanna Spoto, Luca Rosario La Rosa, Claudine Civiale, Manuela Santonocito, Santa Viola, Cristina Zappulla, Maria Cristina Curatolo and Maria Grazia Mazzone

Abstract

Netilmicin is a potent and safe antibiotic with a very low incidence of resistance used as a topical ophthalmic medication in bacterial ocular infections. The aim of this study was to compare netilmicin's Quotient of Inhibitions (QIs) and killing kinetics vs Staphylococci with other ophthalmic antimicrobials. Conjunctival and corneal QIs of netilmicin formulations, in single and multiple doses of administration, were compared with those of tobramycin, ofloxacin, levofloxacin and azithromycin preparations. The same analysis was performed in human tears, comparing netilmicin eye drops solution with tobramycin ofloxacin and levofloxacin. Furthermore, killing kinetics against Staphylococci (ATCC strains and ocular isolates) of the above-cited antibiotics, as well as chloramphenicol, were compared at different time points. QI results showed that in the conjunctiva, netilmicin, in both single and multiple doses of administration, is highly effective against all staphylococcal strains tested, while in the cornea it was particularly active against methicillin-resistant Staphylococci strains. Moreover, in human tears, netilmicin eye drops solution showed a more favourable QI against Staphylococci than tobramycin, ofloxacin and levofloxacin all in single-dose administration regimen. Killing kinetic results showed that netilmicin has a great bactericidal activity vs all the microbe strains tested as netilmicin showed to be almost the most active antibiotic. Results suggest that netilmicin has one of the most favourable killing kinetic and tissue inhibitory effects against Staphylococci than the principal ophthalmic antibiotics on the market.

Keywords: netilmicin, quotient of inhibition, killing curves, Staphylococci, methicillin resistance

1. Introduction

Netilmicin is a third-generation aminoglycoside antibiotic considered a first-line therapy for the treatment of acute bacterial conjunctivitis. It is a semisynthetic 1-N-ethyl derivative of sisomycin, endowed with an excellent *in vitro* and *in vivo* activity against a wide range of ocular pathogens both Gram-positive and Gram-negative bacteria including *Staphylococcus aureus* (*S. aureus*), S. *epidermidis* (*S. epidermidis*) and others *Staphylococcus* Coagulase negative, *Acinetobacter* spp., *Pseudomonas* spp. and *Haemophilus influenzae* [1–3].

The most common causative agents for external ocular infections are *S. aureus* and *S. epidermidis* although the specific causal organisms are frequently unknown [2]. Of particular concern among ocular isolates is the increasing frequency of methicillin-resistant *S. aureus* (*MRSA*) and methicillin-resistant *S. epidermidis* (*MRSE*) [4].

Various classes of topical antibacterial products have been used in the treatment of bacterial conjunctivitis. These include aminoglycosides (e.g. tobramycin, gentamycin and netilmicin), macrolides (e.g. azithromycin), chloramphenicol and, most recently, fluoroquinolones (e.g. ofloxacin and levofloxacin) [4].

Nonetheless, successful therapy for bacterial conjunctivitis continues to be limited by several factors. A primary concern is the development of bacterial resistance that may be impacted not only by widespread antibiotic use but also by antibacterial pharmacokinetics, such as maintenance of insufficient bactericidal concentrations at the site of infection [2, 4].

Importantly, netilmicin is active against strains and resistant to other aminoglycosides, such as tobramycin or gentamicin [2], including methicillin-resistant strains [1, 2, 5, 6]. Indeed, being an antibiotic almost totally dedicated to ophthalmology and not used for systemic route, netilmicin has maintained unchanged its susceptibility and resistance profile over the last 20 years towards the major strains responsible for eye infections [7, 8].

Netilmicin is available on the market in three different topical ophthalmic dosage forms: solution, gel and ointment. Those products are indicated for the treatment of bacterial ocular infections of the anterior segment of the eye and ocular adnexa [2]. Netilmicin ophthalmic formulation is able to cross the cornea of rabbits, reaching aqueous humor levels comparable with the minimal inhibitory concentration (MIC) for usual ocular pathogens [9]. Netilmicin has no toxic effect *in vitro* on human corneal epithelial cells (HCE-T) and human conjunctival epithelial cells (Wong-Kilbourne derivative of Chang conjunctiva) [10]. Bonfiglio *et al*. evaluated the *in vitro* activity of netilmicin of other antibiotics used in ophthalmology against gram-positive and gram-negative microorganisms isolated from ocular infections. The results of this study showed that the activity of netilmicin was superior to that of ofloxacin against both groups of bacteria, with more than 90% of the isolated strains being susceptible to netilmicin [3]. Additionally, in a study carried out on 1333 ocular clinical isolates, netilmicin was revealed to have the best susceptibility profile among aminoglycosides showing the lowest minimum inhibitory concentration (MIC) values against all isolates. Specifically, netilmicin superiority was pronounced against *S. aureus* and coagulase-negative staphylococci (CoNS) [11]. These two Staphylococci strains represent the most diffused clusters of bacteria in ocular infections ranging from 65 to 76.2% of the total isolates under investigation [11, 12].

Moreover, Blanco *et al*. evidenced that netilmicin was effective as vancomycin against both methicillin-resistant *Staphylococcus aureus* (*MRSA*) and methicillin-resistant *Staphylococcus epidermidis* (*MRSE*) clinical-ocular isolates [13]. This result is worthy of note considering that an increasing incidence (55% from 2002 to 2008) of *MRSA* and *MRSE* strains was registered in ophthalmology with few antibiotics capable of being efficacious against these pathogens [14]. Considering this evidence, the aim of the present study was to, directly, compare, within the same experimental setting, anti-staphylococcal activity of netilmicin to those of the main ophthalmic antimicrobials on the market. To this end, two of the most important pharmacological indices for antibiotics, that is, the quotient of inhibition (QI), corresponding to the C_{max}/MIC_{90} ratio [15], and the antibiotic kinetic of killing was investigated. Antibiotic QIs were calculated by mining respective maximum concentration (C_{max}) and MIC_{90} data from peer-reviewed literature and from internal pharmacokinetic studies in rabbits carried out according to Good Laboratory Practice (GLP). The QIs of two netilmicin formulations, eye drops solution and gel, in single and multiple dose administrations (both in cornea and conjunctiva), were compared to those of tobramycin, ofloxacin, levofloxacin and azithromycin. The QI of chloramphenicol was not calculated since no data on C_{max} in the target tissues (cornea and conjunctiva) were found in literature. Moreover, the same analysis was performed in human tears, comparing netilmicin eye drops solution with tobramycin ofloxacin and levofloxacin, all in single-dose administration. Concerning the killing kinetics against two ATCC Staphylococci strains and two Staphylococci methicillin-resistant ocular isolates, netilmicin activity was directly compared to those of the above-cited antibiotics and to chloramphenicol as well.

2. Materials and methods

2.1 QIs determination

Meta-analysis for QIs determination was carried out by scanning scientific literature in search of *in vitro* studies, reporting levofloxacin, ofloxacin, netilmicin, tobramycin and azithromycin MIC_{90} values against the most diffused bacterial species in ocular infections (*MSSA, MRSA, MSCoNS, MRCoNS*), and pre-clinical *in vivo* studies in rabbits, reporting corneal and conjunctival C_{max} values of ophthalmic formulations containing the above antibiotics. In detail, as described in **Tables 1** and **2**, the following eye drops formulations were taken into account: (i) netilmicin 0.3% eye drops solution (Nettacin® eye drops); (ii) Netilmicin 0.3% gel formulation (Xanternet®); (iii) tobramycin 0.3% (Tobrex®); (iv) levofloxacin 1.5% (Iquix® and Cravit®);(v) ofloxacin 0.3% (Tarivid® and Ocuflox®); and (vi) azithromycin 1% (Azasite® and Azimycin®).

As to the MIC_{90}, the selected references adhered to the criteria of encompassing large epidemiological/surveillance studies and including the above-cited groups of bacterial strains. As to the second parameter (C_{max}), only those studies comprising the same animal species and the same regimen of ocular drug administration (single or multiple doses) were considered as eligible and comparable to each other. Then MIC_{90} and C_{max} data were put into ratio and the QI values for the two ocular tissues and regimens were calculated.

Moreover, the same analysis was performed in human tears, comparing netilmicin 0.3% eye drops solution with tobramycin 0.3%, ofloxacin 0.3% and levofloxacin 0.5%, all in single-dose administration.

References for C_{max} values	C_{max} (μg/g) single dose		Antibiotic formulations	References for MIC_{90} values	MIC_{90} μg/ml (strains)
	Cornea	Conjunctiva			
Mazzone M.G., unpublished data	0.35	0.81	NETTACIN EYE DROPS (netilmicin 0.3%)	Sanfilippo CM *et al.* 2016 [11]	0.5 (*MSSA*); 0.5 (*MRSA*); 0.12 (*MSCoNS)*; 0.06 (*MRCoNS*)
	0.98	3.75	NETILMICIN GEL (netilmicin 0.3%)		
Gilbert ML et *al.* 1987* [16]; Owen GR et *al.* 2007** [17]	0	3.1	TOBREX (tobramycin 0.3%)		1 (*MSSA*); 1024 (*MRSA*); 8 (*MSCoNS*); 32 (*MRCoNS*)
Chung JL et *al.* 2013 [18]	10.67	1.99	IQUIX (levofloxacin 1.5%)	Asbell PA *et al.* 2020 [12]	2 (*MSSA*); 128 (*MRSA*); 2 (*MSCoNS*); 256 (*MRCoNS*)
Sakai T et *al.* 2019 [19]	2.21	20.4	TARIVID (ofloxacin 0.3%)		4 (*MSSA);* 16 (*MRSA);* 8 (*MSCoNS*); 32 (*MRCoNS*)
Product Monograph (revision 2013) [20]	3.32	2.95	OCUFLOX (ofloxacin 0.3%)		
Akpek EK et *al.* 2009 [21]	40.4	108	AZASITE (azithromycin 1%)		1024 (*MSSA, MRSA, MSCoNS, MRCoNS*)
Sakai T et *al.* 2019 [19]	79.9	44.2	AZIMYCIN (azithromycin 1%)		

**referring to cornea.*
***referring to conjunctiva.*

Table 1.
C_{max}, MIC_{90} values and relative bibliographic references as to the single dose of antibiotics administration.

2.2 Bacterial strains and killing curves determination

Two eye swabs of bacterial isolates *S. aureus* 801 CT (*MRSA*) and *S. epidermidis* 829 CT (*MRSE*), belonging to SIFI's private collection were used throughout this study. These strains collection comprises different microbial eye isolates collected from 1998 to 2014 from patients with community-acquired ocular infections coming from three different geographical sites (Messina, Catania and Rome (Italy)). The above microorganisms, and their antibiotic resistance patterns, were previously identified by standard laboratory methodologies. Genetic profiles of all *S. aureus* and *S. epidermidis* isolates of the collection were previously determined (data not shown) with the aim of grouping all isolates in 'strain types'. The two methicillin-resistant microorganisms under study were each representative of the most diffused 'strain type' within the collection with regards to species and the geographical provenience. In addition, *S. aureus* ATCC 6538 and *S. epidermidis* ATCC 12228 strains (purchased from Thermo Fisher Scientific, Lenexa, KS, USA) were also included in the experiment. Time kill determination was performed as previously described by Bonfiglio *et al.* [3]. Briefly, microorganisms were grown overnight to reach a density of about 10^8 colony-forming unit (cfu)/ml

References for C_{max} values	C_{max} (µg/g) multiple dose		Antibiotic formulations	References for MIC_{90} values	MIC_{90} µg/ml (*strains*)
	Cornea	Conjunctiva			
Civiale C., unpublished data	0.35	0.77	NETTACIN EYE DROPS (netilmicin 0.3%)	Sanfilippo CM. *et al.* 2016 [11]	0.5 (*MSSA*); 0.5; (*MRSA*); 0.12 (*MSCoNS*); 0.06 (*MRCoNS*)
	0	0.65	TOBREX (tobramycin 0.3%)		1 (*MSSA*); 1024 (*MRSA*); 8 (*MSCoNS*); 32 (*MRCoNS*)
Sugioka K et *al.* 2009 [11]	7.34	1.77	CRAVIT (levofloxacin 0.5%)	Asbell PA *et al.* 2020 [12]	2 (*MSSA*); 128 (*MRSA*); 2 (*MSCoNS*); 256 (*MRCoNS*)
Tarivid -Full Prescribing Info [22]	7.78	34.98	TARIVID (ofloxacin 0.3%)		4 (*MSSA*); 16 (*MRSA*); 8 (*MSCoNS*); 32 (*MRCoNS*)
Product Monograph (revision 2013) [20]	6.5	5.6	OCUFLOX (ofloxacin 0.3%)		
Akpek EK et *al.* 2009 [21]	252	177.4	AZASITE (azithromycin 1%)		1024 (*MSSA, MRSA, MSCoNS, MRCoNS*)

Table 2.
C_{max}, MIC_{90} values and relative bibliographic references to multiple doses of antibiotics administration.

on Mueller Hinton (MH) broth (purchased from Biogenerica, CT, Italy) and then diluted to about 1×10^6 cfu/ml in the same pre-warmed medium containing netilmicin (32 µg/ml; purchased from Zhejiang Zhenyuan Pharmaceutical Co., Ltd, Shaoxing, China), tobramycin (16 µg/ml; purchased from Sigma Aldrich, MI, Italy), ofloxacin, levofloxacin (4 µg/ml; purchased from Sigma Aldrich, MI, Italy), azithromycin (8 µg/ ml, purchased from Sigma Aldrich, MI, Italy) or chloramphenicol (32 µg/ml, Chemo, Spain). These antibiotics concentrations corresponded to the resistance breakpoints values according to CLSI's (2015) interpretative criteria. An antibiotic-free control was similarly inoculated. At 0, 1, 2, 6 and 24 hours after drug exposure, 0.1 ml of the culture was collected, diluted in phosphate buffered saline, inoculated (by inclusion) onto MH agar plates and incubated at 37° C for 24 hours to determine viable cfu/ml. All the experiments were performed in triplicate for three experimental days. Killing curves were constructed by plotting the $\log_{10}$ of cfu/ml versus the established time points (i.e 0, 1, 2, 6 and 24 h). Bactericidal activity was defined as a >3 $\log_{10}$ decrease of the initial inoculum size. A statistical analysis of the area under the curve (AUC) was conducted by the one-way ANOVA statistical test (GraphPad Prism 6; CA, USA).

3. Results

3.1 QIs determination

Corneal and conjunctival C_{max} values for netilmicin, tobramycin, levofloxacin, ofloxacin and azithromycin formulations, in both single and multiple doses administration, were gathered from bibliographic *in vivo* pharmacokinetic studies [16–19, 21, 23] and, as to netilmicin, from two internal GLP studies (M.G. Mazzone and C. Civiale unpublished data). All these studies have been carried out on rabbit and included the same regimen of drug administration. The QI of chloramphenicol was not calculated since no data on C_{max} in the target tissues (cornea and conjunctiva) were found in literature. The values of MIC_{90}, for the five antibiotics under investigation, were retrieved from two studies [11, 12] that fully match the fixed bibliography selection criteria. In the study selected for quinolones (i.e levofloxacin, ofloxacin) and macrolide (i.e azithromycin) antibiotics, MIC_{90} values were calculated from a total of 6091 eye isolates while the second study, for the aminoglycoside antibiotics, considered a total of 734 ocular isolates. C_{max}, MIC_{90} values and their relative bibliographic references were reported in **Tables 1** and **2**. C_{max} values were put into ratio with the above MICs $_{90}$ and the resulting QIs were reported as graphs. Analysis of the QI values showed that, as to the single dose, Nettacin® eye drops (netilmicin 0.3% eye drops solution) were revealed to be the best performing formulation in conjunctiva against *MRSA*, *MRCoNS* and *MSCoNS* (**Figure 1**). Interestingly, under the same conditions, netilmicin 0.3% gel formulation (Xanternet) allowed a general sensible increase of the QIs to make this formulation the best performing one among those studied, also against the *MSSA* (**Figure 2**). In cornea, netilmicin 0.3% eye drops solution showed higher QIs with respect to other formulations *vs MRSA* and *MRCoNS* strains. IQUIX® (levofloxacin 1.5%), due to the fortified formulation, overcame all the other ones in the *MSCoNS* category (**Figure 3**). Also in this case, under the same conditions, the netilmicin 0.3% gel formulation allowed a general sensible increase of the QIs so that netilmicin gel was revealed to be the best performing formulation against the *MSCoNS* and the second best performing one against the *MSSA* category (**Figure 4**). As to the multiple doses of administration, only Nettacin® eye drops were eligible to be included in the analysis. This netilmicin

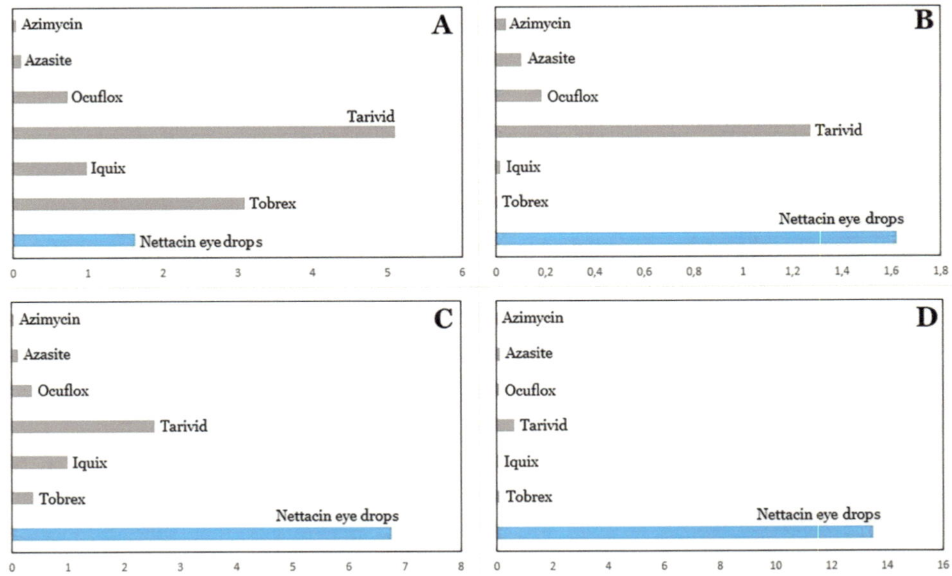

Figure 1.
Netilmicin eye drops (Nettacin eye drops) conjunctival QIs in a single dose against (A) MSSA; (B) MRSA; (C) MSCoNS; and (D) MRCoNS.

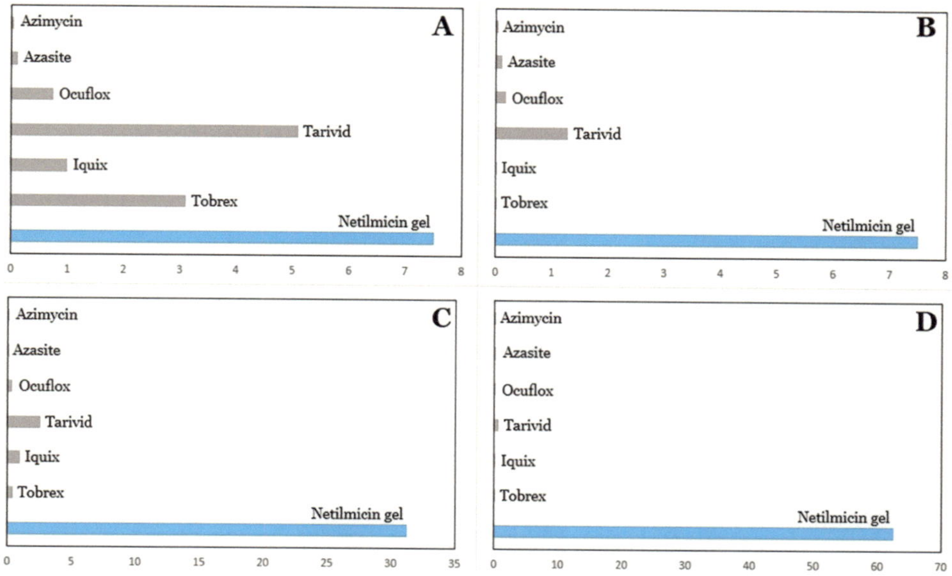

Figure 2.
Netilmicin gel (Xanternet) conjunctival QIs in a single dose against (A) MSSA; (B) MRSA; (C) MSCoNS; and (D) MRCoNS.

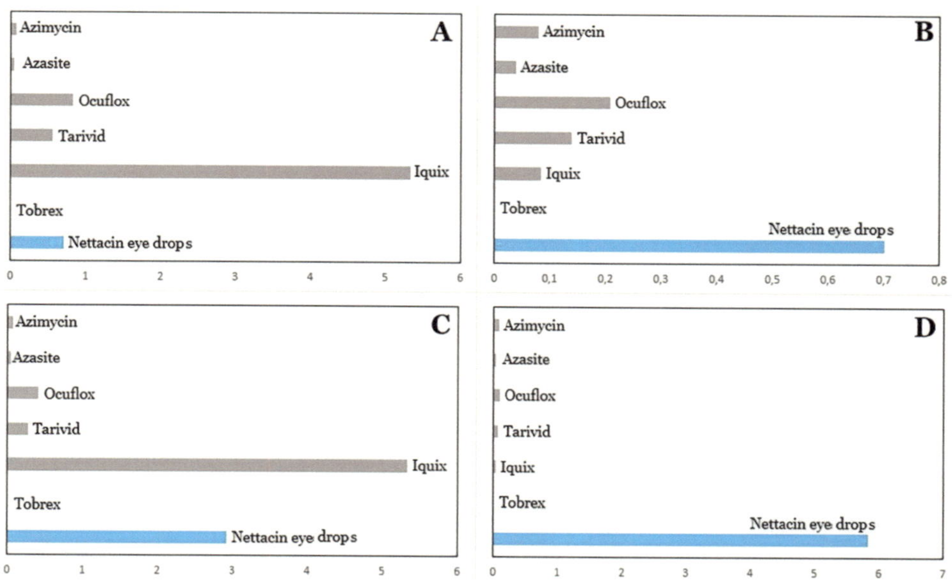

Figure 3.
Netilmicin eye drops (Nettacin eye drops) corneal QIs in a single dose against (A) MSSA; (B) MRSA; (C) MSCoNS; and (D) MRCoNS.

formulation in the conjunctiva was the best performing one among the three antibiotic formulations considered against *MRCoNS* and *MSCoNS* and the second best performing one against the other two strain categories (**Figure 5**). In the cornea, netilmicin in multiple-dose presentation, revealed to be the best performing formulation against *MRCoNS* and *MRSA* (**Figure 6**).

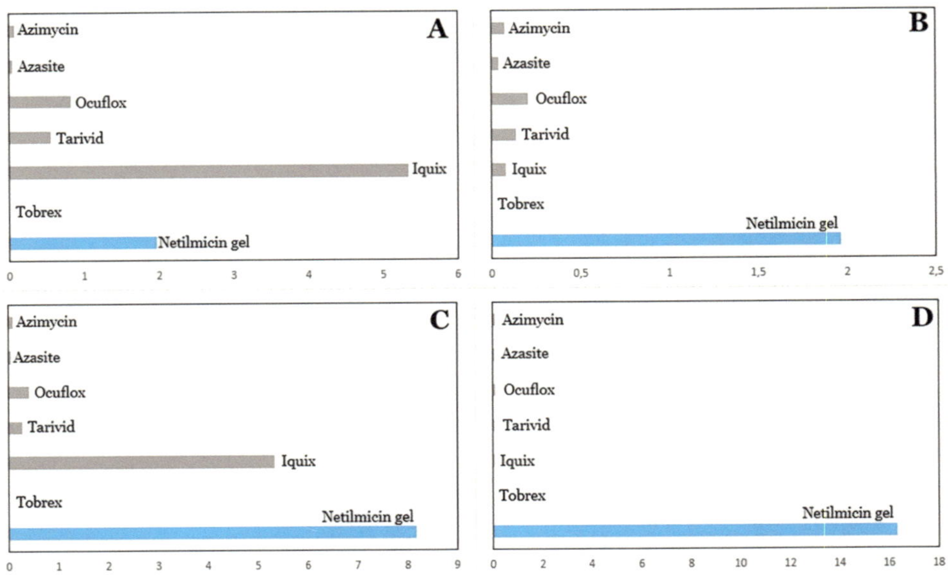

Figure 4.
Netilmicin gel (Xanternet) corneal QIs in a single dose against (A) MSSA; (B) MRSA; (C) MSCoNS; and (D) MRCoNS.

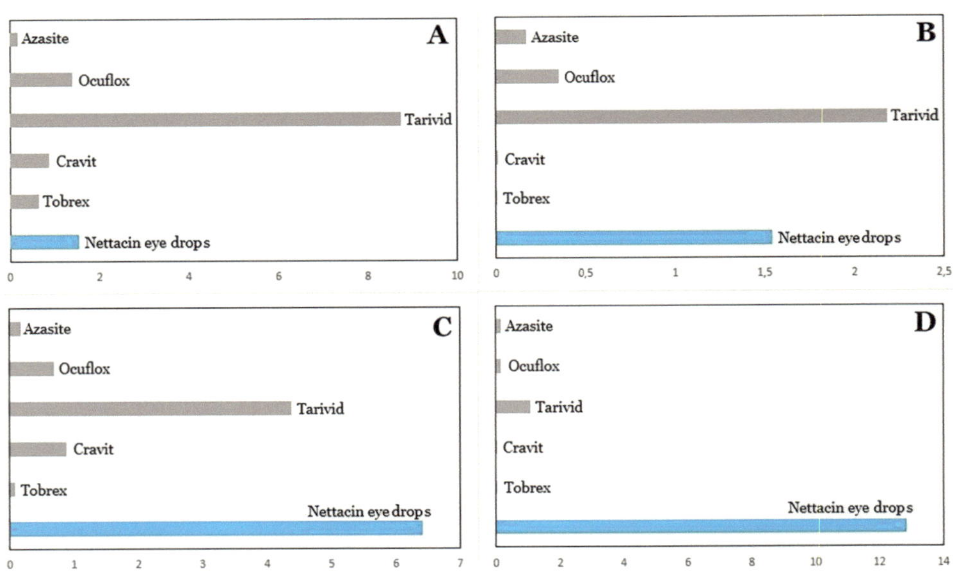

Figure 5.
Netilmicin eye drops (Nettacin eye drops) conjunctival QIs in multiple doses against (A) MSSA; (B) MRSA; (C) MSCoNS; and (D) MRCoNS.

Moreover, QI determination was evaluated in human tear, comparing netilmicin eye drops solution with tobramycin and fluoroquinolones (i.e. ofloxacin and levofloxacin). QIs, were established, using MIC_{90} and C_{max} values retrieved from peer-reviewed literature [11, 24–28]. Results demonstrated that in human tear,

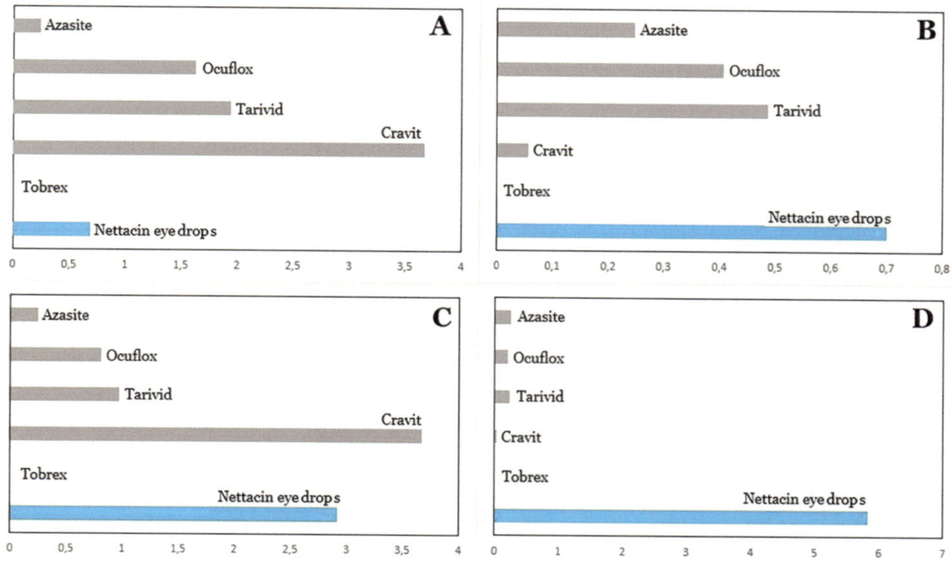

Figure 6.
Netilmicin eye drops (Nettacin eye drops) corneal QIs in multiple doses against (A) MSSA; (B) MRSA; (C) MSCoNS; and (D) MRCoNS.

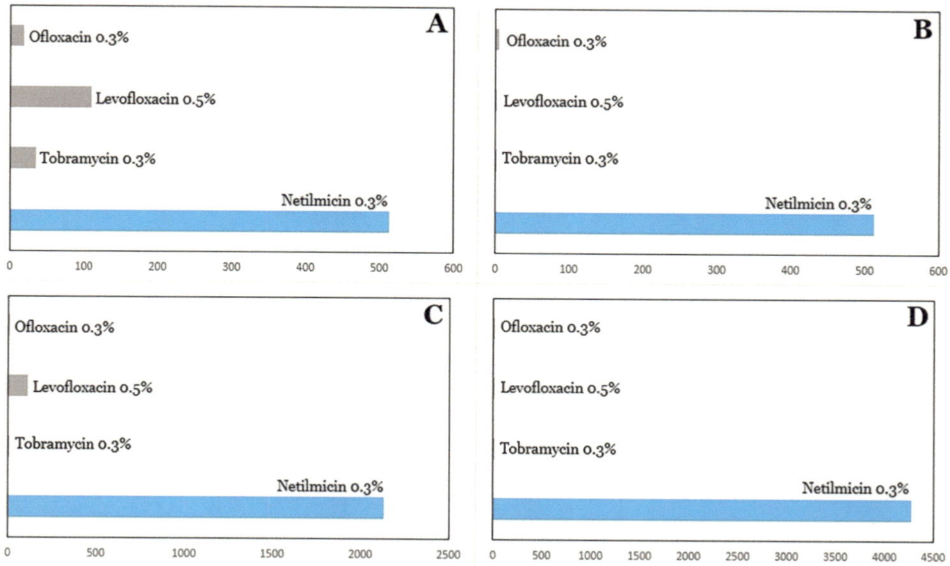

Figure 7.
Netilmicin eye drops tear QIs against (A) MSSA; (B) MRSA; (C) MSCoNS; and (D) MRCoNS.

netilmicin eye drops solution showed a more favourable QI against Staphylococci than tobramycin, ofloxacin and levofloxacin, all evaluated in single-dose administration regimen (**Figure 7**).

Altogether, QI results showed that netilmicin in the conjunctiva, in both single and multiple doses, is a highly effective antibiotic against all staphylococcal categories, while in the cornea it was revealed to be particularly active in single and multiple doses, against methicillin-resistant Staphylococci strains. Importantly, QI data on human tears supports what was found in the cornea and conjunctiva of rabbits, thus confirming the better efficacy of netilmicin with respect to other antibiotics.

3.2 Killing curves

Data showed that netilmicin has a pronounced bactericidal activity against all the four Staphylococci tested strains. For these Staphylococci, netilmicin was revealed to be one of the most active antibiotics achieving, at 24 hours, a > 3 $\log_{10}$ reduction of the initial inoculum (**Figures 8–11**).

In detail, netilmicin, together with tobramycin, showed a bactericidal effect against *S. aureus* 6538 (ATCC strain) with a higher efficacy at 24h (>4 and 6 $\log_{10}$ decrease, respectively) compared to levofloxacin, ofloxacin, azithromycin and chloramphenicol (**Figure 8**).

The same activity was found against *S. aureus* 801 *MRSA* (ocular isolate), where netilmicin, together with tobramycin, showed the best performance reaching the total eradication of the initial inoculum at 24h, (both 6 $\log_{10}$ decreases at 24h) (**Figure 9**). Importantly, this effect is better than levofloxacin, ofloxacin, azithromycin and chloramphenicol that failed to induce a > 3 $\log_{10}$ reduction of the initial inoculum at all time points, with the exception of levofloxacin and ofloxacin that induce a reduction > 3 $\log_{10}$ at 24h (**Figure 9**).

Moreover, netilmicin reduced bacterial growth of *S. epidermidis* 12228 (ATCC strain) with a killing activity from 2h to 24h similar to that of tobramycin (6 $\log_{10}$ decrease, **Figure 10**). Except for levofloxacin which is effective only at 24h (6 $\log_{10}$ decrease), this effect is better than ofloxacin, azithromycin and chloramphenicol that failed to produce a > 3 $\log_{10}$ reduction of the initial inoculum (**Figure 10**).

Surprisingly, it was found that netilmicin was the only antibiotic able to reach the total eradication of the bacterial inoculum of *S. epidermidis* 829 *MRSE* (ocular

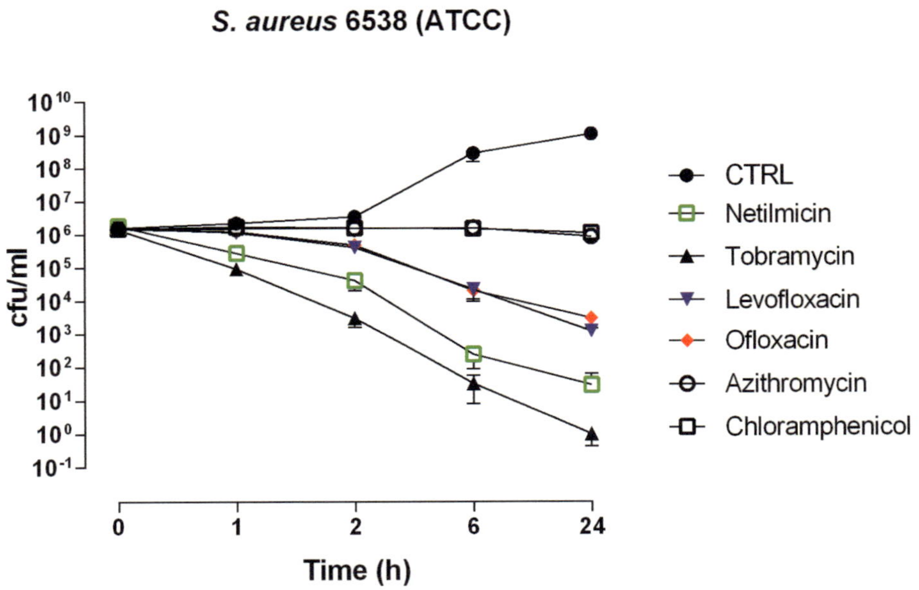

Figure 8.
Time-killing curves of netilmicin (32 µg/ml), tobramycin (16 µg/ml), levofloxacin (4 µg/ml), ofloxacin (4 µg/ml), azitromycin (8 µg/ml) and chloramphenicol against S. aureus (ATCC 6538 strain) exposed for 0, 1, 2, 6 and 24 h. Data represent mean ± S.E.M. of $\log_{10}$ cfu/ml of three replicates.

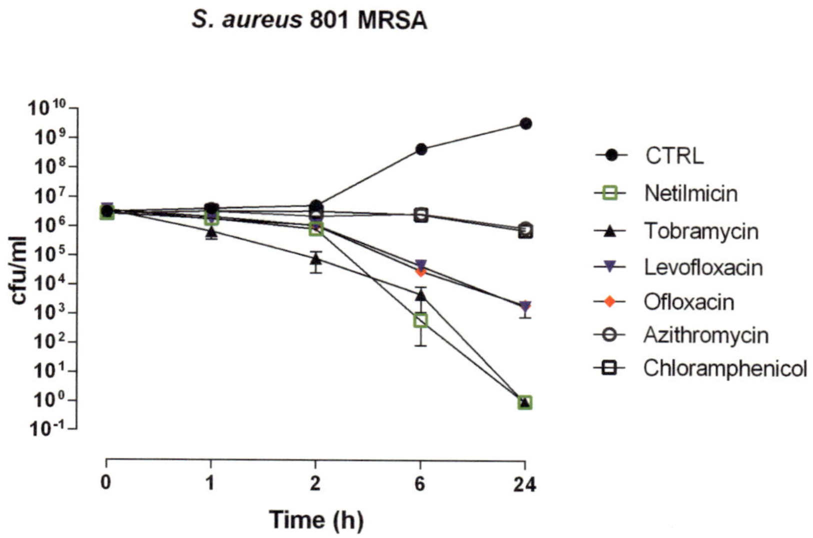

Figure 9.
Time-killing curves of netilmicin (32 μg/ml), tobramycin (16 μg/ml), levofloxacin (4 μg/ml), ofloxacin (4 μg/ml), azitromycin (8 μg/ml) and chloramphenicol against S. aureus 801 isolate (MRSA) exposed for 0, 1, 2, 6 and 24 h. Data represent mean ± S.E.M. of log_{10} cfu/ml of three replicates.

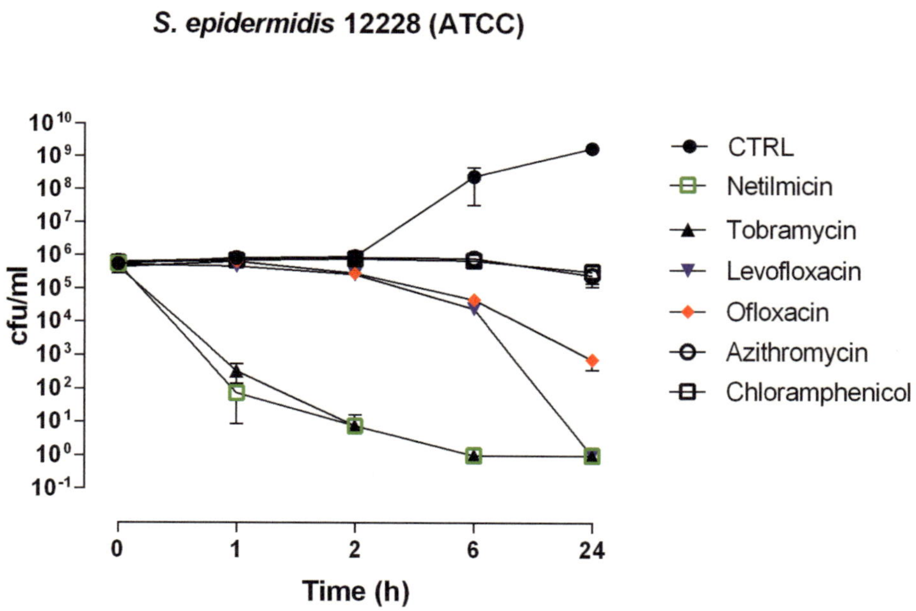

Figure 10.
Time-killing curves of netilmicin (32 μg/ml), tobramycin (16 μg/ml), levofloxacin (4 μg/ml), ofloxacin (4 μg/ml), azitromycin (8 μg/ml) and chloramphenicol against S. epidermidis (ATCC 12228 strain) exposed for 0, 1, 2, 6 and 24 h. Data represent mean ± S.E.M. of log_{10} cfu/ml of three replicates.

isolate) at 24h (6 log_{10} decrease, **Figure 11**) with respect to all other tested antibiotics. Moreover, levofloxacin and ofloxacin showed a bactericidal activity at 24h (3 log_{10} decrease, **Figure 11**) but this effect is lower than netilmicin. Importantly, tobramycin failed to produce a bactericidal effect against *MRSE* ocular isolate (**Figure 11**).

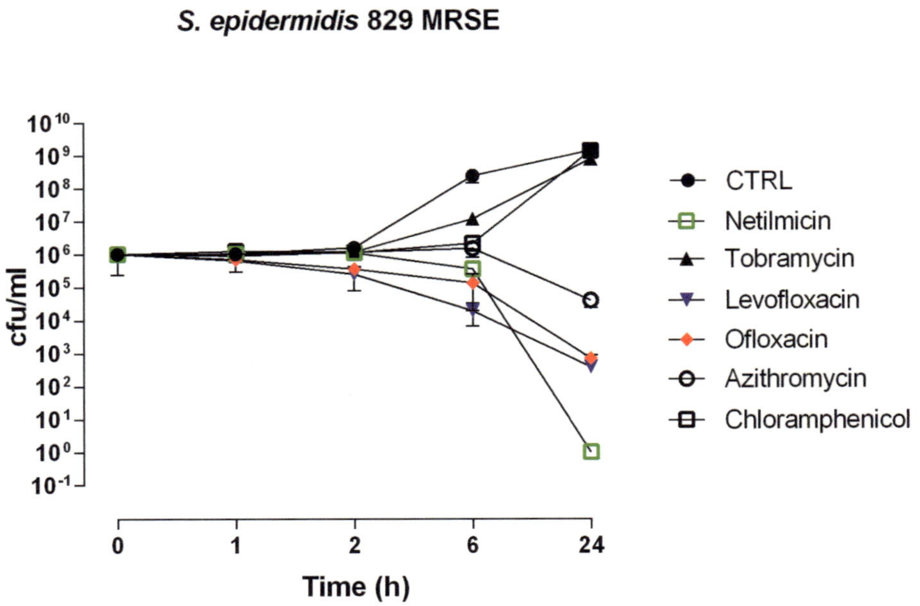

Figure 11.
Time-killing curves of netilmicin (32 μg/ml), tobramycin (16 μg/ml), levofloxacin (4 μg/ml), ofloxacin (4 μg/ml), azitromycin (8 μg/ml) and chloramphenicol against S. epidermidis 829 isolate (MRSE) exposed for 0, 1, 2, 6 and 24 h. Data represent mean ± S.E.M. of $\log_{10}$ cfu/ml of three replicates.

Moreover, in order to better understand and compare the efficacy of the different antibiotics tested, area under the curve (AUC) was calculated for each killing curve obtained and compared to netilmicin AUC for each strain tested (**Table 3**).

Results of the analysis showed that netilmicin has a better activity with respect to tobramycin against *MRSE* strain ($p \leq 0.0001$, **Table 3**).

Moreover, netilmicin is better than azithromycin for three of the total four strains tested, specifically *S. aureus* 6538 and MRSA with $p \leq 0.0001$ and *S. epidermidis* 12228

Antibiotics	**Strains/ocular isolates**			
	S. aureus 6538 (ATCC)	**S. epidermidis 12228 (ATCC)**	**MRSA**	**MRSE**
	Netilmicin	**Netilmicin**	**Netilmicin**	**Netilmicin**
Tobramycin	ns	ns	ns	*
Levofloxacin	ns	ns	ns	ns
Ofloxacin	ns	ns	ns	ns
Azithromycin	****	***	****	ns
Chloramphenicol	****	**	****	***

$^{*}p \leq 0.05$.
$^{**}p \leq 0.01$.
$^{***}p \leq 0.001$.
$^{****}p \leq 0.0001$ vs netilmicin.
One-way ANOVA followed by Dunnett's post-hoc test; ns = no statically significant differences.

Table 3.
Area Under the Curve (AUC) of all antibiotics compared to netilmicin.

($p \leq 0.001$) (**Table 3**). Finally, it was found that netilmicin is better than chloramphenicol for all tested strains ($p \leq 0.01$ for *S. epidermidis* 12228; $p \leq 0.001$ for *MRSE*; $p \leq 0.0001$ for *S. aureus* 6538 and *MRSA*) (**Table 3**).

4. Discussion

Bacterial conjunctivitis affects many people and imposes economic and social burdens [29]. Clinical studies of ocular infections have documented a gradual decline in the effectiveness of many commonly used topical antibacterial agents, creating a continuous demand for newer, effective treatments and better strategies to minimize resistance [4]. Netilmicin is a broad-spectrum, semisynthetic and water-soluble antibiotic of the aminoglycoside group. Compared to gentamicin and tobramycin, netilmicin has a good activity against gentamicin and tobramycin resistant strains, this depending on the N-ethyl substitution of the 2- deoxystreptamine ring [1–3]. Interestingly, netilmicin might also be considered an antibiotic of choice in the preoperative setting thanks to the high *in vitro* susceptibility (>90%) to this antibiotic of those isolates belonging to the normal ocular flora (including also the multi-resistant coagulase-negative Staphylococci) [30]. As to the arising of resistant strains, this antibiotic, when compared to other aminoglycosides and fluoroquinolones, has one of the lowest incidences of resistance among both gram-positive and negative organisms (2% and 3%, respectively) [31]. To truly understand the pharmacology of antimicrobial agents, it's better to go beyond MICs, using metrics that account for the rate of bacterial killing and effects of different dosing regimens and formulations on accumulation in tissues. Appreciation of the pharmacokinetic properties of an antibiotic and its pharmacodynamic measures of efficacy can maximise the utility of these sight-saving drugs. To better understand the antibacterial activity of netilmicin and compare it with that of other ophthalmic antibiotics, two key pharmacological indices, QI and killing kinetic, useful to facilitate this comparison were investigated [15]. QI results showed that netilmicin has more affinity to cornea and conjunctiva with respect to the other molecules studied ensuring, in these tissues, amounts of drug suitable to eradicate Staphylococci (including methicillin-resistant strains). Interestingly, netilmicin 0.3% tested in both solution and gel formulation form, selectively guarantee at the main ocular sites high antibiotic concentrations without neglecting patient's compliance [32]. Particularly, the present study demonstrates that the gel formulation of netilmicin greatly amplifies the potency of the molecule by concurring with the increase of its QIs within target tissues. In fact, the gel formulation of netilmicin contains 1% xanthan gum which affects the retention time of the antibiotic on the ocular surface and, consequently, on the tissues' C_{max} values [24]. Moreover, in human tears, netilmicin eye drops, in single dose, showed to have a more favourable QI against Staphylococci than tobramycin and fluoroquinolones (i.e. ofloxacin and levofloxacin). Also, in this case, to calculate the QIs, MIC_{90} and C_{max} values were retrieved from peer-reviewed literature as above [11, 25–28].

Results of the present study highlight that netilmicin has also a faster killing activity and a more potent antimicrobial effect, against most of the staphylococcal strains tested, including *MRSA* and *MRSE*, than the main ophthalmic antibiotics.

Results demonstrated that netilmicin and tobramycin, both included in the aminoglycosides class, are effective against *S. aureus*, *MRSA* and *S. epidermidis* with a greater effect compared to the other tested antibiotics, that is, azithromycin, ofloxacin, levofloxacin and chloramphenicol. Surprisingly, netilmicin is the only antibiotic able to inhibit the growth of *MRSE* compared to all other molecules including tobramycin although belonging to the same class. Importantly, tobramycin was found to be unable to inhibit the growth of *MRSE* strains, indeed bacterial growth increases as the control (condition without treatment).

These findings are of particular interest considering that among ocular isolates, the frequency of *MRSE* and *MRSA* in bacterial conjunctivitis is increasing [4].

Moreover, the aforementioned susceptibility profile of netilmicin against multi-drug resistant organism (MDRO) like CoNS, including *S. epidermidis* [30], guarantees that its use is beneficial and warranted also to restore the balance of the eye microbiota frequently disrupted in patients suffering from recurrent eye infections who are subjected to repeated, and sometimes empirical, antibiotic treatments.

In fact, normal ocular microbiota could be considered a reservoir of antibiotic resistance and some bacterial strains have the capacity of centralizing and carrying antibiotic resistance genes (belonging to other organisms) so to become MDRO.

It was already proven that empirical antibiotic treatment in eye infections, such as keratitis, leads to an increase in the antibiotic resistome profile of the ocular surface microbiota [33].

As an example of antibiotics leading to multi-drug resistance patterns, it is known that the repeated use of topical antibiotics, e.g. azithromycin or fluoroquinolones, could significantly alter the microbiota composition by increasing the percentage of *S. epidermidis* at the expense of other strains populating the commensal flora. *S. epidermidis* could rapidly emerge after antibiotic exposure acquiring both co-resistance to several classes of antibiotics and alterations in their biofilm formation capacity so to produce considerable clinical implications, such as conjunctivitis, keratitis and endophthalmitis [34].

In this sense, the use of netilmicin in patients where a chronic disruption of the normal balance of the ocular flora occurs as a consequence of the emergence of pathogens like MDRO CoNS should be recommended in order to reconstitute a normal eye surface homeostasis and, therefore, to resolve the aforementioned pathologies.

Moreover, it is worthy of note that in literature there is evidence showing that bactericidal action of netilmicin is maintained for up to 4 hours by its post-antibiotic effect [3]. This evidence could be useful for reducing the antibiotic administration regimen *in vivo*.

5. Conclusions

Netilmicin exhibits superior activity against the most common ocular bacterial strains, with faster and greater inhibitory potency in target tissues than other ophthalmic antibiotics. QI data on cornea and conjunctiva in rabbits demonstrated that netilmicin 0.3% is better than the other products when tested in both dosage forms, that is, eye drops solution and gel. Importantly, netilmicin 0.3% gel, due to the presence of 1% xanthan gum prolongs the retention time on the ocular surface and, consequently, increases the C_{max}. Therefore, based on the severity of the pathology and any other concerns (e.g. corneal healing) associated with bacterial conjunctivitis, it is possible to use netilmicin 0.3% eye drops solution or gel formulation. Moreover, netilmicin offers an excellent broad-spectrum coverage against all tested isolates, including MRSA and MRSE, compared with other ophthalmic antibiotics. These findings are of particular interest considering that among ocular isolates, the frequency of MRSE and MRSA in bacterial conjunctivitis is increasing. Overall, these data support the use of netilmicin as a first-line agent in the treatment of such bacterial ocular infections, due to ocular safety, potency and low resistance.

Conflict of interest

All the authors declare not to have any conflict of interest.

Author details

Andrea Sudano Roccaro*, Carmela Giovanna Spoto, Luca Rosario La Rosa, Claudine Civiale, Manuela Santonocito, Santa Viola, Cristina Zappulla, Maria Cristina Curatolo and Maria Grazia Mazzone
SIFI SpA, Aci Sant'Antonio (CT), Italy

*Address all correspondence to: andrea.sudanoroccaro@sifigroup.com

References

[1] Campoli-Richards DM, Chaplin S, Sayce RH, Goa KL. A review of its antibacterial activity, pharmacokinetic properties and therapeutic use. Drugs. 1989;**38**:703-756

[2] Papa V, Aragona P, Scuderi AC, Blanco AR, Zola P, Di Bella A, et al. Treatment of acute bacterial conjunctivitis with topical netilmicin. Cornea. 2002;**21**:43-47

[3] Bonfiglio G, Scuderi AC, Russo G. Netilmicin: In vitro activity, time-kill evaluation and postantibiotic effect on microorganisms isolated from ocular infections. Chemotherapy. 2001;**47**:117-122

[4] Karpecki P, Paterno MR, Comstock TL. Limitations of current antibiotics for the treatment of bacterial conjunctivitis. Optometry and Vision Science. 2010;**87**(11):908-919

[5] Cagle G, Davis S, Rosenthal A, Smith J. Topical tobramycin and gentamicin sulfate in the treatment of ocular infections: Multicenter study. Current Eye Research. 1981;**1**:723-734

[6] Kallings LO. Resistance factors: Influence on netilmicin activity. Scandinavian Journal of Diseases Supplement. 1980;**23**:54-58

[7] Stefani S. Antibiotic therapy in the multi-drug resistance era. L'Oculista Italiano. 2017. Available from: https://www.oculistaitaliano.it/notizie/antibiotic-therapy-the-multi-drug-resistance/.

[8] Sommer MOA, Dantas G, Church GM. Functional characterization of the antibiotic resistance reservoir in the human microflora. Science. 2009;**28**:1128-1131

[9] Dorigo MT, De Natale R, Miglioli P. Collagen shields delivery of netilmicin: A study of ocular pharmacokinetics. Chemotherapy. 1995;**41**:1-4

[10] Papa V, Leonardi A, Getuli C, Pacelli V, Russo P, Milazzo G. Effect of ofloxacin and netilmicin on human corneal and conjunctival cells in vitro. Journal of Ocular Pharmacology and Therapeutics. 2003;**19**:535-545

[11] Sanfilippo CM, Morrissey I, Janes R, Morris TW. Surveillance of the activity of aminoglycosides and fluoroquinolones against ophthalmic pathogens from Europe in 2010-2011. Current Eye Research. 2016;**41**:581-589

[12] Asbell PA, Sanfilippo CM, Sahm DF, DeCory HH. Trends in antibiotic resistance among ocular microorganisms in the United States From 2009 to 2018. JAMA Ophthalmology. 2020;**138**:1-12

[13] Blanco AR, Sudano Roccaro A, Spoto CG, Papa V. Susceptibility of methicillin-resistant Staphylococci clinical isolates to netilmicin and other antibiotics commonly used in ophthalmic therapy. Current Eye Research. 2013;**38**:811-816

[14] Helzner J, editor. Your role in curbing the rising threat of ophthalmic MRSA. Ophthalmology Management; 2013:45-47. Available online: https://www.ophthalmologymanagement.com/issues/2013/november-2013/your-role-in-curbing-the-rising-threat-of-ophthalm [accessed 15 April 2022]

[15] Barger A, Fuhst C, Wiedemann B. Pharmacological indices in antibiotic therapy. The Journal of Antimicrobial Chemotherapy. 2003;**52**:893-898

[16] Gilbert ML, Wilhelmus KR, Osato MS. Comparative bioavailability and efficacy of fortified topical tobramycin. Investigative Ophthalmology & Visual Science. 1987;**28**:881-885

[17] Owen GR, Brooks AC, James O, Robertson SM. A novel in vivo rabbit model that mimics human dosing to determine the distribution of antibiotics in ocular tissues. Journal of Ocular Pharmacology and Therapeutics. 2007;**23**:335-342

[18] Chung JL, Lim EH, Song SW, Kim BY, Lee JH, Mah FS, et al. Comparative intraocular penetration of 4 fluoroquinolones after topical instillation. Cornea. 2013;**32**:1046-1051

[19] Sakai T, Shinno K, Kurata M, Kawamura A. Pharmacokinetics of azithromycin, levofloxacin, and ofloxacin in rabbit extraocular tissues after ophthalmic administration. Ophthalmology and Therapy. 2019;**8**:511-517

[20] PRODUCT MONOGRAPH—PrOCUFLOX® (ofloxacin)—Ophthalmic Solution 0.3% w/v—Antibacterial Agent. Allergan Inc. Markham, Ontario L6G 0B5. Date of Revision: March 26, 2013

[21] Akpek EK, Vittitow J, Verhoeven RS, Brubaker K, Amar T, Powell KD, et al. Ocular surface distribution and pharmacokinetics of a novel ophthalmic 1% azithromycin formulation. Journal of Ocular Pharmacology and Therapeutics. 2009;**25**:433-439

[22] Tarivid® full prescribing info. Available from: https://www.mims.com/malaysia/drug/info/tarivid%20ophthalmic?type=full [accessed 20 April 2022]

[23] Sugioka K, Fukuda M, Komoto S, Itahashi M, Yamada M, Shimomura Y. Intraocular penetration of sequentially instilled topical moxifloxacin, gatifloxacin, and levofloxacin. Clinical Ophthalmology. 2009;**3**:553-557

[24] Gagliano C, Papa V, Amato R, Malaguarnera G, Avitabile T. Measurement of the retention time of different ophthalmic formulations with ultrahigh-resolution optical coherence tomography. Current Eye Research. 2018;**43**:499-502

[25] Tang-Liu DD, Schwob DL, Usansky JI, Gordon YJ. Comparative tear concentrations over time of ofloxacin and tobramycin in human eyes. Clinical Pharmacology and Therapeutics. 1994;**55**:284-292

[26] Scuderi AC, De Lazzari A, Miano F, Zola P. Residence time of netilmicin in tears. Cornea. 2002;**21**:48-50

[27] Raizman MB, Rubin JM, Graves AL, Rinehart M. Tear concentrations of levofloxacin following topical administration of a single dose of 0.5% levofloxacin ophthalmic solution in healthy volunteers. Thérapie. 2002;**24**:1439-1450

[28] Walters T, Rinehart M, Krebs W, Holdbrook M. Tear concentration and safety of levofloxacin ophthalmic solution 1.5% compared with ofloxacin ophthalmic solution 0.3% after topical administration in healthy adult volunteers. Cornea. 2010;**29**:263-268

[29] Azari AA, Barney NP. Conjunctivitis: A systematic review of diagnosis and treatment. Journal of the American Medical Association. 2013;**310**(16):1721-1729

[30] Papa V, Blanco AR, Santocono M. Ocular flora and their antibiotic susceptibility in patients having cataract surgery in Italy. Journal of Cataract and Refractive Surgery. 2016;**42**:1312-1317

[31] Vanzzini RV, Alcantara-Castro M, Flores V. Susceptibility to netilmicin in 400 bacterial strains isolated from ocular infections. Revista Mexicana de Oftalmologia. 2009;**83**:1-5

[32] Mazzone M, Civiale C, Mattei E, Blanco AR. Netilmicin ocular distribution of three different ophthalmic preparations: Eyedrops, hydrogel and ointment. Investigative Ophthalmology and Visual Science. 2007;**48**:4276

[33] Kang Y, Tian L, Gu X, Chen Y, Ma X, Lin S, et al. Characterization of the ocular surface microbiome in keratitis patients after repeated ophthalmic antibiotic exposure. Microbiological Spectroscopy. 2022;**10**:e0216221

[34] Dave SB, Toma HS, Kim SJ. Changes in ocular flora in eyes exposed to ophthalmic antibiotics. Ophthalmology. 2013;**120**:937-941

Chapter 4

Prevalence of Bacterial Ocular Infections among Patients Attending Eye Clinic of Aminu Kano Teaching Hospital and Murtala Muhammad Specialist Hospital, Kano

Abdulhadi Sale Kumurya and Khadija Abdulaziz Lawan

Abstract

The eye, a functionally and structurally complex organ, experiences a variety of bacterial, viral, fungal and parasitic infections. Bacteria are major causative agents of eye infections that can lead to loss of vision. The objective of this study was to determine the bacterial etiologic agents associated with ocular infections, antimicrobial susceptibility pattern of incriminated isolates and associated factors among patients who visited the eye unit of Aminu Kano Teaching Hospital (AKTH) and Murtala Muhammad Specialist Hospital (MMSH). A hospital-based cross-sectional study was conducted at MMSH and AKTH from 25 May 2021 to 20 July 2021. Specimens from the ocular areas were collected from a total of 88 patients who visited the eye unit. Specimens were inoculated on blood agar, chocolate agar, MacConkey agar and mannitol salt agar. Isolated bacteria were identified by a series of biochemical tests using the standard bacteriological method. Antimicrobial susceptibility test was performed according to the Clinical and Laboratory Standard Institute by disk diffusion method. Factors that could be associated with ocular infection were collected by using structured questionnaire. Data analysis was done using SPSS version 16.0 software package. A P value less than 0.05 was considered statistically significant. Out of the total 88 study participants with ocular infections, 78 (88.6%) were culture-positive. The proportions of Gram-positive and Gram-negative bacteria were 28 (31.8%) and 60 (68.2%), respectively. Among Gram-positive bacteria, *Staphylococcus aureus* were predominant. Among Gram-negative bacteria, *Heamophillus influenzae* were predominant. Most of the isolates were susceptible to ofloxacin and resistant to amoxicillin-clavulanic acid. Majority of ocular infections in this study were caused by bacteria; Gram-negative bacteria were responsible for most cases.

Keywords: ocular infection, bacterial profile, review

1. Introduction

The eye, a functionally and structurally complex organ, experiences a variety of bacterial, viral, fungal and parasitic infections [1]. Bacterial infections are the major contributors of ocular infections worldwide. Infection can be mono or poly-microbial and is associated with many factors including contact lenses, trauma, surgery, age, dry eye state, chronic nasolacrimal duct obstruction and previous ocular infections [2].

Staphylococci are the leading ocular isolates worldwide among the Gram-positive bacteria [3]. Whereas *Pseudomonas aeruginosa, Klebsiella pneumoniae* and *Escherichia coli* are the major Gram-negative bacteria isolated from ocular Infections [4]. The eye may be infected from external sources or through intraocular invasion of microorganisms that are carried out by blood stream [5]. External bacterial infections of the eye are usually localized but may frequently spread to other tissues.

Infection of the eye leads to conjunctivitis, keratitis, blepharitis, dacryocystitis, endophthalmitis and other infections which are responsible for increased incidence of morbidity and blindness worldwide [6].

Ocular infections, if left untreated, can damage the structure of the eye leading to visual impairment and blindness. Even though the eye is rigid and protected by continuous flow of tear which contains antibacterial substances, inflammation and scarring once occurred may not be easily resolved and required immediate management [7].

Ocular infection is a life-threatening condition which needs early diagnosis and treatment to save the patients' eye. In Africa alone, between 1000 and 4000 children are blinded annually by conjunctivitis [8]. Ocular infections are the second most common cause for blindness in developing countries [9].

Ocular infections are common in north-western states in Nigeria. In view of the changing etiological agents documented in other parts of the world and evolving resistance of infective agents to therapeutic agents, which may increase the risk of treatment failure with potentially serious consequences [10]. Therefore, up-to-date information is essential for appropriate antimicrobial therapy and management of ocular infections [11].

The objective of the study to determine the prevalence of bacterial ocular infections, the bacterial etiologic agents associated with ocular infections, the bacterial isolates in patients according to age, sex and other demographic factors and to investigate the antimicrobial susceptibility pattern of incriminated isolates among patients attending eye clinic of Aminu Kano teaching hospital and Murtala Muhammad specialist hospital.

2. Materials and methods

2.1 Sample collection and bacterial identification

A prospective cross-sectional study was conducted at Aminu Kano Teaching Hospital, which is a tertiary hospital situated in Kano state, Nigeria, and Murtala Muhammad Specialist Hospital, a secondary healthcare institution and as well a referral centre for a number of primary healthcare centres, also situated in Kano state. Socio-demographic data collection and relevant clinical evaluations of 88 patients with bacterial ocular infections were done using structured questionnaire. The bacterial ocular infections were clinically defined after patients were examined by an ophthalmologist.

The specimens were collected from eyelids and conjunctiva using sterile cotton swab moistened with sterile saline. The swab was rolled over the eyelid margin from medial to the lateral side and back again. Pus from lacrimal sac (dacryocystitis) and blepharitis was collected using dry sterile cotton-tipped swab either by applying pressure over the lacrimal sac to allow purulent material to reflux punctum or by irrigating the lacrimal drainage system [12]. The swabs were then transported immediately to the laboratory.

Bacterial identifications from eye discharge specimens were performed using standard procedures. Direct gram staining was done for all specimens. The specimens were inoculated on a proper culture media; MacConkey agar, Mannitol Salt Agar, Blood agar and Chocolate agar (Oxoid Ltd. Basingstoke, Hampshire, UK). The inoculated plates was incubated for 24 hours at 37°C. The aerobic atmospheric condition was maintained for the MacConkey agar and mannitol salt agar, while the chocolate agar and blood agar were incubated at 5–10% CO_2 atmosphere.

All the plates were initially examined for growth after 24 hours. After getting pure colonies, further identification was conducted using standard microbiological techniques, which include Gram stain, colony morphology and biochemical tests, namely lactose fermentation, mannitol fermentation catalase, coagulase, oxidase and indole tests.

2.2 Susceptibility testing

Once pure culture was obtained, a loopful of bacteria was taken from colony and transferred to a tube containing 5 ml of physiological saline and mixed gently. The suspension was incubated at 37°C until the turbidity of the suspension becomes adjusted to 0.5 McFarland standards. The suspension was uniformly rapped on to Mueller-Hinton agar for non-fastidious organisms and Mueller-Hinton agar with defibrinated sterile sheep blood (10% V/V) for fastidious organisms. Antimicrobial susceptibility test was carried out on each identified bacterium using the Kirby-Bauer disk diffusion method on Muller Hinton agar (Oxoid Ltd. Basingstoke, Hampshire, UK) based on clinical and laboratory standard institute (CLSI) 2014 guideline. Identifications and antibiotic sensitivity tests were performed according to the manufacturer's instructions. The antimicrobials used include the following: ceftazidime (30 μg), cefuroxime (30 μg), erythromycin (15 μg), cefixime (5 μg), gentamicin (10 μg), ciprofloxacin (5 μg), amoxicillin-clavulanic acid (30 μg), nitrofurantoin (300 μg), ceftriaxone (30 μg), oflaxocin (5 μg) and cloxacillin (10 μg) (Oxoid, England). Reference strains of *E. coli* ATCC 25922 and *Staphylococcus aureus* ATCC 25923 were used as quality control measure for identification criteria and antimicrobial susceptibility tests.

2.3 Quality control

Prior to actual data collection comprehensiveness, reliability and validity of questionnaires were pre-tested on 10 patients at AKTH and MMSH. All specimens were collected following standard operating procedure for ophthalmic specimen collection. The sterility of culture media was ensured by incubating 5% of each batch of the prepared media at 37°C for 24 hours. Performances of all prepared media were also checked by inoculating standard strains such as *E. coli* (ATCC 25922), *S. aureus* (ATCC 25923) and *P. aeruginosa* (ATCC 27853) obtained from AKTH (Ramesh *et al.*, 2010). The qualities of biochemical testing procedures were checked by these reference strains.

2.4 Statistical analysis

The data analysis was done using IBM SPSS software package version 16.0. The results obtained were analyzed using Descriptive Statistics, that is, frequency and percentages. Categorical variables were analyzed using Chi Square test. Finally, the results were presented in tables and figure.

3. Result

The study was conducted in Aminu Kano Teaching Hospital and Murtala Muhammad Specialist Hospital Kano with a total of 88 participants. All participants were examined for bacterial ocular infection. This chapter brings the summary of the study details of bacterial ocular infection and, the result are summarized in tables and figures as follows.

3.1 Prevalence of bacterial ocular infections among ocular infection patients

The prevalence of bacterial ocular infection is shown in **Figure 1**. Out of the 88 study participant who were examined for ocular infection, 78 (88.6%) were culture-positive and 10 (11.4%) have no growth.

3.2 Bacterial etiology of ocular infections

Among the total bacteria isolated, 28 (31.8%) and 61 (68.1%) were Gram-positive and Gram-negative bacteria, respectively. Mixed infection was found in 10 participants (11.3%). *H. influenza* (29.5%) was the predominant bacteria (**Tables 1** and **2**). The predominant bacterium among almost all clinical presentation was *S. aureus* (27.3%) except for conjunctivitis where the predominant bacteria were *H. infleunza* and *S. aureus* (**Table 3**).

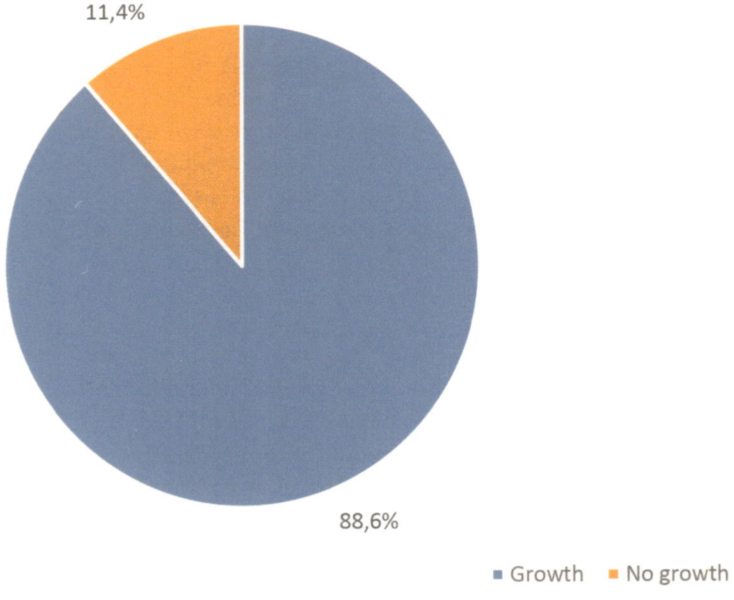

Figure 1.
Prevalence of bacterial ocular infection (n = 78).

Agent	Frequency (n)	Percentage (%)
S. aureus	24	27.3
S. pneumoniae	4	4.5
H. influenzae	26	29.5
P aeruginosa	23	26.1
K. pneumoniae	7	8.0
E. coli	4	4.5
Total	88	100

n = frequency, % = percentage.

Table 1.
Bacterial etiologic agents associated with ocular infections.

Antibiotic	Concentration (μg)	Susceptible n (%)	Intermidiate n (%)	Resistant n (%)
Ceftazidime	30	0	0	26 (100)
Cefuroxime	30	10 (38.5)	0	16 (61.5)
Gentamicin	10	0	1 (4)	25 (96)
Cefixime	5	2 (7.7)	2 (7.7)	22 (84.6)
Nitrofurantoin	300	0	0	26 (100)
Ciprofloxacin	5	19 (73)	1 (4)	6 (23)
Ofloxacin	5	24 (92.3)	0	2 (7.7)
Amoxicillin-clavulanic acid	30	1 (4)	0	25 (96)

Table 2.
Antimicrobial susceptibility pattern of H. influenzae *(n = 26).*

Variables	*S. aureus* n (%)	*S. pneumoniae* n (%)	*H influenzae* n (%)	*P aeruginosa* n (%)	*K pneumoniae* n (%)	*E coli* n (%)	P value
Previous infection							
Yes	3 (3.4)	0	2 (2.3)	4 (4.5)	1 (1.1)	0	0.897
No	21(23.9)	4 (4.5)	22 (25)	19 (21.6)	6	4 (4.5)	
Clinical presentation							
Conjunctivitis	20 (22.7)	4 (4.5)	25 (28.4)	22 (25)	7 (7.9)	4 (4.5)	0.745
Darcryocytitis	2 (2.3)	0	1 (1.1)	0	0	0	
Blephritis	2 (2.3)	0	0	1 (1.1)	0	0	
Immune status							
Immunocompromised	2 (2.5)	0	0	0	0	0	0.363
Non immunocompromised	22 (25)	4 (4.5)	26 (29.5)	23 (26.1)	7 (7.9)	4(4.5)	

KEY: % = Percentage, significance level = $P < 0.005$.

Table 3.
Distribution of bacterial isolates in patients based on clinical data (N = 88).

3.3 Antimicrobial susceptibility profile

From 28 Gram-positive bacteria isolated, 20 (71.4%) and 16 (57.1%) were susceptible to ceftriaxone and ofloxacin, respectively. Among 24 *S. aureus*, 22 (91.6%),21 (87.5%) and 20 (83.3%) were resistant to augmentin, erythromycin and gentamicin, respectively (**Table 4**). All *Streptococcus pneumoniae* isolates were susceptible to erythromycin (**Table 5**). Among 60 Gram-negative bacteria isolated, 50 (83.3%) and 55 (91.6%) were susceptible to ciprofloxacin and ofloxacin, respectively. Three-fourth (75%) of E. coli were susceptible to gentamicin (**Table 6**). 25/26 (96%), 2/4 (50%), 7/7 (100%) and 21/23 (91.3%) of *H. influenza*, *E. coli*, *K. pneumoniae* and *P. aeruginosa* were resistant to amoxicillin-clavulanic acid (augmentin) (**Tables 2, 6–8**).

3.4 Socio-demographic data

In the current study, a total of 88 patients seeking treatment for eye infection at AKTH and MMSH were included; there were no non-respondents. From the total

Antibiotic	Concentration (μg)	Susceptible n (%)	Intermidiate n (%)	Resistant n (%)
Ceftazidime	30	0	1 (4.2)	23 (95.8)
Cefuroxime	30	1 (4.2)	0	23 (95.8)
Gentamicin	10	2 (8.3)	2 (8.3)	20 (83.3)
Ceftriazone	30	15 (62.5)	2 (8.3)	7 (29.2)
Erythromycin	15	2 (8.3)	1 (4.2)	21 (87.5)
Cloxacillin	10	0	2 (8.3)	22 (91.7)
Ofloxacin	5	13 (54.2)	1 (4.3)	10 (41.6)
Amoxicillin-clavulanic acid	30	0	2 (8.3)	22 (91.7)

Table 4.
Antimicrobial susceptibility pattern of S.aureus *(N = 24).*

Antibiotic	Concentration (μg)	Susceptible n (%)	Intermidiate n (%)	Resistant n (%)
Ceftazidime	30	0	0	4 (100)
Cefuroxime	30	1 (25)	0	3 (75)
Gentamicin	10	3 (75)	0	1 (25)
Ceftriazone	30	3 (75)	0	1 (25)
Erythromycin	15	4 (100)	0	0
Cloxacillin	10	1 (25)	0	3 (75)
Ofloxacin	5	2 (50)	0	2 (50)
Amoxicillin-clavulanic acid	30	0	0	4 (100)

Table 5.
Antimicrobial susceptibility pattern of S. pneumoniae *(n = 4).*

Antibiotic	Concentration (μg)	Susceptible n (%)	Intermidiate n (%)	Resistant n (%)
Ceftazidime	30	0	0	4 (100)
Cefuroxime	30	1 (25)	0	3 (75)
Gentamicin	10	3 (75)	0	1 (25)
Cefixime	5	0	0	4 (100)
Nitrofurantoin	300	0	1 (25)	3 (75)
Ciprofloxacin	5	4 (100)	0	0
Ofloxacin	5	2 (50)	0	2 (50)
Amoxicillin-clavulanic acid	30	1 (25)	1 (25)	2 (50)

Table 6.
Antimicrobial susceptibility pattern of E.coli *(n = 4).*

Antibiotic	Concentration (μg)	Susceptible n (%)	Intermidiate n (%)	Resistant n (%)
Ceftazidime	30	5 (21.7)	0	18 (78.3)
Cefuroxime	30	16 (69.6)	0	7 (30.4)
Gentamicin	10	5 (21.7)	1 (4.3)	17 (74)
Cefixime	5	0	0	23 (100)
Nitrofurantoin	300	3 (13)	0	20 (87)
Ciprofloxacin	5	19 (82.6)	1 (4.3)	3 (13)
Ofloxacin	5	22 (95.7)	1 (4.3)	0
Amoxicillin-clavulanic acid	30	2 (8.7)	0	21 (91.3)

Table 7.
Antimicrobial susceptibility pattern of P. aeruginosa *(n = 23).*

Antibiotic	Concentration (μg)	Susceptible n (%)	Intermidiate n (%)	Resistant n (%)
Ceftazidime	30	5 (71.4)	0	2 (28.6)
Cefuroxime	30	2 (28.6)	2 (28.6)	3 (42.9)
Gentamicin	10	4 (57.1)	1 (14.3)	2 (28.6)
Cefixime	5	4 (57.1)	0	3 (42.9)
Nitrofurantoin	300	4 (57.1)	0	3 (42.9)
Ciprofloxacin	5	5 (71.4)	1 (14.3)	1 (14.3)
Ofloxacin	5	5 (71.4)	1 (14.3)	1 (14.3)
Amoxicillin-clavulanic acid	30	0	0	7 (100)

Table 8.
Antimicrobial susceptibility pattern of K.pneumoniae *(n = 7).*

Variables	Frequency (n)	Percentage (%)
Gender		
Male	37	42
Female	51	58
Age group		
0–3	29	33
4–11	16	18.2
12–17	5	5.7
18–39	21	23.9
> 40	17	19.3
Ethnic group		
Hausa	73	83
Fulani	9	10.2
Youruba	3	3.4
Igbo	2	2.3
Others	1	1.1
Residency		
Rural	61	69.3
Urban	27	30.7
Educational level		
Primary	16	18.2
Secondary	21	23.9
Tertiary	8	9.1
Illiterate	11	12.5
Not applicable	32	36.4

n = frequency, % = percentage.

Table 9.
Socio-demographic distribution of the study participants (N = 88).

study participants, 51 (58%), 29 (33%) and 61 (69.3%) were females, in 0–3 years age group and from rural areas, respectively. Most of the study participants were students and from hausa ethinic group 73 (83%) (**Table 9**).

3.5 Clinical presentation

Among 88 study participants assessed, the proportions of clinical finding were as follows: conjunctivitis 82 (93.2%), dacryocystitis 4 (4.5%), blepharitis 2 (2.3%) (**Table 10**).

3.6 Factors associated with ocular infection

None of the factors were significantly associated with ocular infections (P > 0.05). The proportions of bacterial eye infection among study participants with 0–3, 4–11,

Clinical presentation	Frequency (n)	Percent (%)
conjuctivitis	82	93.2
dacryocystitis	4	4.5
blephritis	2	2.3
Total	88	100.0

n = frequency, % = percentage.

Table 10.
Types of clinical presentations.

12–17, 18–39 and ≥ 40 age groups in years were 29 (33%), 16 (18.2%), 5 (5.7%), 21 (23.9%) and 17 (19.3%), respectively. The proportions of bacteria eye infection in rural and urban area were 61 (69.3%) and 27 (30.7%), respectively (**Table 11**). The proportion of bacterial eye infection among participants with repeated infections was 10 (11.36%) and among non-repeated infection was 78 (88.6%). The proportions of bacterial eye infection among participants whom are illiterate, primary, secondary, tertiary and those that are yet to enter school were 11 (12.5%), 16 (18.2%), 21 (23.9%), 8 (9.1%) and 32 (36.4%), respectively (**Table 11**). Conjuctivitis is the predominant clinical presentation (**Table 10**). The proportion of bacterial eye infection among participants with risk of infection was 2 (2.3%) (**Table 3**).

4. Discussion

The prevalence of culture-positive ocular infections caused by bacteria found in this study was 88.6%, and the result is comparable with other previous study reports conducted in India (88%) [13] and Egypt (87.8%) [14]. Our finding is high compared with the report from Southern Ethiopia (74.7%) [15], Bangalore (34.5%) [16], Gondar (47.4%) [17] and Addis Ababa (54.9%) [18]. The difference can be attributed to geographic location, study period, study population, sanitary condition and laboratory method used. Gram-negative bacteria were predominant in our study unlike report from other countries [19]. In the current study, the predominant bacterial isolates were *H. influenzae* (29.5%) followed by *S. aureus* (27.3%). The finding of this study is not comparable with previous studies conducted in Ethiopia [20], Nigeria [21] and India. The proportion of Gram-negative bacteria isolated, (31.8%) in this study is high compared with the report from Ethiopia [22]. Among Gram-negative bacteria isolated in the present study, *H. influenzae* (29.5%) was the most prevalent followed by *P. aeruginosa* (26.1%), *K. pneumoniae* (8%) and *E. coli* (4.5%).

Conjunctivitis was the dominant type of clinical presentation (93.2%) observed in this study followed by dacryocystitis (4.5%) and blepharitis (2.3%). In this study, the majority of bacteria were resistant to ceftazidime and cloxacillin, while most of them were susceptible to ofloxacin. This finding is in agreement with the study conducted in Gondar, Ethiopia [17], Jimma, Ethiopia [23] and Uganda [24]. The reason for increased resistance to ceftazidime and cloxacillin may be prior exposure of the isolates to these antibiotics. Moreover, these antibiotics are common, and patients can access them easily with low price and often can be purchased without prescription over the counter in different pharmacies [16]. Most of the *S. aureus* were resistant to

Variables	*S. aureus* n (%)	*S. pneumoniae* n (%)	*H influenzae* n (%)	*P aeruginosa* n (%)	*K pneumoniae* n (%)	*E coli* n (%)	P value
Gender							
Male	12 (13.6)	2 (2.3)	9 (10.2)	11 (12.5)	2 (2.3)	1 (1.1)	0.757
Female	12 (13.6)	2 (2.3)	17 (19.3)	12 (13.6)	5 (5.7)	3 (3.4)	
Age group							
0–3	9 (10.2)	0	7 (7.9)	7 (7.9)	3 (3.4)	3 (3.4)	0.411
4–11	4 (4.5)	1 (1.1)	4 (4.4)	5 (5.7)	2 (2.3)	0	
12–17	2 (2.3)	0	2 (2.3)	0	1 (1.1)	0	
18–39	3 (3.4)	3 (3.4)	6 (6.8)	8 (9.1)	1 (1.1)	0	
> 40	6 (6.8)	0	7 (7.9)	3 (3.4)	0	1 (1.1)	
Ethnic group							
Hausa	19 (21.6)	3 (3.4)	20	21 (23.9)	7 (7.9)	3 (3.4)	0.946
Fulani	3 (3.4)	1 (1.1)	3 (3.4)	1 (1.1)	0	1 (1.1)	
Yoruba	2 (2.3)	0	1 (1.1)	0	0	0	
Igbo	0	0	1 (1.1)	0	0	0	
Others	0	0	1 (1.1)	0	0	0	
Residency							
Rural	16 (18.2%)	2 (2.3%)	17 (19.3%)	19 (21.6)	5 (5.7)	2 (2.3)	0.609
Urban	8 (9.1%)	2 (2.3%)	9 (10.2%)	4 (4.5)	2 (2.3)	2 (2.3)	
Educational level							
Primary	4 (4.5)	1 (1.1)	5 (5.7)	3 (3.4)	3 (3.4)	0	0.228
Secondary	3 (3.4)	1 (1.1)	10 (11.4)	5 (5.7)	1 (1.1)	1 (1.1)	
Tertiary	3 (3.4)	2 (2.3)	1 (1.1)	2 (2.3)	0	0	
Illiterate	5 (5.7)	0	3 (3.4)	3 (3.4)	0	0	
Not apllicable	9 (10.2)	0	7 (7.9)	10 (11.4)	3 (3.4)	3 (3.4)	

KEY: % = Percentage, significance level = P < 0.005.

Table 11.
Distribution of bacterial isolates in patients based on age gender and other socio-demographic data (N = 88).

ceftazidime (95.8%) and cloxacillin (91.7%); however, 70.8% were susceptible to ceftriaxone. A similar finding was reported from other parts of Ethiopia [18]. However, low susceptibility (87.5%) to gentamicin was reported from other parts of Ethiopia [22]. Like *S. aureus, S. pneumoniae* (75%) were resistant to cloxacillin; similarly high resistance to penicillin was reported from Ethiopia [20]. *S. pneumoniae* isolated in this study were susceptible to erythromycin and gentamicin; this is not in line with other studies [22], in contrast to another study from Ethiopia [20].

H. influenzae and *P. aeroginosa* isolates in this study were susceptible to ciprofloxacin, ofloxacin and were resistant to gentamicin, nitrofurantoin and amoxicillin-clavulanic acid. *E. coli* isolates in this study were susceptible to ciprofloxacin, ofloxacin and gentamicin and were resistant to amoxicillin-clavulanic acid, ceftazidime and cefuroxime. *K. pneumoniae* isolates in this study were susceptible to ciprofloxacin, ofloxacin and ceftazidime. All of them were resistant to amoxicillin-clavulanic acid; this is in partial agreement with the Getahun *et al.* report.

In the present study, the sensitivity to antibiotics was variable in bacterial ocular infections and increased resistance to most antibiotics. The fluoroquinolones (ciprofloxacin and ofloxacin) were highly effective against all bacterial isolates, followed by ceftriaxone.

In conclusion, in the current study, the most prevalent clinical presentation was conjunctivitis followed by dacryocystitis. From 88 study participants with ocular infections, 88.6% were culture-positive. Gram-negative bacteria were the most prevalent with *H. influenzae* taking the largest share. Most of the isolates are susceptible to ofloxacin and resistant to amoxicillin-clavulanic acid. And none of the factors were significantly associated with ocular infections ($P > 0.05$).

The following recommendations are made based on the findings of the study: To mitigate the burden of bacterial ocular infections, physicians should regard risk reduction and comply with etiologic approach of diagnosis. Antibiotic resistance among ocular pathogens is a challenge to the ophthalmologists. Resistance to most groups of antibiotics is increasing with resultant decline in the effectiveness of many commonly used topical antibiotics. It remains to be seen whether newer antibiotics such as besifloxacin will outlive the others before it, especially because of lack of systemic use. A strategy including judicious use of antibiotics in humans, animals and agriculture fields along with development of new products having low-resistance potential is required to end or at least reign in the current trend. Health education and personal hygiene should be practiced, and additional studies are needed in this study area.

4.1 Limitation of the study

The limitation of the study was that the lack of reagents limited the diagnosis of Chlamydia infections.

Acknowledgements

All thanks and Honors go to Almighty Allah (S.W.T) for my health, strength and guidance throughout this period.

I wish to express my profound gratitude to the supervisor of this work, Professor Abdulhadi Sale Kumurya of the Department of Medical Laboratory Science, Bayero University, Kano, for his due contributions, fatherly advices and assistance towards the completion of this research project.

My earnest appreciation to all lecturers of the Department of Medical Laboratory Science, Bayero University, Kano, headed by my respected Head of Department Dr. Jamilu Abubakar Bala. Special thanks to the staff of Medical bacteriology Unit of the Medical Laboratory Science Department, Bayero University, Kano. And also my special gratitude goes to my mentor, Malama Rahinatu S. Sharfadi.

My sincere gratitude also goes to all members of staff of the Department of Medical Microbiology, Aminu Kano Teaching Hospital, Kano, and everybody who contributed in one way or the other to the completion of this project.

With much and sincere humility, my deepest gratitude goes to my beloved parents Haj. Afiya bashir and Alh Abdulaziz Lawan, my aunties and uncles especially Alh Abdulhadi Lawan, Kawu Aminu, Kawu Mahdi, aunty Binta and aunty Sadiya as well as to my relatives and friends for their continuous moral support and encouragement, and also my sincere appreciation goes to my father's best friend who has also been a great father to me Dr. Auwal Baba Ahmad and to my sarang Sauban M. Jibril. I would also like to thank my quadruple squad Bilkisu B., Maryam B and Rukkayya M. May Allah SWT reward you all with Jannatul Firdaus Ameen.

Lastly, I will be forever indebted to everybody who shared knowledge, a moment, classroom and laboratory with me during my undergraduate programme.

Additional information

This study replicates the original research reported in: Mohammed AA, Ali MM, Zenebe MH. Bacterial etiology of ocular and periocular infections, antimicrobial susceptibility profile and associated factors among patients attending eye unit of Shashemene comprehensive specialized hospital, Shashemene, Ethiopia [Internet]. Vol. 20, BMC Ophthalmology. Springer Science and Business Media LLC; 2020. Available from: http://dx.doi.org/10.1186/s12886-020-01398-w.

Abbreviation

AKTH	Aminu Kano Teaching Hospital
MMSH	Murtala Muhammad Specialist Hospital

Author details

Abdulhadi Sale Kumurya and Khadija Abdulaziz Lawan*
Bayero University Kano, Kano State, Nigeria

*Address all correspondence to: khadijaabdulaziz10@gmail.com

References

[1] Long C, Liu B, Xu C, Jing Y, Yuan Z, Lin X. Causative organisms of post-traumatic endophthalmitis: A 20-year retrospective study. BioMed Central Ophthalmology. 2014; **14**(1):1-7

[2] Galvis V, Tello A, Guerra A, Acuña MF, Villarreal D. Antibiotic susceptibility patterns of bacteria isolated from keratitis and intraocular infections at Fundación Oftalmológica de Santander (FOSCAL), Floridablanca, Colombia. Biomédica. 2014;**34**:23-33

[3] Kaliamurthy J, Kalavathy CM, Parmar P, Nelson Jesudasan CA, Thomas PA. Spectrum of bacterial keratitis at a tertiary eye care Centre in India. BioMed Research International. 2013:181564

[4] Rahimi F, Hashemian MN, Khosravi A, Moradi G, Bamdad S. Bacterial keratitis in a tertiary eye Centre in Iran: A retrospective study. Middle East African Journal of Ophthalmology. 2015;**22**(2):238

[5] Williams-Noble FA, Sorsby A, Conrad B. Etiology of the eye diseases; developmental defects; heredity. The Eye and its Diseases. 1950;**309**:321

[6] Juárez-Verdayes MA, Reyes-López MÁ, Cancino-Díaz ME, Muñoz-Salas S, Rodríguez-Martínez S, De la Serna FJ, et al. Isolation, vancomycin resistance and biofilm production of Staphylococcus epidermidis from patients with conjunctivitis, corneal ulcers, and endophthalmitis. Rev Latinoam Microbial. 2006;**48**(3-4):238-246

[7] Ubani UA. Common bacterial isolates from infected eye. J Niger Optom Assoc. 2009;**15**:40-47

[8] Mohammed A, Asani M, Ibrahim M. Bacterial agents and sensitivity pattern of neonatal conjunctivitis in Aminu Kano teaching hospital. Nigerian Journal of Paediatrics. 2013;**40**(4):360-363

[9] Ashaye A, Aimola A. Keratitis in children as seen in a tertiary hospital in Africa. Journal of the National Medical Association. 2008;**100**(4):386-393

[10] Sharma S. Antibiotic resistance in ocular bacterial pathogens. Indian Journal of Medical Microbiology. 2011; **29**(3):218

[11] Brown L. Resistance to ocular antibiotics: An overview. Clinical and Experimental Optometry. 2007;**90**(4): 258-262

[12] Mah FS, Davidson R, Holland EJ, Hovanesian J, John T, Kanellopoulos, J. ... and ASCRS Cornea Clinical Committee. Current knowledge about and recommendations for ocular methicillin-resistant Staphylococcus aureus. Journal of Cataract and Refractive Surgery. 2014;**40**(11): 1894-1904

[13] Bharathi MJ, Ramakrishnan R, Shivakumar C, Meenakshi R, Lionalraj D. Etiology and antibacterial susceptibility pattern of community-acquired bacterial ocular infections in a tertiary eye care hospital in South India. Indian Journal of Ophthalmology. 2010; **58**(6):497

[14] Nofal FA, El-Baz NA, Ismail MA, Hadhoud NA. Bacteriological and immunological study of mucopurulent conjunctivitis (MPC) in Sharkia Govamate. Az. J. Microbiol. 1990;**10**:108

[15] Mshangila B, Paddy M, Kajumbula H, Ateenyi-Agaba C,

Kahwa B, Seni J. External ocular surface bacterial isolates and their antimicrobial susceptibility patterns among pre-operative cataract patients at Mulago National Hospital in Kampala, Uganda. BioMed Central Ophthalmology. 2013; **13**(1):1-6

[16] Hemavathi PS, Shenoy P. Profile of microbial isolates in ophthalmic infections and antibiotic susceptibility of the bacterial isolates: A study in an eye care hospital, Bangalore. Journal of Clinical and Diagnostic Research: JCDR. 2014;**8**(1):23

[17] Anagaw B, Biadglegne F, Belyhun Y, Mulu A. Bacteriology of ocular infections and antibiotic susceptibility pattern in Gondar University hospital, north West Ethiopia. Ethiopian Medical Journal. 2011;**49**(2):117-123

[18] Aklilu A, Bitew A, Dessie W, Hailu E, Asamene N, Mamuye Y. Prevalence and drug susceptibility pattern of bacterial pathogens from ocular infection in St. Paul's hospital millennium medical college, Ethiopia. Journal Bacteriol Mycol. 2018; **5**(8):1085

[19] Mohammed AA, Ali MM, Zenebe MH. Bacterial etiology of ocular and periocular infections, antimicrobial susceptibility profile and associated factors among patients attending eye unit of Shashemene comprehensive specialized hospital, Shashemene, Ethiopia. BioMed Central Ophthalmology. 2020;**20**(1):1-8

[20] Getahun E, Gelaw B, Assefa A, Assefa Y, Amsalu A. Bacterial pathogens associated with external ocular infections alongside eminent proportion of multidrug resistant isolates at the University of Gondar Hospital, Northwest Ethiopia. BMC Ophthalmology. 2017;**17**(1):1-10

[21] Iwalokun BA, Oluwadun A, Akinsinde KA, Niemogha MT, Nwaokorie FO. Bacteriologic and plasmid analysis of etiologic agents of conjunctivitis in Lagos, Nigeria. Journal of Ophthalmic Inflammation and Infection. 2011;**1**(3):95-103

[22] Shiferaw B, Gelaw B, Assefa A, Assefa Y, Addis Z. Bacterial isolates and their antimicrobial susceptibility pattern among patients with external ocular infections at Borumeda hospital, Northeast Ethiopia. BioMed Central Ophthalmology. 2015;**15**(1):1-8

[23] Tesfaye T, Beyene G, Gelaw Y, Bekele S, Saravanan M. Bacterial profile and antimicrobial susceptibility pattern of external ocular infections in Jimma University specialized hospital, Southwest Ethiopia. American Journal of Infectious Diseases and Microbiology. 2013;**1**(1):13-20

[24] Aweke T, Dibaba G, Ashenafi K, Kebede M. Bacterial pathogens of exterior ocular infections and their antibiotic vulnerability pattern in southern Ethiopia. African Journal of Immunology Research. 2014;**1**(1): 019-025

Chapter 5

Ocular Manifestations of COVID-19

Giulia Regattieri, Gabriela Belem and Jordana Sandes

Abstract

The SARS-CoV-2 is a highly infective virus, which is transmitted by exposure to infectious respiratory fluids. Ocular manifestations occur in 10% of the patients. The main ophthalmologic manifestation described so far has been conjunctivitis with mild follicular reaction. The clinical signals usually are conjunctival hyperemia, foreign body sensation, tearing, dry eye, and photophobia, but there is a wide range of ocular signals and symptoms described. Fragments of viral RNA could be detected in the tears of some of these patients. The virus recognizes the ACE-2 receptor in the corneal epithelium and then gains circulation and spreads to other sites. That would demonstrate that there may be a tropism from the new SARS-COV-2 with the eye.

Keywords: coronavirus infections, pandemics, signs and symptoms, ophthalmology, conjunctivitis

1. Introduction

COVID-19 is caused by SARS-CoV2 an enveloped, single-stranded RNA virus of the *Coronaviridae* family that emerged in China in 2019 with rapid worldwide spread becoming a pandemic within months. SARS-CoV-2 is a highly infectious virus, transmitted by exposure to contaminated respiratory fluids.

Laboratory diagnosis of COVID is usually done by detecting viral fragments in the upper respiratory tract, but in some patients, these fragments can be detected in the tear that confirms the ocular route as a possible route of viral inoculation. It has even been found that detection of viral fragments on the ocular surface can occur earlier than systemic symptoms (D2 of infection) and remain up to day 29, even with a negative nasopharyngeal swab.

2. Physiopathology

There are some theories proposed to explain the pathophysiology of viral inoculation into the human conjunctiva. The main ones are direct inoculation of infected droplets on the ocular surface (cornea and conjunctiva); migration of the virus from the upper respiratory tract through the nasolacrimal duct to the ocular surface; and hematogenous infection of the lacrimal gland. All these theories are based on the presence of the ACE2 receptor, essential for the entry of SARS-CoV2 into human cells, in several structures of the human eye [1–3].

IntechOpen

Figure 1 shows an illustration of the theory of direct inoculation of the virus on the ocular surface by binding to the ACE2 receptor.

SARS-CoV-2 enters the target cells by binding the viral Spike (S) protein to the ACE2 receptor, followed by its initiation by the (TMPRSS2) protein. The ACE2 receptor is present in several organs of the body, including various structures of the human eye such as the cornea, conjunctiva, iris, ciliary body, and aqueous humor.

Note in **Figure 2** this distribution in different tissues of the body.

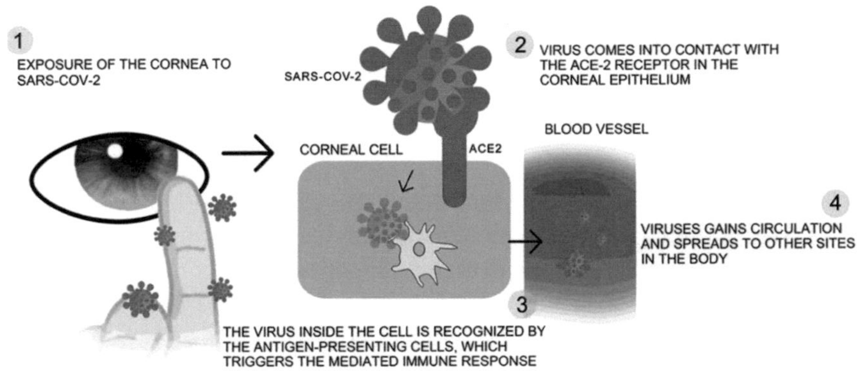

Figure 1.
Source: Cortesy by Cunha CEX, 2020. This figure was designed using freepik.com resources (https://br.freepik.com/). The physiopathology illustrated was described by Napoli et al.

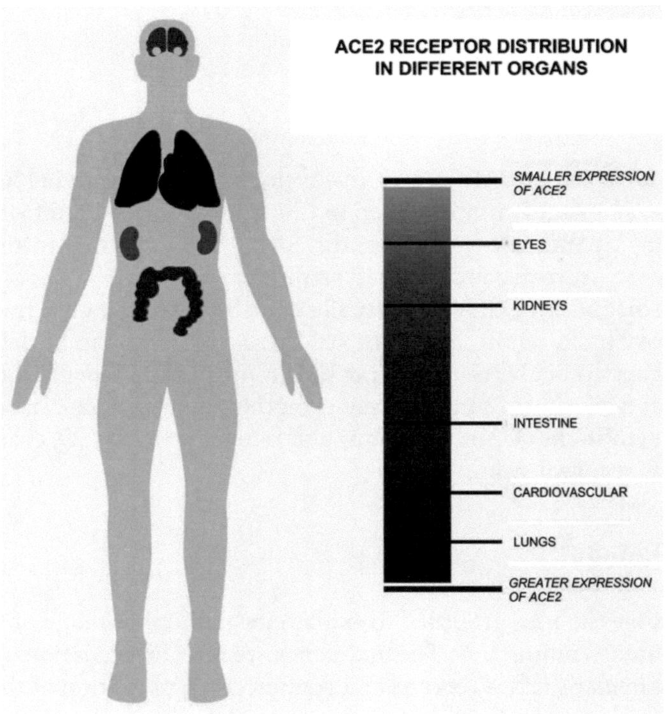

Figure 2.
Source: Cortesy by Cunha CEX, 2020. This figure was designed using freepik.com resources (https://br.freepik.com/). Distribution of the ACE2 receptor in different tissues of the body as presented by Amesty et al.

3. Ocular manifestations

In general, ocular manifestations of COVID-19 are rare. The prevalence of ocular disease is about 11.03% (ranging from 2% to 32%) [4–7].

This data suggest that approximately one out of 10 patients shows at least one ocular symptom.

According to Nasiri et al., the weighted mean between the onset of ocular manifestations and systemic disease was 0.04 days (range, 1–3 days). However, the weighted mean between systemic disease and ocular manifestations was 1.5 days (range, 2–21 days) [5].

The most prevalent ocular manifestation in patients with COVID-19 is follicular conjunctivitis, corresponding to 90% of ocular findings [5, 8]. Most frequent symptoms are dry eye or foreign body sensation (16%), eye redness (13.3%), tearing (12.8%), and itching (12.6%) (see **Table 1**).

Characteristics	**N (%)**
Symptom and sign (n = 932)	
Dry eyes or foreign body sensation	138 (16.0)
Redness	114 (13.3)
Tearing	111 (12.8)
Itching	109 (12.6)
Eye pain	83 (9.6)
Discharge	76 (8.8)
Blurred vision or decreased vision	71 (8.2)
Photophobia	62 (7.2)
Chemosis	42 (4.9)
Irritation	21 (2.4)
Gritty feeling	14 (1.6)
Burning sensation	8 (0.9)
Lid edema	8 (0.9)
Subconjunctival hemorrhage	3 (0.3)
Pseudomembrane and hemorrhage	2 (0.2)
Pseudodendrite	1 (0.1)
Subepithelial Infiltrates	1 (0.1)
Water secretion	1 (0.1)
Disease (n = 89)	
Conjunctivitis	79 (88.8)
Keratitis	2 (2.2)
Episcleritis	2 (2.2)
Keratoconjunctivitis	2 (2.2)
Pingueculitis	1 (1.1)
Hordeolum	2 (2.2)
Posterior ischemic optic neuropathy	1 (1.1)

Table 1.
Symptoms and diseases of ocular manifestation in COVID-19 infection included in the reviewed studies (n = 1,021).

The association between COVID and dry eye is uncertain because this condition might be related to wearing face masks and the stream of air against the ocular surface as well as the overuse of digital devices leading to an evaporative dry eye.

Since conjunctivitis is a common eye condition, ophthalmologists may be the first medical professionals to evaluate a patient with COVID-19. Therefore, attention to ocular manifestations, especially conjunctivitis, could increase the sensitivity of COVID-19 detection among patients during pandemic. As said before, SARS-CoV-2 can be transmitted by tear, so ophthalmologists (mainly given their close contact) and healthcare providers should wear protective devices, such as protective gears and face masks while examining a patient [9].

Other less common conditions are keratitis, episcleritis, keratoconjunctivitis, hordeolum, pingueculitis, and posterior ischemic optic neuropathy. Reports show associations of COVID-19 with uveitic, retinovascular, and neuro-ophthalmic disease due to microvascular injury and inflammation [4, 5, 10–16].

3.1 Cornea and conjunctiva

Unspecific signs of mild viral conjunctivitis: unilateral or bilateral bulbar conjunctiva injection, follicular reaction of the palpebral conjunctiva, watery discharge, and mild eyelid edema [4].

Bilateral chemosis alone may represent third-spacing in a critically ill patient rather than a true ocular manifestation of the virus [4].

Cheema et al. described the first case of keratoconjunctivitis: corneal findings that developed rapidly over 3 days, including transient pseudodendritic lesions and diffuse subepithelial infiltrates with overlying epithelial defects [8].

Navel et al. observed a case of severe hemorrhagic conjunctivitis and pseudomembrane formation [17].

3.2 Sclera and episclera

Cases of episcleritis, anterior scleritis, and necrotizing anterior scleritis have been reported [18–20].

3.3 Anterior chamber

Acute anterior uveitis has also been reported both in isolation and in association with COVID-19-related multi-system inflammatory disease [10, 11].

3.4 Retina and choroid

Vascular, inflammatory, and neuronal changes induced by the virus cause posterior segment manifestations. These are less frequent than anterior segment findings.

There are some case reports showing that the most common retinal involvements are microvascular changes, such as cotton wool spots and microhemorrhages. Usually, these patients had normal visual acuity and pupillary reflexes. Physiopathology is related to a complement-induced prothrombic and inflammatory state causing endothelial damage and microangiopathic injury [6, 21].

Deep retinal capillary plexus ischemia is involved in acute macular neuro-retinopathy (AMN) and paracentral acute middle maculopathy (PAMM), both observed as hyperreflective changes at the level of the outer plexiform and inner nuclear layers [22–25].

Increased tortuosity of retinal vessels has also been described, but a true relation between such occurrences and COVID-19 has yet to be established [26].

Central vein occlusion is an important complication of COVID-19 and can occur in healthy patients as SARS-CoV-2 infection causes endothelial damage and increases the risk of thrombosis. However, retinal artery occlusion occurred mostly in patients with additional underlying conditions, such as hypertension, obesity, and coronary artery disease [26].

In addition, some studies showed hyper-reflective lesions at the level of ganglion cell and inner plexiform layers more prominently at the papilomacular bundle in patients with COVID-19 [27].

Other studies evaluated changes in retinal microvasculature and retinal layers in patients who recovered from COVID-19 with spectral domain optical coherence tomography (OCT) and optical coherence tomography angiography (OCTA).

OCT-A was performed in patients 6 months post SARS-CoV-2 pneumonia and revealed a significant reduction in vessel density of the superficial capillary plexus and deep capillary plexus as well as retinal nerve fiber layer (RNFL) thinning. These findings are probably related to thrombotic microangiopathy events [28, 29]. There is evidence that retinal layers can be affected, especially in patients with headache and ocular pain symptoms during the COVID-19 period [29].

Other retinal findings were seen in patients with COVID-19: Vitritis; hyper-reflective lesions at the level of the inner plexiform and ganglion cell layers in OCT (optical coherence tomography); cotton wool spots, microhemorrhages, dilated veins, and tortuous vessels (due to vascular damage); Purtscher-like retinopathy and acute retinal necrosis (ARN) in immunocompromised patients (probably related to a reactivation of latent herpesvirus and breakdown of blood–retinal barrier allowing an increased inflammatory response) [6, 14–16, 21–23].

Posterior uveitis was observed following COVID-19 infection and vaccine. Cases of serpiginous, ampiginous, and multifocal choroiditis also have been reported. It is believed that autoimmunity is involved in these manifestations [22–25, 30].

3.5 Neuro-ophthalmologic manifestations

Several neuro-ophthalmologic manifestations have been observed: Optic neuritis, papillophlebitis (only one case reported), Adie's tonic pupil, cranial nerve palsy, neurogenic ptosis, Miller Fisher syndrome, and ocular myasthenia gravis [4, 6, 31–37].

It is already known that the SARS-CoV-2 virus has a neurotropism. Some cases of bilateral optic neuritis have been described, but it is possible that this is a consequence of an immune-mediated insult caused by the virus as these patients presented with anti-myelin oligodendrocyte glycoprotein (MOG) antibodies and cerebrospinal fluid (CSF) did not reveal virus presence. There have also been reports of acute optic neuritis following vaccination for COVID-19 [4, 6, 31, 38–41].

A case of multiple sclerosis following COVID-19 infection was reported by Palao et al. These cases suggest that SARS-CoV-2 can either trigger or exacerbate the inflammatory and demyelinating disease [39].

3.6 Orbital manifestations

There have been reports of sinusitis, orbital cellulitis, mucormycosis, orbital myositis, and dacryoadenitis. The most significant of those is mucormycosis as it is an opportunistic pathogen. The hypoxic respiratory environment induced by

SARS-CoV-2 added to an immunocompromised state induced by high-dose steroids and immunosuppressive therapies creates the perfect environment for this fungal infection [42–48].

Singh et al. published a systematic review of 101 reported cases of COVID-19 patients with mucormycosis; these patients were predominantly male (79%), 80% of which had diabetes and 15% with concomitant diabetic ketoacidosis [49].

4. Differential diagnosis

COVID has several features that are highly unspecific and can simulate a lot of other common conditions and most of the time indistinguishable from other etiologies.

Differential diagnoses are those which present red eye and tearing, for example:

- Other viral conjunctivitis (e.g., adenovirus)
- Bacterial conjunctivitis
- Allergic conjunctivitis
- Herpes simplex virus keratitis
- Anterior uveitis
- Corneal abrasion
- Foreign body
- Dry eye syndrome
- Exposure keratopathy in an intubated patient
- Chemosis in a critically ill patient

5. Ophthalmologic evaluation

A thorough history is necessary regarding the onset, duration, and characteristics of symptoms. All patients should be questioned about recent fever and respiratory symptoms. Ophthalmologic evaluation must be complete to rule out other differential diagnoses. Measurement of visual acuity, intraocular pressure, pupil and dilated fundus examination, color testing to evaluate patients for evidence of optic neuropathy, extraocular motility (searching for nystagmus or cranial neuropathies), visual field testing (to investigate deficits related to stroke or optic neuropathy).

In the presence of optic neuritis or neurologic symptoms, neuroimaging must be done. Additional serum or cerebrospinal fluid testing may be useful [6].

6. Treatment/Management

As with other viral infections, COVID-19 conjunctivitis is presumed to be self-limited and can be managed with symptomatic care. In the absence of mild symptoms, patients can be managed remotely with preservative-free artificial tears and cold compresses [6].

7. Guidance and screening recommendations for corneal transplantation (Eye Bank Association of America, Updated Guidance – March 14, 2022)

EBAA guidance and screening recommendations for COVID-19 pandemic are based on the latest guidelines from the FDA and CDC as well as available scientific evidence [50].

The most current set of guidelines specifies criteria for:

1. Donor ineligibility – Donors should be considered ineligible who in the 10 days prior to death:

   a. Were diagnosed with acute COVID-19; OR

   b. Tested positive for COVID-19 by direct viral testing methods (e.g., NAAT and/or antigen); OR

   c. Had close contact with a person diagnosed with or suspected to have COVID-19 and developed signs and symptoms of COVID-19, regardless of a plausible alternative etiology or vaccination history

2. Donors eligibility – Donors should be evaluated for eligibility by a Medical Director who:

   a. In the 10 days prior to death, without a known close contact with a person diagnosed with or suspected to have COVID-19, developed new signs and/or symptoms consistent with acute COVID-19 not explained by a plausible alternative etiology; OR

   b. In the 10 days prior to death, had known close contact with a person diagnosed with or suspected to have COVID-19 AND was asymptomatic; OR

   c. In the 11 to 20 days prior to death had a positive test for SARS-CoV-2 AND had ongoing signs and/or symptoms of COVID-19

EBAA contraindications to transplant are active ocular or intraocular inflammations, such as conjunctivitis, keratitis, scleritis, iritis, vitritis choroiditis, or retinitis.

Current EBAA Medical Standards require that 5% povidone–iodine solution shall contact the entire surface of any ocular tissue intended for transplantation at least twice between the time of the donor's death and tissue preservation, as povidone–iodine has been documented *in vitro* viricidal activity against coronaviruses.

Global Alliance of Eye Bank Associations (GAEBA) declared on November 12, 2020 that there is no evidence that coronaviruses can be transmitted by human tissue or cell transplantation and therefore measures in this response are precautionary, as there have been no reported cases of transmission of SARS-CoV-2, MERS-CoV, or any other coronavirus via transplantation of human ocular tissue [6, 51].

The European Eye Bank Association (EEBA) and European Association of Tissue and Cell Banks (EATCB) refer to guidance provided by the ECDC (European Centre for Disease Prevention and Control 1st update, April 2020): corneal transplants are usually disinfected with povidone (PVP) iodine and then stored in organ culture at 30–37°C for at least 14 days. The presence of viruses capable of reproduction after this procedure seems very unlikely. These data and the absence of known ocular transmission cases indicate that the risk of COVID-19 cases entering the eye donor pool and subsequent transmission is theoretical [52, 53].

8. Discussion

SARS-CoV-2 is a highly infectious virus, transmitted by exposure to contaminated respiratory fluids causing mainly respiratory illness. Transmission by tear is not unlikely, and the eye can be a way for viral infection. This can be explained by the ACE2 coronaviruses receptor in the eye cells and that is why protecting the eyes is essential, especially for healthcare providers.

One out of 10 COVID-19 patients presents at least one ocular manifestation. The most prevalent ocular manifestation in patients with COVID-19 is follicular conjunctivitis, corresponding to 90% of ocular findings. The most frequent symptoms are dry eye or foreign body sensation, eye redness, tearing, itching, eye pain, and discharge.

It is important to know that the mechanism of dry eye or foreign body sensation is uncertain as during the pandemic screen time and face masks could also contribute to tear evaporation.

Attention to ocular manifestations, especially when combined with other COVID-19 manifestations like respiratory symptoms or fever, could help improve COVID-19 diagnosis, although ocular involvements are rare and nonspecific. There is evidence showing that conjunctivitis-related symptoms may occur prior to the onset of respiratory symptoms and could be the precursors for early diagnosis. Loffredo and colleagues reported that conjunctivitis in COVID-19 patients was significantly correlated with disease severity.

Posterior segment findings are less common than anterior segment manifestation. A few studies showed retinal layer attenuation in OCT. It should be noted that there is an important correlation between COVID-19 and Central Retinal Vein Occlusion, even in patients without comorbidities.

Ophthalmic manifestations are varied in terms of presentation, severity, and timing. Usually, ocular symptoms are mild and improve without further complications.

9. Conclusion

In general, ocular manifestations of COVID-19 are rare but can be the first symptom of the disease. Follicular conjunctivitis is the most common eye condition, but there are described manifestations of COVID-19 in all eye segments. Attention to ocular manifestations in combination with other COVID-19 manifestations could help improve COVID-19 diagnosis. SARS-Cov-2 can be transmitted by tear, so ophthalmologists (mainly given their close contact) should wear protective devices while examining a patient.

Author details

Giulia Regattieri, Gabriela Belem and Jordana Sandes*
Federal University of Goiás, Goiania, Brazil

*Address all correspondence to: jordana.oftalmo@gmail.com

References

[1] Torres BRS, Cunha CEX da, Castro LR, Brito LMP de, Ferreira CVO, Ribeiro MVMR. Ocular manifestations of COVID-19: A literature review. Revista da Associação Médica Brasileira. 2020;**66**(9):1296-1300

[2] Ho D, Low R, Tong L, Gupta V, Veeraraghavan A, Agrawal R. COVID-19 and the ocular surface: A review of transmission and manifestations. Ocular Immunology and Inflammation. 2020;**28**(5):726-734

[3] Salz AK, Acharya M, Hofmann N, et al. Risk of SARS-CoV-2 virus transmission from donor corneal tissue: A review. Indian Journal of Ophthalmology. 2021;**69**(6):1592-1597. DOI: 10.4103/ijo.IJO_3249_20

[4] Sen M, Honavar SG, Sharma N, Sachdev MS. COVID-19 and eye. Indian Journal of Ophthalmology. 2021;**69**(3):488-509

[5] Nasiri N, Sharifi H, Bazrafshan A. Ocular manifestations of COVID-19: A systematic review and meta-analysis. JOVR. 2021;**16**(1):103-112

[6] Hu K, Patel J, Swiston C, et al. Ophthalmic Manifestations of Coronavirus (COVID-19). Treasure Island: StatPearls; 2022

[7] Wu P, Duan F, Luo C. Characteristics of ocular findings of patients with coronavirus disease 2019 (COVID-19) in Hubei Province, China. JAMA Ophthalmology. 2020;**138**(5):575-578

[8] Cheema M, Aghazadeh H, Nazarali S. Keratoconjunctivitis as the initial medical presentation of the novel coronavirus disease 2019 (COVID-19). Canadian Journal of Ophthalmology. 2020;**55**(4):e125-e129

[9] Napoli PE, Nioi M, d'Aloja E. The ocular surface and the coronavirus disease 2019: Does a dual 'Ocular Route' exist? Journal of Clinical Medicine. 2020;**9**(5):1269. DOI: 10.3390/jcm9051269

[10] Mazzotta C, Giancipoli E. Anterior acute uveitis report in a SARS-CoV-2 patient managed with adjunctive topical antiseptic prophylaxis preventing 2019-nCoV spread through the ocular surface route. International Medical Case Report Journal. 2020;**13**:513-520

[11] Bettach E, Zadok D, Weill Y, Brosh K, Hanhart J. Bilateral anterior uveitis as a part of a multisystem inflammatory syndrome secondary to COVID-19 infection. Journal of Medical Virology. 2021;**93**(1):139-140

[12] Walinjkar JA, Makhija SC, Sharma HR. Central retinal vein occlusion with COVID-19 infection as the presumptive etiology. Indian Journal of Ophthalmology. 2020;**68**(11):2572-2574

[13] Yahalomi T, Pikkel J, Arnon R. Central retinal vein occlusion in a young healthy COVID-19 patient: A case report. American Journal of Ophthalmological Case Report. 2020;**20**:100992

[14] Gascon P, Briantais A, Bertrand E. Covid-19-associated retinopathy: A case report. Ocular Immunology and Inflammation. 2020;**28**(8):1293-1297

[15] Bottini AR, Steinmetz S, Blinder KJ. Purtscher-like retinopathy in a patient with COVID-19. Case Report Ophthalmological Medicine. 2021;**2021**:6661541

[16] Invernizzi A, Torre A, Parrulli S. Retinal findings in patients with COVID-19: Results from the SERPICO-19 study. EClinicalMedicine. 2020 Oct;**27**:100550

[17] Navel V, Chiambaretta F, Dutheil F. Haemorrhagic conjunctivitis with pseudomembranous related to SARS-CoV-2. American Journal of Ophthalmology Case Reports. 2020;**19**:100735

[18] Otaif W, Al Somali AI, Al HA. Episcleritis as a possible presenting sign of the novel coronavirus disease: A case report. American Journal of Ophthalmological Case Report. 2020;**20**:100917

[19] Méndez Mangana C, Barraquer Kargacin A, Barraquer RI. Episcleritis as an ocular manifestation in a patient with COVID-19. Acta Ophthalmologica. 2020;**98**(8):e1056-e1057

[20] Feizi S, Meshksar A, Naderi A, Esfandiari H. Anterior Scleritis manifesting after coronavirus disease 2019: A report of two cases. Cornea. 2021;**40**(9):1204-1206

[21] Vinores SA, Wang Y, Vinores MA. Blood-retinal barrier breakdown in experimental coronavirus retinopathy: Association with viral antigen, inflammation, and VEGF in sensitive and resistant strains. Journal of Neuroimmunology. 2001;**119**(2):175-182

[22] Providência J, Fonseca C, Henriques F. Serpiginous choroiditis presenting after SARS-CoV-2 infection: A new immunological trigger? European Journal of Ophthalmology. 2020;**2**:11206

[23] Tom ES, McKay KM, Saraf SS. Bilateral ampiginous choroiditis following presumed SARS-CoV-2 infection. Case Report Ophthalmological Medicine. 2021;**2021**:1646364

[24] de Souza EC, de Campos VE, Duker JS. Atypical unilateral multifocal choroiditis in a COVID-19 positive patient. American Journal of Ophthalmological Case Report. 2021;**22**:101034

[25] Goyal M, Murthy SI, Annum S. Bilateral multifocal choroiditis following COVID-19 vaccination. Ocular Immunology and Inflammation. 2021;**29**(4):753-757

[26] Zhang Y, Stewart JM. Retinal and choroidal manifestations of COVID-19. Current Opinion in Ophthalmology. 2021;**32**(6):536-540

[27] Marinho PM, Marcos AAA, Romano AC. Retinal findings in patients with COVID-19. Lancet. 2020;**395**(10237):1610

[28] Abrishami M, Emamverdian Z, Shoeibi N. Optical coherence tomography angiography analysis of the retina in patients recovered from COVID-19: A case-control study. Canadian Journal of Ophthalmology. 2021;**56**(1):24-30

[29] Dag Seker E, Erbahceci Timur IE. COVID-19: More than a respiratory virus, an optical coherence tomography study. International Ophthalmology. 2021;**41**(11):3815-3824

[30] Soni A, Narayanan R, Tyagi M, Belenje A, Basu S. Acute retinal necrosis as a presenting ophthalmic manifestation in COVID 19 recovered patients. Ocular Immunology and Inflammation. 2021;**29**(4):722-725

[31] Sawalha K, Adeodokun S, Kamoga GR. COVID-19-induced acute bilateral optic neuritis. Journal of Investigative Medicine High Impact Case Reports. 2020;**8**:2324

[32] Insausti-García A, Reche-Sainz JA, Ruiz-Arranz C. Papillophlebitis in a COVID-19 patient: Inflammation and hypercoagulable state. European Journal of Ophthalmology. 2020;**11**:2067

[33] Ortiz-Seller A, Martínez Costa L, Hernández-Pons A, Valls Pascual E, Solves Alemany A, Albert-Fort M. Ophthalmic and neuro-ophthalmic manifestations of coronavirus disease 2019 (COVID-19). Ocular Immunology and Inflammation. 2020;**28**:1285-1289

[34] Dinkin M, Gao V, Kahan J. COVID-19 presenting with ophthalmoparesis from cranial nerve palsy. Neurology. 2020;**95**:221-223

[35] Huber M, Rogozinski S, Puppe W. Postinfectious onset of myasthenia gravis in a COVID-19 patient. Frontiers in Neurology. 2020;**11**:576153

[36] Theophanous C, Santoro JD, Itani R. Bell's palsy in a pediatric patient with hyper IgM syndrome and severe acute respiratory syndrome coronavirus 2 (SARS-CoV-2). Brain & Development. 2021;**43**:357-359

[37] Gutiérrez-Ortiz C, Méndez-Guerrero A, Rodrigo-Rey S. Miller Fisher Syndrome and polyneuritis cranialis in COVID-19. Neurology. 2020;**95**:e601

[38] Leber HM, Santna L, Konichi da Silva NR. Acute thyroiditis and bilateral optic neuritis following SARS-CoV-2 vaccination with CoronaVac: A case report. Oculate Immunological Inflammation. 2021;**17**:1

[39] Palao M, Fernández-Díaz E, Gracia-Gil J. Multiple sclerosis following SARS-CoV-2 infection. Multiple Sclerosis and Related Disorders. 2020;**45**:102377

[40] Zhou S, Jones-Lopez EC, Soneji DJ. Myelin oligodendrocyte glycoprotein antibody-associated optic neuritis and myelitis in COVID-19. Journal of Neuro-Ophthalmology. 2020;**40**(3):398-402

[41] de Ruijter NS, Kramer G, Gons RAR. Neuromyelitis optica spectrum disorder after presumed coronavirus (COVID-19) infection: A case report. Multiple Sclerosis and Related Disorders. 2020;**46**:102474

[42] Turbin RE, Wawrzusin PJ, Sakla NM. Orbital cellulitis, sinusitis and intracranial abnormalities in two adolescents with COVID-19. Orbit. 2020;**39**(4):305-310

[43] Mekonnen ZK, Ashraf DC, Jankowski T. Acute invasive rhino-orbital mucormycosis in a patient with COVID-19-associated acute respiratory distress syndrome. Ophthalmic Plastic & Reconstructive Surgery. 2021;**37**(2):e40-e80

[44] Mehta S, Pandey A. Rhino-orbital mucormycosis associated with COVID-19. Cureus. 2020;**12**(9):e10726

[45] Sen M, Lahane S, Lahane TP. Mucor in a viral land: A tale of two pathogens. Indian Journal of Ophthalmology. 2021;**69**(2):244-252

[46] Armstrong BK, Murchison AP, Bilyk JR. Suspected orbital myositis associated with COVID-19. Orbit. 2021;**40**(6):532-535

[47] Eleiwa T, Abdelrahman SN, ElSheikh RH. Orbital inflammatory disease associated with COVID-19 infection. Journal of AAPOS. 2021;**25**(4):232-234

[48] Martínez Díaz M, Copete Piqueras S, Blanco MC. Acute dacryoadenitis in a patient with SARS-CoV-2 infection. Orbit. 2021;**2021**:1-4

[49] Singh AK, Singh R, Joshi SR. Mucormycosis in COVID-19: A systematic review of cases reported worldwide and in India. Diabetes Metabolism Syndrome. 2021;**15**(4):102146

[50] [updated 2020 Jan 10; cited 2021 Febr 07]. https://www.eeba.eu/news/news-details/ coronavirus-ocular-tissue-donation

[51] [updated 2020 Nov 12; cited 2021 Feb 07]. https://www.gaeba.org/2020/alertcoronavirus-2019-ncov-and-ocular-tissue-donation/

[52] [updated 2020 Mar 23; cited 2021 Feb 07]. https://eatb.org/updates/106-covid-21

[53] Loffredo L, Pacella F, Pacella E. Conjunctivitis and COVID-19: A meta-analysis. Journal of Medical Virology. 2020;**92**:1413-1414

Chapter 6

Trachoma

Alada Joel James

Abstract

Trachoma is the most common infectious cause of blindness worldwide. In children, repeated episodes of infection within cohorts and family with *Chlamydia trachomatis* would lead to severe conjunctival inflammation, scarring, and potentially blinding trichiasis or entropion in later life. Trachoma is a disease associated with poverty, poor hygiene, and sanitation as well inadequate water supply. Collaborative control programs are implementing the "SAFE" strategy: surgery for trichiasis, mass distribution of antibiotics, promotion of facial cleanliness, and environmental improvement. The SAFE strategy has remained the cornerstone of WHO's plan to eliminate trachoma as public health problem, and many countries and districts have eliminated trachoma by this means.

Keywords: trachoma, poverty, Trichiasis, chlamydia, sanitation, azithromycin, water, corneal opacity

1. Introduction

Trachoma has been recognized as a cause of blindness since antiquity [1–3]. Early Egyptian and Chinese manuscripts described its manifestation, therapy, and complications. Trachoma remains the leading cause of infectious blindness worldwide [4]. The intracellular bacterium *Chlamydia trachomatis* (*C. trachomatis*) is the causative agent, and it causes chronic keratoconjunctivitis [5].

C. trachomatis can spread either directly through interpersonal contact with secretions from the eyes and noses of infected individuals or indirectly via contact with pieces of clothing or flies that have picked up the bacterium from an infected person [6]. It has been demonstrated that poor sanitation, overcrowding, and insufficient clean water and toilets significantly increase the rate of spread [4].

Episodes of repeated reinfection within cohorts and families cause intense conjunctival inflammation described as *active trachoma*, which leads to conjunctival scarring. Scarring from trachoma distorts the normal anatomy of the upper tarsal plate leading to entropion and trichiasis also known as *cicatricial trachoma* [7].

The World Health Organization (WHO) along with its partners in 1996 adopted surgery (S), antibiotics (A), facial cleanliness (F), and environmental improvement (E) strategy as the best approach for the control of trachoma [8].

The Neglected Tropical Disease Road map 2021–2030 has set 2030 as the target year for the global elimination of trachoma as a public health problem. Recently, the Global Trachoma Mapping Project and its successor Tropical Data established communities across the globe where elimination efforts should be concentrated to achieve the goal of eliminating trachoma [9].

2. Epidemiology

Trachoma is endemic in 44 countries, and the highest prevalence are in sub-Saharan Africa, Asia, Latin America, and the Middle East [4, 6, 10]. *C. trachomatis* infection occurs mostly in children, and in areas where trachoma is endemic, the first infection usually occurs in the first 2 years of life. Even though initial infections may resolve spontaneously, they are frequently followed by reinfection or superimposed bacterial conjunctivitis [11]. However, the prevalence generally declines to low levels in adults [12].

Complications arising from trachoma may result in severe ocular pains and loss of vision with its attendant poor quality of life and loss of economic productivity [13]. In 2021, approximately 1.9 million people were blind or suffer significant visual impairment from trachoma with over 136 million people living in communities requiring trachoma elimination programs [14].

2.1 Morbidity and mortality

Approximately, 1.9 million people are blind because of trachoma [8]. The risk of mortality in endemic communities is increased among those blinded by the disease [14].

2.2 Poverty

Trachoma is a disease of the poor and deprived [4, 15]. The risk of active trachoma is higher in households with crowed living spaces and poor sanitation. Trachoma persists in low- and middle-income countries (LMICs) where resources are scarce and shared within households [16]. Additionally, the disability that results from the sequelae of chronic infection with C. trachomatis such trichiasis and corneal opacities may lead to reduced productivity and unemployment. Demonstrably, trachoma remains a good proxy of inequality in a population [16, 17]. A study in Ethiopia found that within communities afflicted with trachoma, individuals and households affected by trachomatous trichiasis (TT) are significantly poorer economically than those that are not affected [18]. Trachoma therefore creates a vicious cycle of poverty that traps those affected.

2.3 Race and sex

Trachoma remains a disease of poverty and poor hygiene. Consequently, trachoma has no racial predilection [19]. The disease affects the marginalized and deprived members of the communities [20]. The disease persists in communities with inadequate access to water and sanitation and in dry, dusty, and hot climates [15, 21, 22]. Other agents of transmission include dirty faces, eye-seeking flies (particularly, *Musca sorbens*), and fomites such as clothing.

Women are usually affected by severe trachoma more than twofold compared to men [19, 23]. Because women carry the burden of childcare in most endemic communities, they tend to be more at risk. School age children harbor the active forms of the disease, thereby increasing exposure to C trachomatis [19].

2.4 Age

It has been established that active trachoma is a disease of school age children [24–26]. However, young adults especially mothers have trachomatous scarring. Older patients and grandparents tend to have trichiasis and corneal opacity [21]. In hyper-endemic communities, these forms of presentation can occur concurrently [27].

3. Pathophysiology

C. trachomatis serovars A, B, Ba, and C predominate as causative agents of trachoma. Serovars D-K may rarely cause a subacute follicular conjunctivitis that except for scarring, may indistinguishable clinically from trachoma [27–29].

Trachomatous inflammation begins with the recruitment and activation of a host of leukocytes in the conjunctival tissue [30]. Increased expression of certain proteases like matrix metalloproteinases (MMPS), e.g. MMP7, MMP9, and MMP12, and pro-inflammatory agents like chemokines and cytokines are associated with severe disease. Research has shown that the predominant cellular constituents of trachoma follicles are macrophages, plasma cells with lymphocytic and monocytic infiltrate [27]. Typically, the follicles are made up of germinal centers with clumps of intense B-cell proliferation that are surrounded by multiple T cells. Scarring ensues when conjunctival epithelium lose goblet cells and compact collagen bands replace the normally freely mobile and vascular subepithelial stroma [7, 31].

3.1 Histopathology/immunology

Histology of conjunctival tissue will reveal a diffuse mixed inflammatory cell infiltrate of the conjunctiva with mild to moderate epithelial hyperplasia [32]. The hallmark of trachoma is the presence of lymphoid follicles in the stroma. In late stages of the disease known as cicatricial trachoma, the conjunctiva will show chronic inflammatory infiltrate in the substantia propria with lymphocytes predominating [27, 32, 33]. Additionally, the conjunctival epithelium may show squamous metaplasia with multiple denuded areas where the underlying stroma may be replaced with thick, compact scar tissue [34].

Trachoma evades host immune responses through intracellular invasion. Therefore, the leading sequalae are a result of inflammation rather than infection by C. Trachomatis. It is now clear that host immunity plays a significant role in clinical presentation and disease severity [34, 35]. The most likely pathway is that increased chemokine responses lead to neutrophil activation, chemotaxis, and fibrosis. This is mediated by the activities of TH1 as a pro-inflammatory as well as TH2 serving as a potent inducer of anti-inflammatory responses [27, 31].

Blindness from trachoma occurs from conjunctival scarring which is attributed to recurrent infection. Subconjunctival fibrotic bands eventually cause scar contraction leading to entropion, trichiasis, and finally corneal opacification [34].

4. Clinical presentation

Trachoma presents in two phases: the active phase and the cicatricial or scarring phase; however, both phases can coexist concurrently [6]. Active trachoma is characterized by a mucopurulent keratoconjunctivitis [36]. The conjunctival surface of the upper eyelid shows a follicular and inflammatory response. The cornea may have limbal follicles, superior neovascularization also known as pannus, and punctate keratitis [31]. *C trachomatis infection* may occur concurrently with that of other extraocular mucous membranes, e.g. the nasopharynx, leading to a nasal discharge.

Most patients with active trachoma are relatively asymptomatic [11].

The cicatricial phase has characteristic clinical features, which can lead to definitive diagnosis in most cases [7, 37].

4.1 Grading

The most widely used grading system for trachoma is the WHO grading (**Figure 1**) [38]:

4.1.1 Trachomatous inflammation Folliculla r (TF)

Follicular trachoma indicates active disease. It is defined as the presence of five or more follicles at least 5 mm in diameter in the central part of the upper tarsal conjunctiva.

4.1.2 Trachomatous inflammation (TI)

Trachomatous inflammation is defined as pronounced inflammatory thickening of the upper tarsal conjunctiva that obscures more than one half of the normal deep tarsal vessels.

4.1.3 Trachomatous scarring (TS)

Trachomatous scarring is defined as the presence of easily visible scars in the tarsal conjunctiva.

Grade	Description
TF	Trachomatous inflammation – follicular: the presence of 5 or more follicles (>0.5 mm) in the upper tarsal conjunctiva
TI	Trachomatous inflammation – intense: pronounced inflammatory thickening of the tarsal conjunctiva that obscures more than half of the deep normal vessels
TS	Trachomatous scarring: the presence of scarring in the tarsal conjunctiva
TT	Trachomatous trichiasis: at least one lash rubs on the eyeball
CO	Corneal opacity: easily visible corneal opacity over the pupil

Figure 1.
The simplified WHO grading system of trachoma.

4.1.4 Corneal opacity

Corneal opacity is defined as easily visible corneal opacity over the pupil that is so dense that it blurs at least part of the pupillary margin when it is viewed through the opacity.

Corneal opacity or scarring reflects the prevalence of vision loss and blindness resulting from trachoma.

4.2 Differential diagnosis

- Allergic conjunctivitis
- Viral conjunctivitis
- Bacterial conjunctivitis
- Acute chlamydial infection
- Neonatal conjunctivitis
- Toxic follicular conjunctivitis

5. Diagnosis

Trachoma diagnosis is usually determined clinically using a x2.5 binocular magnifying loupe to examine the everted upper tarsal conjunctiva. In non-endemic areas, the laboratory methods of diagnosis are usually preferred [39].

However, the laboratory detection of c trachomatis is problematic. Firstly, it requires sophisticated equipment that are hard to acquire or even maintain in trachoma endemic communities. Secondly, the services of a specialist microbiologist or pathologist is often required in order to make accurate and consistent diagnosis of C trachomatis [40]. Thirdly and most importantly is the fact that clinical signs of trachoma are poorly correlated with actual evidence of infection demonstrable in the laboratory [41, 42].

For operational purposes, any modality of *C. trachomatis* diagnosis will have to be cheap and reliable and provide rapid results. It becomes apparent, therefore, that trachoma control programs overwhelmingly rely on clinical signs of trachoma for diagnosis [43–46].

Even though laboratory tests are not commonly used in the field of the diagnosis of *C. trachoma*, they are useful in non-endemic areas as well as in research laboratories. Frequently performed laboratory tests include the following:

1. Polymerase chain reaction (PCR), specifically nucleic acid amplification tests (NAATs) are most sensitive.
2. Direct fluorescent antibody assay.
3. Enzyme immunoassay.

6. Treatment and control

Trachoma remains a major public health problem in many endemic countries. A multifaceted strategy has been advocated as the best approach if success is to be had beyond the ophthalmology clinic [15]. Following a resolution by the World Health Assembly in 1998, the World Health Organization (WHO) recommended the "SAFE" strategy as the most effective means of managing trachoma [38]. It has been operationalized in all programs aimed at eliminating trachoma. Elimination has been successfully achieved in hitherto endemic countries such as Gambia, Morocco, Mexico, Laos, and Nepal [47–49]. Control programs utilize a four-step approach as follows:

S: Surgery for trichiasis.

A: Antibiotics for chlamydia trachomatis infection.

F: Facial cleanliness.

E: Environmental change to improve sanitation and increase access to clean water.

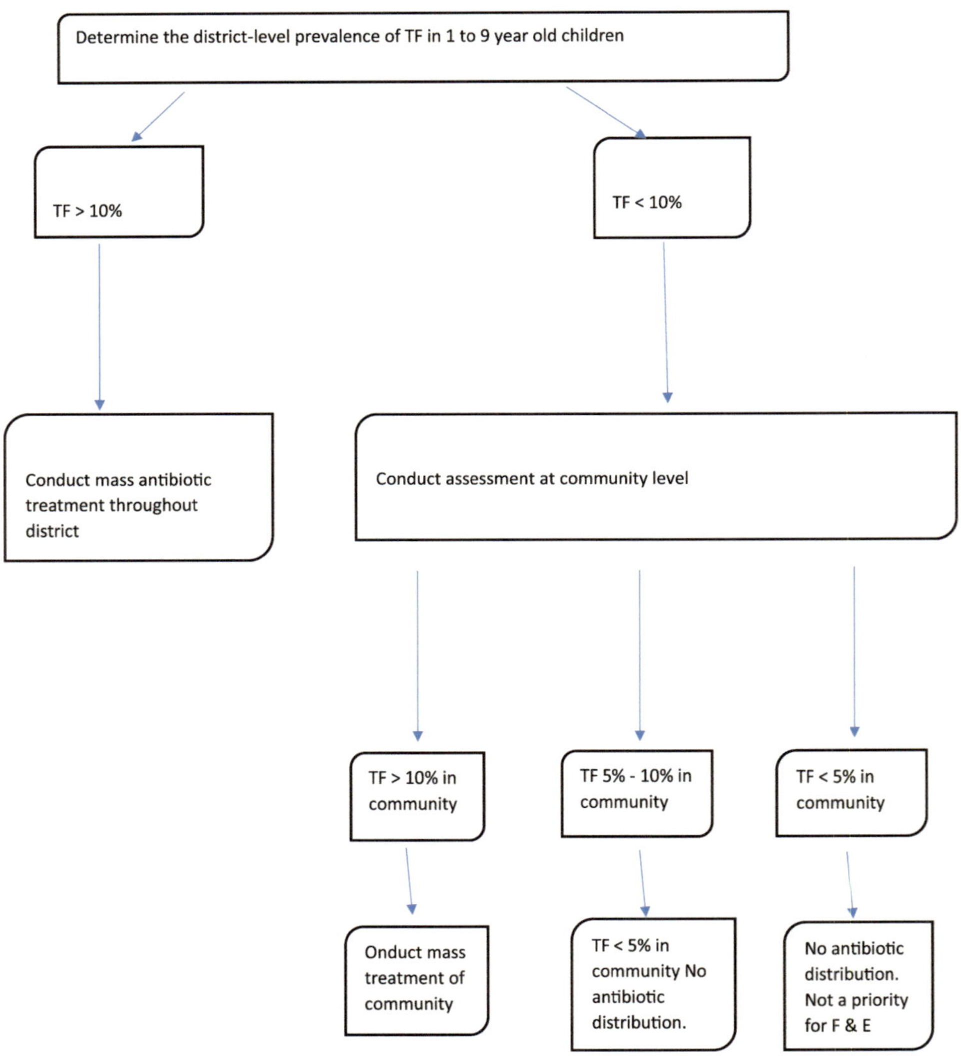

Figure 2.
WHO recommendations for initiating antibiotic treatment for trachoma.

6.1 Surgery for Trichiasis

Trachomatous trichiasis (TT) afflicts about 8 million people worldwide [50]. Untreated TT will ultimately lead to blinding corneal opacity which is an irreversible sequela. Eyelid surgeries to avert complications from trichiasis have been extensively studied. Varying success rates have been reported with several surgical techniques used in several control programs. The WHO endorsed the bilamellar tarsal rotation because of its low TT recurrence rate.

6.2 Antibiotics

The WHO recommends mass distribution of antibiotics in communities where follicular trachoma is >10% in children [12]. In 1940, sulfonamide was the first antibiotic to be used at a large scale to treat trachoma. Over the ensuing decades, several other antibiotics were evaluated with little success until in 1990 when tetracycline became the drug of choice.

In more recent decades, azithromycin has been adopted as the drug of choice by many trachoma control programs because of its many advantages over tetracycline ointment [51]. For example, azithromycin is a single-dose regime and treatment can be directly observed to improve compliance significantly.

The WHO has developed guidelines for determining how community treatment of trachoma based solely on the prevalence of trachoma follicles in children aged 1–9 (**Figure 2**) [52]. It is recommended that trachoma control programs use either 6 weeks' regimen of tetracycline eye ointment instilled into the lower conjunctival sacs two times a day or a single dose of azithromycin (20 mg/kg up to 1 g) [53, 54]. The duration of treatment remains a subject of debate and further research. The WHO recommends three annual rounds of mass treatment endemic communities after which a reassessment of active disease will determine whether another round of treatment will be needed or discontinued [55].

6.3 Face washing

Face washing plays a crucial role in the control of trachoma because it disrupts the transmission of C. trachomatis by removing potentially infected ocular secretions [56].

6.4 Environmental improvements

Trachoma control programs advocate for improved water supply which is essential for face washing and sanitation as major contributors of successful control efforts. Latrine building is particularly advocated and incorporated because in trachoma control programs, because it limits the preferred breeding ground of the mechanical vector of *C. trachomatis, Musca sorbens*. It is to be noted that most of the changes that tend to improve the control of trachoma will also benefit the general health of the community [19, 53].

6.5 Prognosis

If the risk of reinfection is eliminated, early identification and treatment lead to resolution and full recovery [11]. Surgery may have a limited role once corneal scarring develops.

7. Conclusion

There is a real chance that trachoma will be eliminated as a public health problem in our lifetime [14, 20]. Following over two decades of sustained "SAFE" strategy, the disease burden of trachoma has been substantially reduced. As we near the end, research efforts are now geared toward accurate diagnosis of trachoma infection and monitoring of symptoms. Several studies have shown that mass distribution of azithromycin antibiotic also provides ancillary benefits such as the reduction infectious diseases and childhood mortality [55]. For these efforts to be sustainable, integrating trachoma programs with other neglected tropical diseases (NTDs) may prove cost-effective in many ways [44].

Acknowledgements

I will like to acknowledge the brilliant suggestions of Dr. Ruth J. alfin and Dr. Nievel Maigida.

Conflict of interest

"The authors declare no conflict of interest."

Notes/thanks/other declarations

Special thanks to Prof. Caleb Mpyet for kindling my interest in ophthalmic epidemiology and being a mentor per excellence.

Author details

Alada Joel James
Jos University Teaching Hospital, Plateau State, Nigeria

*Address all correspondence to: joel.alada@gmail.com

References

[1] Taylor HR. Doyne lecture: Trachoma, is it history? Eye (London, England). 2009;**23**(11):2007-2022

[2] Al-Rifai K. Trachoma through history. International Ophthalmology. 1988;**12**(3):9-14

[3] Taylor HR. Trachoma: A Blinding Scourge from the Bronze Age to the Twenty-First Century. Australia: Centre for Eye Research; 2008

[4] Burton MJ. Trachoma: An overview. British Medical Bulletin. 2007;**84**:99-116

[5] Solomon A, Peeling R. Diagnosis and assessment of trachoma. Clinical microbiology. 2004;**17**(4):982-1011

[6] Solomon A, Mabey D. Trachoma. BMJ Clin Evid. 2007;**2007** (Published online 2007 Dec 6) [Accessed: April 20, 2022]

[7] Rajak SN, Collin JRO, Burton MJ. Trachomatous trichiasis and its management in endemic countries. Survey of Ophthalmology. 2014;**57**(2):105-135

[8] World Health Organization. Planning for the Global Elimination of Trachoma (GET): Report of a WHO Consultation (WHO/PBL/97.60). Geneva: World Health Organization; 1997

[9] Solomon AW, Kurylo E. The global trachoma mapping project. Community eye health/International Centre for Eye Health. 2014;**27**(85):18

[10] Polack S, Brooker S, Kuper H, Mariotti S, Mabey D, Foster A. Mapping the global distribution of trachoma. Bulletin of the World Health Organization. 2005;**83**(12):913-919

[11] Kuper H, Solomon AW, Buchan J, Zondervan M, Foster A, Mabey D. A critical review of the SAFE strategy for the prevention of blinding trachoma. Lancet Infectious Diseases. 2003;**3**:372-381

[12] Burton MJ, Mabey DCW. The global burden of trachoma: A review. PLoS Neglected Tropical Diseases. 2009;**3**:e460

[13] Frick KD, Hanson CL, Jacobson GA. Global burden of trachoma and economics of the disease. The American Journal of Tropical Medicine and Hygiene. 2003;**69**(5 Suppl):1-10

[14] Burton MJ, Ramke J, Marques AP, Bourne RRA, Congdon N, Jones I, et al. The lancet Global Health Commission on global eye health: Vision beyond 2020. The Lancet Global Health. 2021;**9**(4):e489-e551

[15] Hu VH, Harding-Esch EM, Burton MJ, Bailey RL, Kadimpeul J, Mabey DCW. Epidemiology and control of trachoma: Systematic review. Tropical Medicine and International Health. 2010;**15**:673-691

[16] Gilbert CE, Shah SP, Jadoon MZ, Bourne R, Dineen B, Khan MA, et al. Poverty and blindness in Pakistan: Results from the Pakistan national blindness and visual impairment survey. BMJ British Medical Journal. 2008;**336**(7634):29

[17] Habtamu E, Wondie T, Aweke S, Tadesse Z, Zerihun M, Zewdie Z, et al. Trachoma and relative poverty: A case-control study. PLoS Neglected Tropical Diseases. 2015;**9**(11):e0004228

[18] Rajak SN, Habtamu E, Weiss HA, Kello AB, Abera B, Zerihun M, et al.

The outcome of trachomatous Trichiasis surgery in Ethiopia: Risk factors for recurrence. PLoS Neglected Tropical Diseases. 2013;**7**(8):1-11

[19] Courtright P, West SK. Contribution of sex-linked biology and gender roles to disparities with trachoma. Emerging Infectious Diseases. 2004;**10**(11):2012-2016

[20] Malecela MN, Ducker C. A road map for neglected tropical diseases 2021-2030. Transactions of the Royal Society of Tropical Medicine and Hygiene. 2021;**115**:121-123. DOI: 10.1093/trstmh/traa118

[21] Haddad D. Trachoma: The beginning of the end? Community eye health/International Centre for Eye Health. 2012;**25**(77):18

[22] Mpyet C, Tagoh S, Boisson S, Willis R, Muhammad N, Bakhtiari A, et al. Prevalence of trachoma and access to water and sanitation in Benue state, Nigeria: Results of 23 population-based prevalence surveys. Ophthalmic Epidemiology. 2018;**25**(sup1):79-85

[23] Cromwell EA, Courtright P, King JD, Rotondo LA, Ngondi J, Emerson PM. The excess burden of trachomatous trichiasis in women: A systematic review and meta-analysis. Transactions of the Royal Society of Tropical Medicine and Hygiene. 2009;**103**(10):985-992. DOI: 10.1016/j.trstmh.2009.03.012

[24] Nash SD, Chernet A, Moncada J, Stewart AEP, Astale T, Sata E, et al. Ocular chlamydia trachomatis infection and infectious load among pre-school aged children within trachoma hyperendemic districts receiving the SAFE strategy, Amhara region, Ethiopia. PLoS Negl Trop Dis. 2020;**14**(5):e0008226. DOI: 10.1371/journal.pntd.0008226

[25] Muhammad N, Mohammed A, Isiyaku S, Adamu MD, Gwom A, Rabiu MM. Mapping trachoma in 25 local government areas of Sokoto and Kebbi states, northwestern Nigeria. The British Journal of Ophthalmology. 2014;**98**(4):432-437

[26] Smith AG, Broman AT, Alemayehu W, Munoz BE, West SK, Gower EW. Relationship between trachoma and chronic and acute malnutrition in children in rural Ethiopia. Journal of Tropical Paediatrics. 2007;**53**(5):308-312

[27] Hu VH, Holland MJ, Burton MJ. Trachoma: Protective and pathogenic ocular immune responses to chlamydia trachomatis. PLoS Neglected Tropical Diseases. 2013;**7**:e2020

[28] Mariotti SP, Pascolini D, Rose-Nussbaumer J. Trachoma: Global magnitude of a preventable cause of blindness. The British Journal of Ophthalmology. 2009;**93**(5):563-568

[29] Baneke A. Review: Targeting trachoma: Strategies to reduce the leading infectious cause of blindness. Travel Medicine and Infectious Disease. 2012;**10**(2):92-96

[30] Gambhir M, Gloria BM, Turner F, Kumaresan J, Grassly NC. Trachoma: Transmission, infection, and control. The Lancet Infectious Diseases. 2007;**7**(June):420-427

[31] Burton MJ, Rajak SN, Bauer J, Weiss HA, Tolbert SB, Shoo A, et al. Conjunctival transcriptome in scarring trachoma. Infection and Immunity. 2011;**79**(1):499-511

[32] Guzey M, Ozardali I, Basar E, Aslan G, Satici A, Karadede S. A survey of trachoma: The histopathology and the mechanism of progressive cicatrization of eyelid tissues. Ophthalmologica

Journal international d'ophtalmologie International journal of ophthalmology Zeitschrift fur Augenheilkunde. 2000;**214**(4):277-284

[33] Hu VH, Weiss HA, Massae P, Courtright P, Makupa W, Mabey DCW, et al. In vivo confocal microscopy in scarring trachoma. Ophthalmology. 2011;**118**(11):2138-2146

[34] Burton MJ, Ramadhani A, Weiss HA, Hu V, Massae P, Burr SE, et al. Active trachoma is associated with increased conjunctival expression of IL17A and profibrotic cytokines. Infection and Immunity. 2011;**79**(12):4977-4983

[35] Bailey R, Duong T, Carpenter R, Whittle H, Mabey D. The duration of human ocular chlamydia trachomatis infection is age dependent. Epidemiology and Infection. 1999;**123**(3):479-486

[36] Allen HF. Chlamydial eye disease. International Ophthalmology Clinics. 1975;**15**:257-268

[37] Melese M, Alemayehu W, Bejiga A, Adamu Y, Worku A. Modified grading system for upper eyelid trachomatous trichiasis. Ophthalmic Epidemiology. 2003;**10**(2):75-80

[38] Thylefors B, Dawson CR, Jones BR, West SK, Taylor HR. A simple system for the assessment of trachoma and its complications. Bulletin of the World Health Organization. 1987;**65**(4):477-483

[39] Martin DL, Saboya-Diaz MI, Abashawl A, Alemayeh W, Gwyn S, et al. The use of serology for trachoma surveillance: Current status and priorities for future investigation. PLoS Neglected Tropical Diseases. 2020;**14**(9):e0008316

[40] Yang JL, Schachter J, Moncada J, Habte D, Zerihun M, House JI, et al. Comparison of an rRNA-based and DNA-based nucleic acid amplification test for the detection of chlamydia trachomatis in trachoma. The British Journal of Ophthalmology. 2007;**91**(3):293-295

[41] Michel CEC, Roper KG, Divena MA, Lee HH, Taylor HR. Correlation of clinical trachoma and infection in aboriginal communities. PLoS Neglected Tropical Diseases. 2011;**5**(3):e986

[42] Macleod CK, Bailey RL, Dejene M, Shafi O, Kebede B, Negussu N, et al. Practice of epidemiology estimating the Intracluster correlation coefficient for the clinical sign "trachomatous inflammation-follicular" in population-based trachoma prevalence surveys: Results from a meta-regression analysis of 261 standardized Preintervention surveys carried out in Ethiopia, Mozambique, and Nigeria. American Journal of Epidemiology World Health Organization. 2020;**189**(1):68-76

[43] Morberg DP, Amza A, Gebresillasie S, Tadesse Z, Yu SN, Stoller NE, et al. Follicle size in trachoma: Assessment of a well-known trachoma grading diagram. The British Journal of Ophthalmology. 2014;**98**(5):706-708

[44] Solomon AW, Engels D, Bailey RL, Blake IM, Brooker S, Chen JX, et al. A diagnostics platform for the integrated mapping, monitoring, and surveillance of neglected tropical diseases: Rationale and target product profiles. PLoS Neglected Tropical Diseases. 2012;**6**(7):e1746

[45] Rashid A, Jakobiec FA. Avoiding the major complication of ophthalmic pathology: Misdiagnosis. A Review of Three Common Diagnostic Challenges. 2014;**29**(August):468-474

[46] Bird M, Dawson CR, Schachter JS, Miao Y, Shama A, Osman A, et al. Does

the diagnosis of trachoma adequately identify ocular chlamydial infection in trachoma-endemic areas ? The Journal of Infectious Diseases. 2003;**187**:1669-1673

[47] Aboe A, Joof BM, Kanyi SK, Hydara A, Downs P, Bush S, et al. The Gambia has eliminated trachoma as a public health problem. Challenges and successes. PLoS Neglected Tropical Diseases. 2022;**16**(3):e0010282

[48] Friedrich MJ. Two southeast Asian countries eliminate trachoma. Journal of the American Medical Association. 2017;**318**(19):1857-1857

[49] Hammou J, el Ajaroumi H, Hasbi H, Nakhlaoui A, Hmadna A, el Maaroufi A. In Morocco, the elimination of trachoma as a public health problem becomes a reality. The Lancet Global Health. 2017;**5**(3):e250-e251

[50] Lietman TM, Francisco-San, Catherine Oldenburg CE, San Francisco M, Jeremy Keenan CD. Editorial trachoma: Time to talk eradication. Ophthalmology. 2020;**127**:11-13. DOI: 10.1016/j.ophtha.2019.11.001

[51] Evans JR, Solomon AW, Kumar R, Perez A, et al. Antibiotics for trachoma. Cochrane Database of Systematic Review. 2019;**9**:1-138 [Accessed: July 19, 2022]

[52] World Health Organization G. World Health Organization. Report of the 2nd Global Scientific Meeting on Trachoma. Geneva: WHO; 2003

[53] Alexander NDE, Ph D, Massae PA, Aguirre A, West SK, Bailey RL, et al. Mass treatment with single-dose azithromycin for trachoma. The New England Journal of Medicine. 2004;**351**(19):1962-1971

[54] Bhosai SJ, Bailey RL, Gaynor BD, Lietman TM. Trachoma: An update on prevention, diagnosis, and treatment. Current Opinion in Ophthalmology. 2012;**23**(4):288-295

[55] Mahmud H, Landskroner E, Amza A, Aragie S, Godwin WW, de Hostos BA, et al. Stopping azithromycin mass drug administration for trachoma: A systematic review. PLoS Neglected Tropical Diseases. 2021;**15**(7):e0009491

[56] Zack R, Mkocha H, Zack E, Munoz B, West SK. Issues in defining and measuring facial cleanliness for national trachoma control programs. Transactions of the Royal Society of Tropical Medicine and Hygiene. 2008;**102**(5):426-431

Section 2

Uveitis and Inmunomediated Diseases

Chapter 7

Multimodal Imaging of White Dot Syndromes

Cristian de los Santos, Lidia Cocho and José María Herreras

Abstract

White dot syndromes are an uncommon group of posterior uveitis affecting the outer retina, retinal pigment epithelium, choriocapillaris, and/or choroidal stroma. Multimodal imaging, including fundus fluorescein angiography, indocyanine green angiography, autofluorescence, and optical coherence tomography angiography, has improved our understanding regarding their pathophysiology, helping us to rename or even regroup some of these disorders as one disease in opposition to the historical description. It also provides useful information to evaluate disease activity and monitor response to treatment. This chapter will review the different findings on multimodal imaging of these heterogenous disorders and classify them according to their primary anatomic involvement.

Keywords: white dot syndromes, noninfectious choroiditis, Choriocapillaritis, multimodal imaging, autofluorescence, optical coherence tomography angiography (OCT-A), fundus fluorescein angiography (FFA), Indocyanine green angiography (ICGA)

1. Introduction

White dot syndromes are an uncommon group of posterior uveitis affecting the outer retina, retinal pigment epithelium (RPE), choriocapillaris, and/or choroidal stroma. However, the clinical finding of white spots itself is variably present, the pathophysiology, as supported by multimodal imaging, may differ between them and the clinical course is different. For this reason, the term "noninfectious choroiditis" has been suggested to be more appropriate [1–4].

These noninfectious choroiditis are the result of autoimmune infiltration of the choroidal stroma (primary stromal choroiditis) such as birdshot retinochoroiditis (BRC) or immune-mediated choriocapillaris non-perfusion (primary choriocapillaritis) [3] which includes conditions self-resolving as multiple evanescent white dot syndrome (MEWDS) or sight threatening as acute posterior multifocal placoid pigment epitheliopathy (APMPPE), multifocal choroiditis (MFC)/punctate inner choroidopathy (PIC), and serpiginous choroiditis (SC).

Multimodal imaging includes several imaging modalities, such as fundus fluorescein angiography (FFA), indocyanine green angiography (ICGA), fundus autofluorescence (FAF), and optical coherence tomography (OCT) and optical coherence tomography angiography (OCT-A), that play a key role, in determining the primary level of tissue involvement, evaluate disease activity, and monitor response to

IntechOpen

treatment. The aim of this chapter is to describe the different findings on multimodal imaging of these heterogenous disorders.

2. Primary stromal choroiditis with additional independent retinitis: birdshot retinochoroiditis (BRC)

It is also known as vitiliginous chorioretinitis [5], and it is a bilateral, asymmetric, and progressive disease without known systemic involvement first described in 1980 by Ryan and Maumenee [6] that predominates in Caucasian women past the fourth decade of life and presents a strong association with HLA-A29 (90–95%) [7]. Because of this strong association, the disease should be better called HLA-A29 BRC [3]. Early symptoms include floaters, decreased vision, and photopsias, and later, it can present with nyctalopia, decreased color vision, and diminished contrast sensitivity. All these complaints may be related to vitritis, macular or optic disk edema and/or outer retina atrophy, or other complications. Multimodal imaging shows a dual and independent retinal and choroidal inflammation in BRC.

Fundus photography is useful in documenting retinal vasculitis of large veins, papillitis, and the classic depigmented ovoid spots that are more prominent inferonasal to the optic disk (**Figure 1**) and radiate to the equator. These choroidal spots typically indicate stromal scars and may never appear if the disease is treated early [3].

FAF exhibits hypoautofluorescent spots if RPE atrophy occurs more numerous than clinically and sometimes is not uniformly correspondent with the birdshot choroidal lesions suggesting a dual independent RPE damage by inner retina and choroid. A placoid macular hypoautofluorescence which correlates with poor visual outcome may also be seen [8].

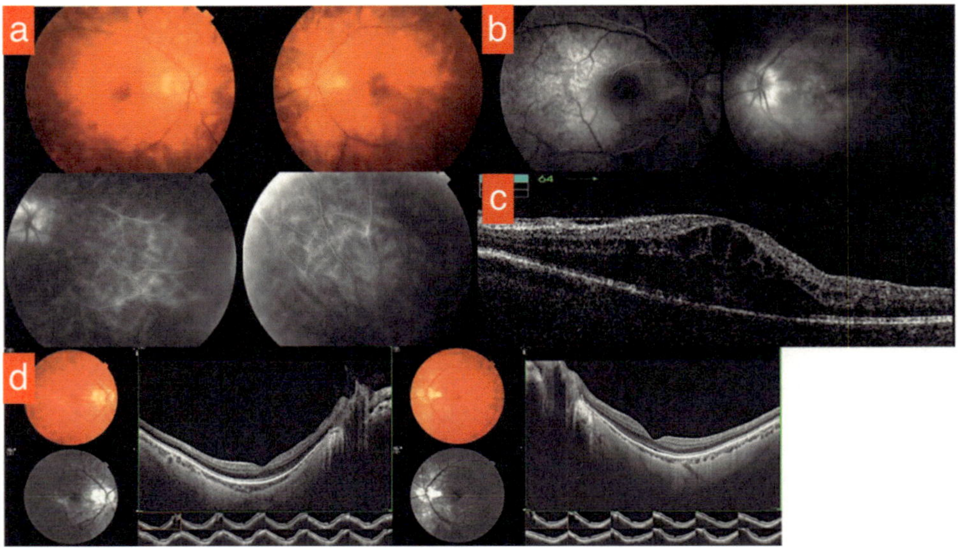

Figure 1.
This patient presents mild vitritis, birdshot choroidal depigmented spots. (a) FAF shows optic nerve leakage and phlebitis in both eyes. Petaloid macular leakage is seen in late phase in the left eye. There is also "quenching" of the dye in the right eye. (b) Optical coherence tomography (OCT) in the left eye demonstrates ERM and CME. (c) In advanced stage, there is choroidal thinning in both eyes on OCT. (d) ERM: Epiretinal membrane; CME: Cystoid macular edema.

FFA shows optic nerve hyperfluorescence, vascular leakage (predominantly phlebitis), and macular leakage (**Figure 1**) [9]. Moreover, circulation times are called to be "delayed" in the venous circulation but in fact is a pseudo-delay or "quenching" of the dye due to diffuse capillary leakage of fluorescein into the surrounding tissue so that there is not enough dye to normally mark the veins (**Figure 1**) [10]. Active choroidal inflammatory lesions are not generally visible until they affect the overlying RPE appearing hypofluorescent in early phases with subtle late staining [11].

ICGA shows more numerous choroidal lesions and even before than clinical examination or FFA. They are seen as multiple hypofluorescent round spots in the early and mid-phases becoming isofluorescent in the late angiographic phase if active, probably, partial thickness granulomas, indicating non-penetration of the dye only at the site of inflammatory choroidal infiltrates. If the lesions remain hypofluorescent in late phase, it may be due to full thickness lesions or that the lesions have become atrophic [12, 13]. Also, there may be seen fuzzy vessels in active disease showing choroidal vasculitis during the intermediate and late phases [11–13].

OCT may show cystoid macular edema (CME), secondary epiretinal membrane (ERM) (**Figure 1**), loss of ellipsoid zone (EZ) with RPE degeneration beneath the areas of photoreceptor involvement, as well as other complications, such as macular atrophy, optic atrophy, and rarely, choroidal neovascularization (CNV). Enhanced-depth OCT imaging may be useful to evaluate choroidal thickening early in the disease and thinning in advanced disease (**Figure 1**).

En-face OCT-A has identified areas of flow void in the Haller layer corresponding to those hypofluorescent spots on ICGA with initial sparing of the choriocapillaris, thereby supporting the primary involvement of choroidal stroma in the disease with secondary involvement of choriocapillaris and the RPE [14]. It also demonstrates retinal capillary density reduction at the deep retinal capillary plexus level, which may indicate that ischemia, in addition to inflammation, may play a role in the development of retinal neovascularization (NV), retinal thinning, and reduction of visual function [15]. Other changes in both the superficial and deep capillary plexus that may explain the common finding of CME in BRC have been documented such as capillary dilatations and loops, telangiectatic vessels, increased intercapillary space, and decreased capillary density without a change in the size of the foveal avascular zone (FAZ) [16–18], and alternatively, it has been found a larger area of FAZ [19].

3. Primary choriocapillaritis

3.1 Acute posterior multifocal placoid pigment epitheliopathy (APMPPE)/acute multifocal ischemic choriocapillaritis (AMIC)

APMPPE is an idiopathic, commonly bilateral although asymmetric, disorder affecting young healthy adults who complain of having visual loss, photopsias, and paracentral scotomas of acute onset. However, there have been some unilateral cases or delayed involvement of the second eye by several weeks [20].

The disease origin was first attributed to the RPE by Gass in 1968 [21]; hence the name, however, Deutman and coworkers [22], in the same period, hypothesized that it is a disease primarily affecting the choriocapillaris; therefore, they suggested the name acute multifocal ischemic choroidopathy (AMIC). This last term seems to be more proper as multimodal imaging has demonstrated [9].

Fundus photography shows multifocal, yellowish creamy, or pale discolored placoid chorioretinal lesions [23], located posterior to the equator (generally at the posterior pole) (**Figure 2**) that tend to progressively fade over the weeks, although new lesions may appear more peripherally later without extending beyond the equator, resulting in hyperpigmentation (clumping of pigment) and chorioretinal atrophy with potential damage to visual function.

FFA shows hypofluorescent lesions in early phases due to choriocapillaris non-perfusion, becoming hyperfluorescent by exudation and pooling in late frames due to increased permeability of retinal vascular plexuses induced by the massive ischemia in choriocapillaris and therefore in the overlying outer retina (**Figure 2**), which correspond to the yellow discolored plaques seen on fundus examination [3]. Inactive lesions appear hyperfluorescent due to window defects derived from RPE atrophy and blocked fluorescence from pigment clumping [24].

ICGA exhibits geographic hypofluorescent spots across all phases due to choriocapillaris non-perfusion. Acute lesions are more numerous or extensive than those seen clinically or on FFA [23] suggesting a primary choroid involvement. Inactive lesions tend to become smaller, probably due to the absence of swollen outer retina and RPE secondary to choroidal ischemia, and thus, less blockage [24]. When healed, hypofluorescence can also completely resolve except for a few areas of persistent hypofluorescence due to chorioretinal atrophy.

FAF shows hypoautofluorescence in acute lesions due to the blocking effect of overlying retinal edema [25] and hyperautofluorescence in areas where loss of photoreceptor outer segments has occurred causing increased exposure of RPE lipofuscin (**Figure 2**). Healed lesions develop increased central hyperpigmentation appearing hyperautofluorescent and a surrounding depigmentation zone that shows hypoautofluorescence due to RPE dysfunction/damage/atrophy in areas with severe vascular drop out that do not always correlate with the fundus lesions and/or FFA, and are fewer in number, implicating a primary choroidal alteration. These patterns in advanced lesions suggest centripetal contraction of the placoid lesions with atrophy and depigmentation of surrounding RPE cells [13].

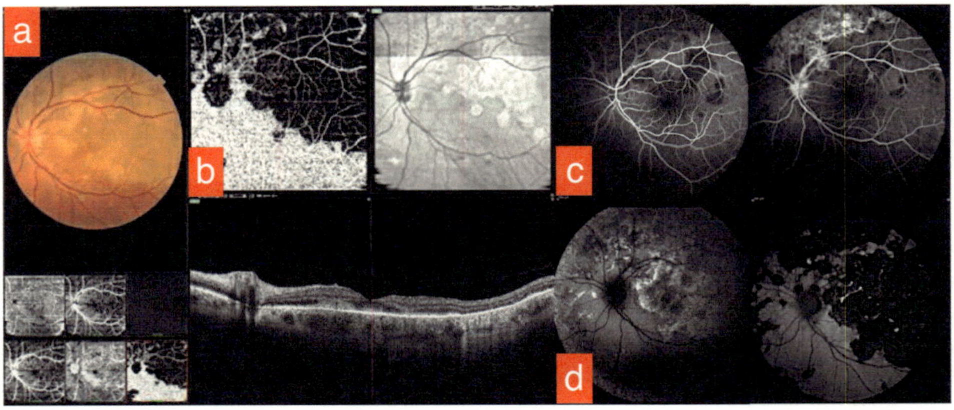

Figure 2.
Patient presents a yellowish confluent placoid chorioretinal lesion. (a) On optical coherence tomography (OCT), there is loss of outer retina and EZ with a hyperreflectivity lesion nasal to the fovea. Optical coherence tomography angiography (OCT-A) demonstrates flow deficit at the level of choriocapillaris. (b) Later, FFA was made showing early hypofluorescence and late hyperfluorescence. (c) FAF shows mixed areas with hypo/hyperautofluorescence at the initial visit and hypoautofluorescence in follow-up. (d) EZ: Ellipsoid zone.

On OCT, there may be hyperreflectivity probably due to ischemic edema or presence of inflammatory cell infiltrates (**Figure 2**) [24, 26, 27] with subsequent disruption or loss of the outer retina and EZ, and sometimes subretinal fluid. As the lesions resolve, RPE disruption or atrophy may also occur. OCT-A demonstrates that this changes correlate with greater areas of hypoperfusion at the level of choriocapillaris being detected also on FFA and ICGA [9].

All these findings thus support the theory that APMPPE/AMIC is a disorder primarily caused by ischemic events occurring in the choriocapillaris and secondarily affecting the outer retina and RPE.

3.2 Serpiginous choroiditis (SC)

SC is a bilateral, although asymmetric, progressive, and recurrent ocular disorder, representing the most severe form of primary choriocapillaritis, probably because the vaso-occlusive involvement occurs in the larger arterioles producing a more widespread choriocapillaris non-perfusion with secondary involvement of the outer retina and RPE, and leading to an extensive and irreversible chorioretinal scarring if not treated promptly, in contrast to MEWDS, which involves the more distal end-choriocapillary vessels, causing less ischemia and consequently less damage that frequently is reversible [4]. Patients report decreased vision, metamorphopsias, scotomas, and photopsias.

Fundus photography shows gray-white-yellow choroidal active lesions [28] which start from the peripapillary region and spread centrifugally in a serpiginous pattern, hence the name. Rarely, macular may present without peripapillary involvement. Over time, these lesions become pigmented chorioretinal scars and recurrences can occur at the border of these atrophic lesions, weeks to years after prior episodes of inflammation (**Figure 3**).

FFA reveals active lesions with early diffuse hypofluorescence probably by blockage of the underlying choroidal fluorescence by swollen outer retina and RPE cells and/or impaired perfusion of choriocapillaris [24, 29] with late hyperfluorescence at the borders [28] by leakage of surrounding intact choriocapillaris [29]. Gradually,

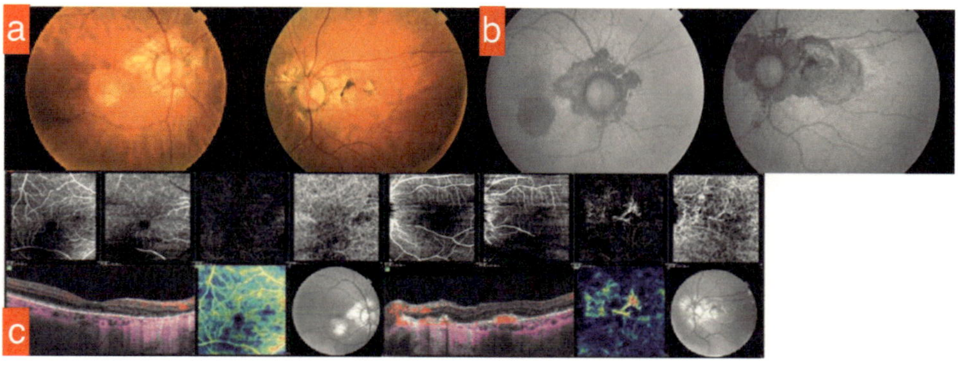

Figure 3.
This patient presents a peripapillary chorioretinal scar affecting also the macula. (a) On FAF, lesions appear hypoautofluorescent. (b) OCT shows outer retina/RPE loss and choroidal thinning in the atrophic areas. In the left eye, there is also a subretinal hyperreflective lesion suggestive of CNV which is better defined by optical coherence tomography angiography (OCT-A) in the outer retina and choriocapillaris and with flow signals in the B-scan. OCT-A also shows flow deficit in choriocapillaris in both eyes. (c) RPE: Retinal pigment epithelium; CNV: Choroidal neovascularization.

there is profuse leakage of the dye from larger choroidal vessels which is observed as hyperfluorescence of the lesion [30]. Early hyperfluorescence with late leakage may represent CNV, usually at the edge of lesions. Older atrophic lesions appear early hypofluorescent by the choriocapillaris atrophy and in late phases hyperfluorescent by diffuse staining of the chorioretinal scar [29]. Some areas show hypofluorescence by blockage (masking effect) from pigment clumping [3].

On ICGA, lesions appear hypofluorescent throughout all phases and are more extensive than FFA or clinically, as it represents both atrophic and active choriocapillaris non-perfusion which explains the pathophysiology. In addition, there may be a diffuse perilesional hyperfluorescent halo that indicates progression of disease [3].

OCT-A demonstrates areas of flow deficit at the level of the choriocapillaris which correlate the hypofluorescence on ICGA, what confirms the choriocapillaris non-perfusion as a primary alteration. Also, it is helpful in detecting CNV and monitoring treatment (**Figure 3**).

OCT shows outer retinal/RPE loss and choroidal thinning in the center of atrophic lesions (**Figure 3**), and at the border there is hyperreflectivity and thickening of the outer retina corresponding with ICGA halo around atrophic lesion and disruption of the EZ representing active lesions.

On FAF, active lesions appear with central hypoautofluorescence, when choriocapillaris and RPE are lost, surrounded by a hyperautofluorescent halo as choriocapillaris and RPE are still present but there is loss of photoreceptor outer segments (**Figure 3**).

3.3 Relentless placoid chorioretinitis (RPC)/ampiginous choroiditis (AC)

Ampiginous choroiditis is an uncommon variant that overlap features of both APMPPE/AMIC and SC [9]. It is characterized by chronic and recurrent clinical course as SC unlike APMPPE/AMIC. Fundus photography shows an atypical distribution of lesions in the mid-periphery and posterior pole in contrast to APMPPE/AMIC or SC which are usually limited to the posterior pole (**Figure 4**) and are smaller than SC and APMPPE/AMIC, approximately 1/2 disk area and more numerous than APMPPE/AMIC (50 or more). There is often active disease in both eyes simultaneously with white placoid lesions present throughout the fundus [31] in contrast to serpiginous chorioretinitis in which usually only one eye is active at a time [24].

Angiographic changes are comparable to SC [9, 23], but active lesions may start distant from previous lesions, but in SC they usually start at margin of an atrophic scar [31]. FAF shows a marked hypoautofluorescence in areas of chorioretinal atrophy (**Figure 4**) [24] and OCT-A detects flow reduction at the level of the choriocapillaris which is also the pathophysiology of both SC and APMPPE/AMIC [32].

3.4 Idiopathic multifocal choroiditis (MFC)/punctate inner choroidopathy (PIC)

MFC is a chronic and recurrent bilateral inflammatory disease that predominantly affects healthy myopic White women in their third to fifth decade of life with no known associated systemic or ocular diseases [9, 33]. It was first called multifocal uveitis and panuveitis [34], although the panuveitis finding in most cases is absent or rarely seen with minimal vitreous or anterior inflammation. Therefore, a group of experts merged different sub-entities that have been described separately in the past, such as PIC, pseudo-POHS (presumed ocular histoplasmosis syndrome) in

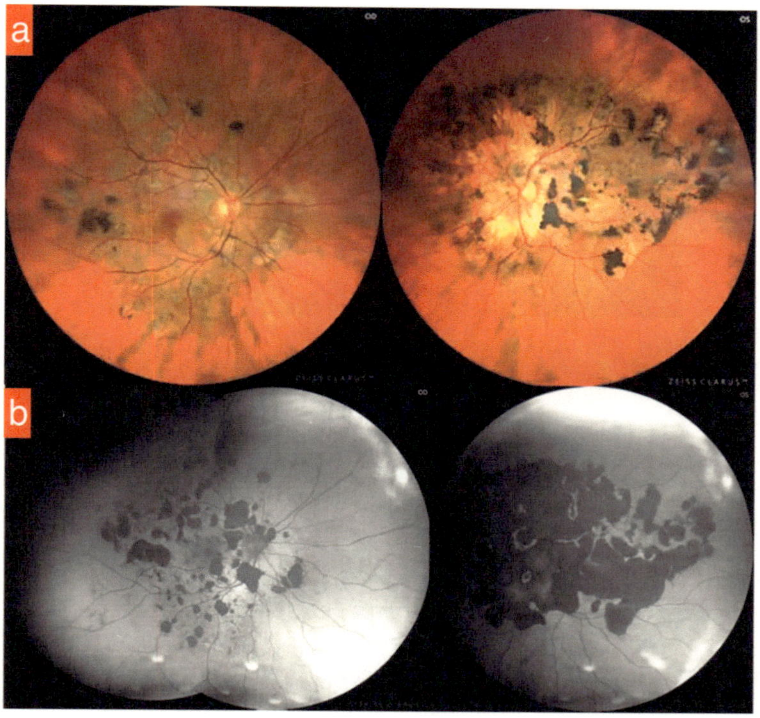

Figure 4.
This patient has an initial presentation as APMPPE/AMIC in the right eye and as SC in the left eye, but then the lesions were extending and affecting both the posterior pole and the mid-periphery leaving chorioretinal atrophy (a) seen as hypoautofluorescence on fundus autofluorescence (FAF). (b) APMPPE/AMIC: Acute posterior multifocal placoid pigment epitheliopathy (APMPPE)/acute multifocal ischemic choriocapillaritis; SC: Serpiginous choroiditis.

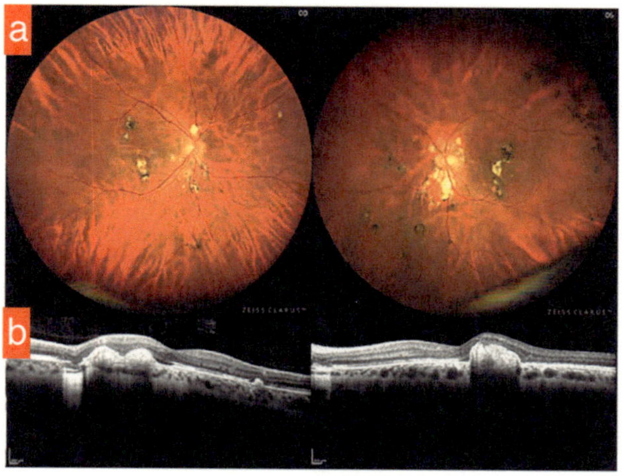

Figure 5.
Atrophic chorioretinal lesions. (a) Optical coherence tomography (OCT) shows sub-RPE hyperreflective lesions with overlying outer retina disruption and thinning of choroid. There is also disruption of RPE/Bruch complex with hyperreflectivity beneath. (b) RPE: Retinal pigment epithelium.

non-endemic areas, progressive subretinal fibrosis, and others, with the single term of idiopathic multifocal choroiditis, regarding them as the same disease [35]. Symptoms include photopsias, blurred vision, and scotomas.

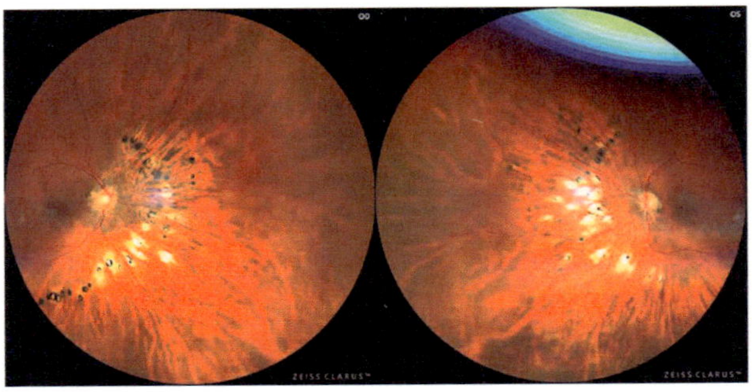

Figure 6.
Schlaegel lines.

Fundus photography shows numerous randomly distributed yellow-white chorioretinal lesions that leave atrophic scars with variable degree of pigmentation in the posterior pole around the disk and/or the mid-periphery (**Figure 5**) that may cluster forming curvilinear chorioretinal streaks (Schlaegel lines) (**Figure 6**) [33]. In as much as one third of cases, there may be seen CNV due to repeated ischemic attacks, which is more frequent than in other primary choriocapillaritis.

FFA identifies recurrences or acute lesions, even in the absence of clinical scars, as early hypofluorescence [9, 36], although early hyperfluorescence can also occur [37–39], and late hyperfluorescence by retinal and subretinal leakage and/or staining due to severe hypoperfusion of the choriocapillaris causing ischemia of outer retina as for APMPPE/AMIC [3, 40]. Early hyperfluorescence with late leakage may represent CNV. Atrophic scars show early hyperfluorescence due to atrophy of the RPE and outer retina (window defect) [9] and areas of hypofluorescence by blockage (masking effect) from pigment deposition (**Figure 7**) [40].

ICGA demonstrates hypofluorescence in new lesions reflecting choriocapillaris hypo or non-perfusion, sometimes in the absence of clinical signs or changes on FFA and helps in detecting progression or regression following inflammation suppressive treatment. Old scarred chorioretinal lesions appear hypofluorescent in all phases [40].

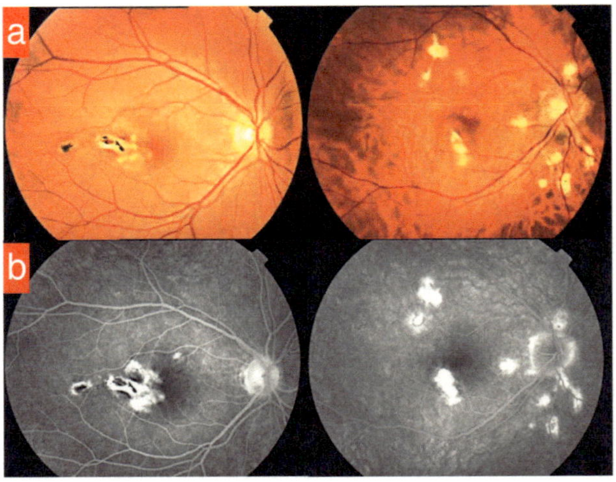

Figure 7.
Atrophic chorioretinal lesions (a) with mixed hype/hypoautofluorescence on fundus autofluorescence (FAF) (b).

OCT-A identifies reduced flow in the choriocapillaris co-localizing with FFA and ICGA findings but less extensive, and it is also useful to identify CNV [9, 40, 41]. OCT shows drusen-like sub-RPE material corresponding to fibrosis with overlying outer retinal disruption and choroidal hyperreflectivity beneath them (**Figure 5**). Chorioretinal atrophic areas can also be seen [9, 40].

FAF shows hyperautofluorescence (exposure of RPE lipofuscin due to loss of outer segments of photoreceptors) and hypoautofluorescence by blockage in cicatricial areas [9, 40].

3.5 Multiple evanescent white dot syndrome

MEWDS is an idiopathic and unilateral inflammatory disorder first described by Lee Jampol et al. in 1984 [42] with a predilection for women in their second to fourth decade of life [27]. As the name indicates, it is self-limited, resolving within 8–10 weeks without sequelae and no need for treatment [43].

Flu-like symptoms may precede ocular manifestations in about half of cases, and there is also association with influenza and other vaccinations [3, 44]. Patients refer sudden visual loss, photopsias, dyscromatopsia, and scotomas.

Fundus photography depicts yellowish-white deep chorioretinal lesions, commonly located at the posterior pole and extending to mid-periphery (**Figure 8**). Foveal granularity is seen, and mild intraocular inflammation can be present in the form of vitritis and/or optic disk edema.

FAF shows hyperautofluorescence produced by exposure of RPE due to loss of outer segments photoreceptors/ellipsoid zone and co-localize with ICGA findings (**Figure 8**). A particular finding of MEWDs is the presence of foveal granularity seen as irregular hyperautofluorescence in near-infrared FAF that remains a little longer than other imaging modalities or clinically [45].

ICGA shows early- to mid-phase hypofluorescence [44] better seen in the late phase due to lesions in the ellipsoid zone causing thickening of RPE resulting in abnormal indocyanine green uptake by the RPE [9] or by choriocapillaris non-perfusion of end-capillary portions [3] which can explain both the self-limited

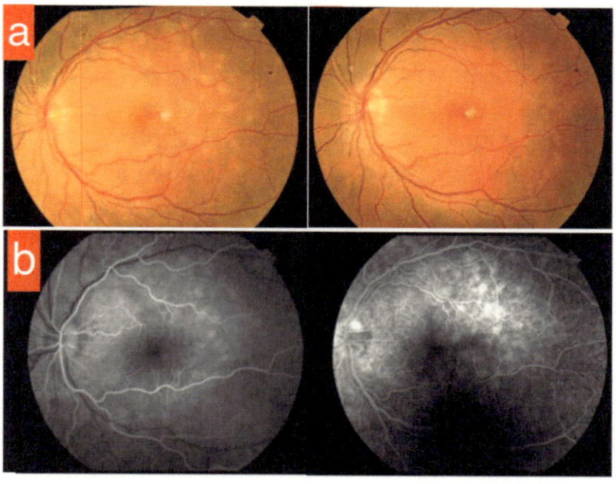

Figure 8.
Yellowish-white chorioretinal lesions that later resolved. (a) On acute lesions, FFA shows early hyperfluorescence than persists in late phases and a mild hot disk (b).

damage and the reversibility of the disease in contrast to other primary choriocapillaritis [4, 26].

OCT shows loss of EZ zone which corresponds to FAF and ICGA lesions, and accumulation of hyperreflective material over RPE that may extend anteriorly through the interdigitation zone, EZ, and outer nuclear layer (ONL) [27, 45].

OCTA does not typically detect areas of flow deficit in the choriocapillaris [41, 46] unless severe damage has occurred showing discrete areas of dropout [47, 48]. Nevertheless, OCTA is probably unable to show end-capillary circulation in contrast to larger vessels such as in APMPPE/AMIC, MFC, and SC [26] and needs sufficient flow to identify the presence or absence of vessels, in contrast to ICGA [3, 49].

FFA shows early faint hyperfluorescence (**Figure 8**) that persists in late phases in wreath-like configuration [44] probably due to lesions involving the EZ/RPE or by outer retinal ischemia that in comparison to APMPPE/AMIC is less pronounced because smaller vessels are affected [3, 26]. Less frequently, optic disk hyperfluorescence and focal retinal vascular stain can be seen [44, 50, 51].

Therefore, there is an ongoing debate about pathophysiology of this disorder whether it is a primary phtoreceptoritis [46] or a primary choriochapillaritis leading to secondary ischemic damage at the outer retina and RPE [49], and more studies are needed.

4. Secondary choriocapillaritis: acute zonal occult outer retinopathy (AZOOR)

AZOOR is a primary disease of the outer retina (photoreceptoritis) with a secondary choriocapillaris involvement. It was first described by JD Gass in 1992 [52] and affects young- to middle-aged patients (13–63 years), predominantly myopic women which present an acute onset of scotomas and photopsias in one or both eyes, sometimes associated with mild vitritis. Furthermore, there may be recurrences in one-third of cases [53].

Fundus photography is normal at presentation, but later can present zonal or multizonal retinochoroidal atrophy, often seen as peripapillary depigmentation, occasionally with a demarcation line if there is active disease expansion or pigment clumping, retinal arteriolar attenuation, and focal perivenous sheathing in later stages (**Figure 9**).

FAF shows a trizonal distribution (**Figure 9**) of normal autofluorescence outside the lesion (zone 1), speckled hyperautofluorescence in the rim of the expanding lesion (zone 2) which correspond to loss of photoreceptor outer segments and increased exposure of RPE lipofuscin and/or the result of accumulated lipofuscin in RPE cells due to metabolic overactivity as a response of photoreceptor outer segment turnover [54, 55], and a central area of hypoautofluorescence within the lesion (zone 3) that indicates RPE and choriocapillaris atrophy [56].

OCT also demonstrates a trizonal pattern corresponding to FAF characterized by normal retina outside the lesion (zone 1), subretinal hyperreflective deposits and loss or irregularity of EZ (zone 2) in the rim of the lesion, and EZ, RPE and choriocapillaris atrophy (zone 3) inside the lesion (**Figure 9**), although thinning can also extend to the inner retina [56].

OCT-A detects markedly reduced flow in choriocapillaris in areas of retinochoroidal atrophy [57]. Active lesions may present an increase in the deep flow density which may be the source of mediators of inflammation, in contrast to inactive phase where it is decreased, but further studies are needed [55]. En-face OCTA demonstrates hyperreflective dot structures at the level of ellipsoid zone that might represent degenerating photoreceptor segments (**Figure 9**) [58].

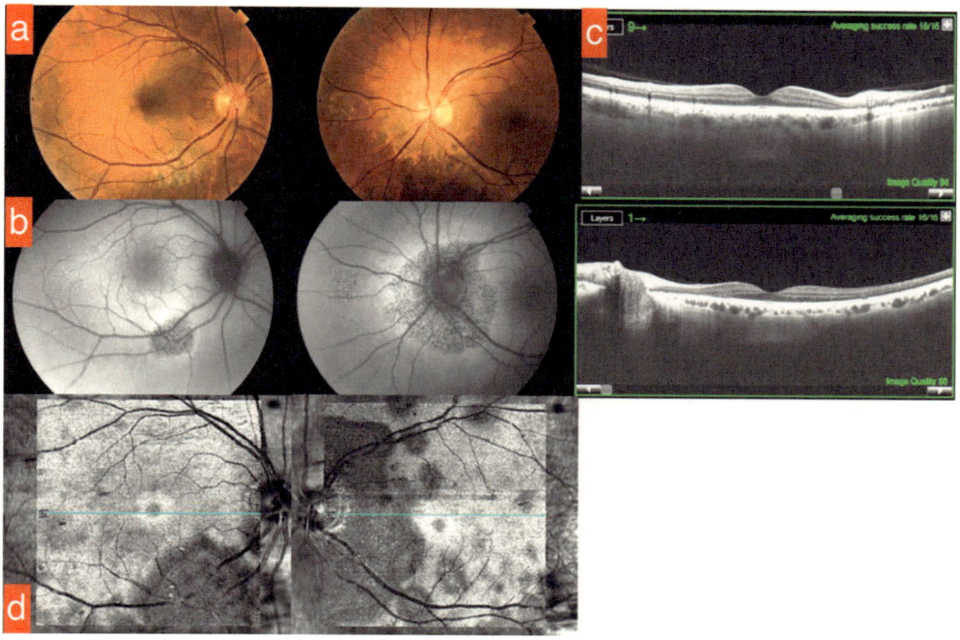

Figure 9.
This patient present a retinochoroidal atrophic lesion inferotemporal to the disk in right eye and two lesions in the left eye located in peripapillary area and another nasal to the optic disk. (a) Fundus autofluorescence (FAF) shows hypoautofluorescence inside the lesions and a rim with faint hyperautofluorescence. (b) Optical coherence tomography (OCT) shows outer retina/EZ atrophy and choroidal thinning, (c) and en-face optical coherence tomography angiography (OCT-A) at the level of EZ shows hyperreflective dots (more evident in the left eye) in a hyporreflective background. (d) EZ: Ellipsoid zone.

ICGA also shows a trizonal pattern of preserved fluorescence (zone 1) indicating choriocapillaris integrity, a late hyperfluorescence with minimal leakage in subacute areas demarcating the lesion (zone 2), and an inner area of hypofluorescence due to retinochoroidal atrophy [56].

FFA depicts faint late hyperfluorescence indicating loss of photopigment of outer segments, except in those areas with retinochoroidal atrophy that are early and late hyperfluorescent due to window effect. Retinal arteriolar narrowing in the areas of involvement may be seen. Retinal vessel staining and leakage may be present [24].

5. Conclusion

In summary, combining multiple imaging modalities, including OCT, FFA, ICGA, FAF, and OCT-A, may help us in classifying better this heterogenous group of diseases according to their pathophysiological process and therefore differentiate between one another, detect ocular complications, and monitor response to treatment.

Conflict of interest

The authors declare no conflict of interest.

Author details

Cristian de los Santos[1*], Lidia Cocho[1,2] and José María Herreras[1,2]

1 IOBA (Instituto de Oftalmobiologia Aplicada), University of Valladolid, Valladolid, Spain

2 Ophthalmology Department, Hospital Clinico Universitario de Valladolid, Valladolid, Spain

*Address all correspondence to: hes.oftalmologia.cs@gmail.com

References

[1] Neri P, Herbort CP, Hedayatfar A, et al. "White dot syndromes", an inappropriate and outdated misnomer. International Ophthalmology. 2022;**42**: 1-6. DOI: 10.1007/s10792-021-02121-4

[2] Papasavvas I, Tugal-Tutkun I, Herbort CP Jr. Mechanisms, pathophysiology and current immunomodulatory/immunosuppressive therapy of non-infectious and/or immune-mediated choroiditis. Pharmaceuticals. 2022;**15**:398. DOI: 10.3390/ph15040398

[3] Herbort CP Jr, Mantovani A, Tugal-Tutkun I, Papasavvas I. Classification of non-infectious and/or immune mediated choroiditis: A brief overview of the essentials. Diagnostics. 2021;**11**:939. DOI: 10.3390/diagnostics11060939

[4] Herbort CP Jr, Neri P, Papasavvas I. Clinicopathology of non-infectious choroiditis: Evolution of its appraisal during the last 2-3 decades from "white dot syndromes" to precise classification. Journal of Ophthalmic Inflammation and Infection. 2021;**11**:43. DOI: 10.1186/s12348-021-00274-y

[5] Gass JD. Vitiliginous chorioretinitis. Archives of Ophthalmology. 1981;**99**:1778-1787. DOI: 10.1001/archopht.1981.03930020652006

[6] Ryan SJ, Maumenee AE. Birdshot retinochoroidopathy. American Journal of Ophthalmology. 1980;**89**:31-45. DOI: 10.1016/0002-9394(80)90226-3

[7] Standardization of Uveitis Nomenclature (SUN) Working Group. Classification criteria for birdshot Chorioretinitis. American Journal of Ophthalmology. 2021;**228**:65-71. DOI: 10.1016/j.ajo.2021.03.059

[8] Koizumi H, Pozzoni MC, Spaide RF. Fundus autofluorescence in birdshot chorioretinopathy. Ophthalmology. 2008;**115**:e15-e20. DOI: 10.1016/j.ophtha.2008.01.025

[9] Testi I, Modugno RL, Pavesio C. Multimodal imaging supporting the pathophysiology of white dot syndromes. Journal of Ophthalmic Inflammation and Infection. 2021;**11**:32. DOI: 10.1186/s12348-021-00261-3

[10] Guex-Crosier Y, Herbort CP. Prolonged retinal arterio-venous circulation time by fluorescein but not by indocyanine green angiography in birdshot chorioretinopathy. Ocular Immunology and Inflammation. 1997;**5**:203-206. DOI: 10.3109/09273949709116895

[11] Vitale AT. Birdshot retinochoroidopathy. In: Foster CS, Vitale AT, editors. Diagnosis and Treatment of Uveitis. 2nd ed. New Delhi: Jaypee Brothers Medical Publishers (P) Ltd; 2013. pp. 982-1004. DOI: 10.5005/jp/books/11822_69

[12] Pavesio CE, Lehoang P. Birdshot chorioretinopathy. In: Zierhut M, Pavesio C, Ohno S, Oréfice F, Rao NA, editors. Intraocular Inflammation. Berlin: Springer; 2016. pp. 929-939. DOI: 10.1007/978-3-540-75387-2_83

[13] Baharani A, Errera MH, Jhingan M, Samanta A, Agarwal A, Singh SR, et al. Choroidal imaging in uveitis: An update. Survey of Ophthalmology. 2022;**67**:965-990. DOI: 10.1016/j.survophthal.2022.01.001

[14] Pepple KL, Chu Z, Weinstein J, Munk MR, Van Gelder RN, Wang RK. Use of En face swept-source optical coherence tomography angiography in identifying

choroidal flow voids in 3 patients with birdshot Chorioretinopathy. JAMA Ophthalmology. 2018;**136**:1288-1292. DOI: 10.1001/jamaophthalmol.2018.3474

[15] Phasukkijwatana N, Iafe N, Sarraf D. Optical coherence tomography angiography of A29 birdshot chorioretinopathy complicated by retinal neovascularization. Retinal Cases and Brief Reports. 2017;**11**:S68-S72. DOI: 10.1097/ICB.0000000000000418

[16] Pohlmann D, Macedo S, Stübiger N, Pleyer U, Joussen AM, Winterhalter S. Multimodal imaging in birdshot retinochoroiditis. Ocular Immunology and Inflammation 2017;**25**:621-632. DOI: 10.1080/09273948.2017.1375532

[17] de Carlo TE, Bonini Filho MA, Adhi M, Duker JS. Retinal and choroidal vasculature in birdshot chorioretinopathy analyzed using spectral domain optical coherence tomography angiography. Retina. 2015;**35**:2392-2399. DOI: 10.1097/IAE.0000000000000744

[18] Roberts PK, Nesper PL, Goldstein DA, Fawzi AA. Retinal capillary density in patients with birdshot chorioretinopathy. Retina. 2018;**38**:387-394. DOI: 10.1097/IAE.0000000000001543

[19] Pichi F, Sarraf D, Arepalli S, Lowder CY, Cunningham ET Jr, Neri P, et al. The application of optical coherence tomography angiography in uveitis and inflammatory eye diseases. Progress in Retinal and Eye Research. 2017;**59**:178-201. DOI: 10.1016/j.preteyeres.2017.04.005

[20] Palestine AG. White dot syndromes. In: Whitcup SM, Sen NH, editors. Uveitis. Fundamental and Clinical Practice. 5th ed. India: Elsevier; 2022. pp. 378-394. DOI: 10.1016/B978-0-323-48014-7.00030-0

[21] Gass JD. Acute posterior multifocal placoid pigment epitheliopathy. Archives of Ophthalmology. 1968;**80**:177-185. DOI: 10.1001/archopht.1968.00980050179005

[22] Deutman AF, Oosterhuis JA, Boen-Tan TN. Aan de Kerk AL. Acute posterior multifocal placoid pigment epitheliopathy. Pigment epitheliopathy of choriocapillaritis? The British Journal of Ophthalmology. 1972 Dec;**56**:863-874. DOI: 10.1136/bjo.56.12.863

[23] Standardization of Uveitis Nomenclature (SUN) Working Group. Classification criteria for acute posterior multifocal Placoid pigment Epitheliopathy. American Journal of Ophthalmology. 2021;**228**:174-181. DOI: 10.1016/j.ajo.2021.03.056

[24] Mirza RG, Jampol LM. White spot syndromes and related diseases. In: Schachat AP, editor. Ryan's Retina. 6th ed. Vol. 2. China: Elsevier; 2018. pp. 4559-4702

[25] Khanamiri HN, Rao NA. Multifocal choroiditis/serpiginous choroiditis and related entities. In: Rao NA, Schallhorn J, Rodger DC, editors. Posterior Uveitis, Essentials in Ophthalmology. Cham: Springer; 2019. pp. 57-75. DOI: 10.1007/978-3-030-03140-4_4

[26] Papasavvas I, Herbort CP Jr. Diagnosis and treatment of primary inflammatory Choriocapillaropathies (PICCPs): A comprehensive overview. Medicina. 2022;**58**:165. DOI: 10.3390/medicina58020165

[27] Raven ML, Ringeisen AL, Yonekawa Y, Stem MS, Faia LJ, Gottlieb JL. Multi-modal imaging and anatomic classification of the white dot syndromes. International Journal of Retina and Vitreous. 2017;**3**:12. DOI: 10.1186/s40942-017-0069-8

[28] Standardization of Uveitis Nomenclature (SUN) Working Group. Classification criteria for serpiginous choroiditis. American Journal of Ophthalmology. 2021;**228**:126-133. DOI: 10.1016/j.ajo.2021.03.038

[29] Rodriguez-Garcia A. Serpiginous choroiditis. In: Foster CS, Vitale AT, editors. Diagnosis and Treatment of Uveitis. 2nd ed. New Delhi: Jaypee Brothers Medical Publishers (P) Ltd; 2013. pp. 1077-1089. DOI: 10.5005/jp/books/11822_69

[30] Dutta Majumder P, Biswas J, Gupta A. Enigma of serpiginous choroiditis. Indian Journal of Ophthalmology. 2019;**67**:325-333. DOI: 10.4103/ijo.IJO_822_18

[31] Thomas AS. Noninfectious intermediate, posterior, and panuveitis. In: Lin P, editor. Uveitis, Current Practices in Ophthalmology. Singapore: Springer; 2020. pp. 43-99. DOI: 10.1007/978-981-15-0331-3_3

[32] Klufas MA, Phasukkijwatana N, Iafe NA, Prasad PS, Agarwal A, Gupta V, et al. Optical coherence tomography angiography reveals Choriocapillaris flow reduction in Placoid Chorioretinitis. Ophthalmology Retina. 2017;**1**:77-91. DOI: 10.1016/j.oret.2016.08.008

[33] Tavallali A, Yannuzzi LA. Idiopathic multifocal choroiditis. J. Ophthalmic Vis. Res. 2016;**11**:429-432. DOI: 10.4103/2008-322X.194141

[34] Krill AE, Chishti MI, Klien BA, Newell FW, Potts AM. Multifocal inner choroiditis. American Academy of Ophthalmology and Otolaryngology. 1969;**73**:222-245

[35] Essex RW, Wong J, Jampol LM, Dowler J, Bird AC. Idiopathic multifocal choroiditis: A comment on present and past nomenclature. Retina. 2013;**33**:1-4. DOI: 10.1097/IAE.0b013e3182641860

[36] Choi EY, Kim M. Multifocal choroiditis and panuveitis. In: Yu HG, editor. Inflammatory and Infectious Ocular Disorders, Retina Atlas. Singapore: Springer; 2020. pp. 29-37. DOI: 10.1007/978-981-13-8546-9_4

[37] Standardization of Uveitis Nomenclature (SUN) Working Group. Classification criteria for punctate inner choroiditis. American Journal of Ophthalmology. 2021;**228**:275-280. DOI: 10.1016/j.ajo.2021.03.046

[38] Ahnood D, Madhusudhan S, Tsaloumas MD, Waheed NK, Keane PA, Denniston AK. Punctate inner choroidopathy: A review. Survey of Ophthalmology. 2017;**62**:113-126. DOI: 10.1016/j.survophthal.2016.10.003

[39] Dolz-Marco R, Fine HF, Freund KB. How to differentiate myopic choroidal neovascularization, idiopathic multifocal choroiditis, and punctate inner Choroidopathy using clinical and multimodal imaging findings. Ophthalmic Surgery, Lasers & Imaging Retina. 2017;**48**:196-201. DOI: 10.3928/23258160-20170301-01

[40] Papasavvas I, Neri P, Mantovani A, Herbort CP Jr. Idiopathic multifocal choroiditis (MFC): Aggressive and prolonged therapy with multiple immunosuppressive agents is needed to halt the progression of active disease. An offbeat review and a case series. Journal of Ophthalmic Inflammation and Infection. 2022;**12**:2. DOI: 10.1186/s12348-021-00278-8

[41] Mebsout-Pallado C, Orès R, Terrada C, Dansingani KK, Chhablani J, Eller AW, et al. Review of the current literature and our experience on the value of OCT-angiography in white dot syndromes. Ocular Immunology and Inflammation. 2022;**30**(2):364-378. DOI: 10.1080/09273948.2020.1837185

[42] Jampol LM, Sieving PA, Pugh D, Fishman GA, Gilbert H. Multiple evanescent white dot syndrome. I. Clinical findings. Archives of Ophthalmology. 1984;**102**:671-674. DOI: 10.1001/archopht.1984.01040030527008

[43] Papasavvas I, Mantovani A, Tugal-Tutkun I, Herbort CP Jr. Multiple evanescent white dot syndrome (MEWDS): Update on practical appraisal, diagnosis and clinicopathology; a review and an alternative comprehensive perspective. Journal of Ophthalmic Inflammation and Infection. 2021;**11**:45. DOI: 10.1186/s12348-021-00279-7

[44] Standardization of Uveitis Nomenclature (SUN) Working Group. Classification criteria for multiple evanescent white dot syndrome. American Journal of Ophthalmology. 2021;**228**:198-204. DOI: 10.1016/j.ajo.2021.03.050

[45] Mantovani A, Invernizzi A, Staurenghi G, Herbort CP Jr. Multiple evanescent white dot syndrome: A multimodal imaging study of foveal granularity. Ocular Immunology and Inflammation. 2019;**27**:141-147. DOI: 10.1080/09273948.2017.1353104

[46] Pichi F, Srvivastava SK, Chexal S, Lembo A, Lima LH, Neri P, et al. En face optical coherence tomography and optical coherence tomography angiography of multiple evanescent white dot syndrome: New insights into pathogenesis. Retina. 2016;**36**(Suppl 1):S178-S188. DOI: 10.1097/IAE.0000000000001255

[47] Wang JC, Laíns I, Sobrin L, Miller JB. Distinguishing white dot syndromes with patterns of choroidal Hypoperfusion on optical coherence tomography angiography. Ophthalmic Surgery, Lasers & Imaging Retina. 2017;**48**(8):638-646. DOI: 10.3928/23258160-20170802-06

[48] Khochtali S, Dridi T, Abroug N, Ksiaa I, Lupidi M, Khairallah M. Swept-source optical coherence tomography angiography shows Choriocapillaris flow reduction in multiple evanescent white dot syndrome. Journal of Current Ophthalmology. 2020;**32**(2):211-215. DOI: 10.4103/JOCO.JOCO_107_20

[49] Lages V, Mantovani A, Papadia M, Herbort CP. MEWDS is a true primary choriocapillaritis and basic mechanisms do not seem to differ from other choriocapillaritis entities. Journal of Current Ophthalmology. 2018;**30**(4):281-286. DOI: 10.1016/j.joco.2018.09.009

[50] Lee JE. Multiple evanescent white dot syndrome. In: Yu HG, editor. Inflammatory and Infectious Ocular Disorders, Retina Atlas. Singapore: Springer; 2020. pp. 39-44. DOI: 10.1007/978-981-13-8546-9_5

[51] Herbort CP Jr. Multiple evanescent white dot syndrome (MEWDS). In: Zierhut M, Pavesio C, Ohno S, Oréfice F, Rao NA, editors. Intraocular Inflammation. Berlin: Springer; 2016. pp. 997-1005. DOI: 10.1007/978-3-540-75387-2_91

[52] Gass JD. Acute zonal occult outer retinopathy. Donders lecture: The Netherlands ophthalmological society, Maastricht, Holland, June 19, 1992. Journal of Clinical Neuro-Ophthalmology. 1993;**13**:79-97

[53] Gass JD, Agarwal A, Scott IU. Acute zonal occult outer retinopathy: A long-term follow-up study. American Journal of Ophthalmology. 2002;**134**:329-339. DOI: 10.1016/s0002-9394(02)01640-9

[54] Herbort CP Jr, Arapi I, Papasavvas I, Mantovani A, Jeannin B. Acute zonal

occult outer retinopathy (AZOOR) results from a Clinicopathological mechanism different from Choriocapillaritis diseases: A multimodal imaging analysis. Diagnostics. 2021;**11**:1184. DOI: 10.3390/diagnostics11071184

[55] Pichi F, Sarraf D, Morara M, et al. Pearls and pitfalls of optical coherence tomography angiography in the multimodal evaluation of uveitis. Journal of Ophthalmic Inflammation and Infection. 2017;7:20. DOI: 10.1186/s12348-017-0138-z

[56] Mrejen S, Khan S, Gallego-Pinazo R, Jampol LM, Yannuzzi LA. Acute zonal occult outer retinopathy: A classification based on multimodal imaging. JAMA Ophthalmology. 2014;**132**(9):1089-1098. DOI: 10.1001/jamaophthalmol.2014.1683

[57] Roberts PK, Jampol L, Fawzi AA. White dot syndromes. In: Huang D, Lumbroso B, Jia Y, et al., editors. Optical Coherence Tomography Angiography of the Eye. Thorofare (NJ): Slack Inc; 2017. pp. 229-234

[58] Naik AU, Ezhilvathani N, Biswas J. Acute zonal occult outer retinopathy: Is optical coherence tomography angiography useful? Indian Journal of Ophthalmology. 2018;**66**(11):1637-1639. DOI: 10.4103/ijo.IJO_966_18

Chapter 8

Immunotherapy-Associated Uveitis

Erick Rivera-Grana and Stephanie M. Llop

Abstract

Novel immunotherapies used to treat some cancers, such as checkpoint inhibitors and target therapies of B-RAF protooncogene and mitogen-activated protein kinase (BRAF/MEK), have been strongly associated with adverse events related to immune dysregulation. These effects are known as immune-related adverse events (irAEs). Uveitis is among the known irAEs, and it occurs in approximately 1% of patients using these therapies. The uveitis observed in these patients ranges from anterior, intermediate, to panuveitis. If irAEs are severe, current recommendations are to stop immunotherapy treatment and simultaneously treat the uveitis with steroids (local or systemic). These oncologic immunotherapies have proved to show positive results in cancer treatment. Their use has increased with time, showing ocular side effects that were not reported previously. It is important that ophthalmologists and non-ophthalmologists are aware of these agents and their potential ocular side effects for timely diagnosis and adequate management. This chapter will review different immunotherapies and their potential ocular manifestations and how to diagnose, monitor, and manage these patients.

Keywords: immune-therapy, uveitis, immune checkpoint inhibitors, BRAF-/MEK-inhibitor, immune-related adverse events

1. Introduction

Our immune system not only works to fight infections and produce inflammation but also has the ability to adequately recognize self-antigens to prevent autoimmunity. As part of our adaptive immune system, T-cells have a selection process in the thymus in which cells that react too strongly to self-peptides are eliminated to prevent autoreactivity in a process called central tolerance [1]. Only cells with some response to MHC complexes and self-peptides are released into the bloodstream. To prevent autoimmunity, numerous immune checkpoint pathways regulate the activation of T cells at multiple steps during an immune response, in a process called peripheral tolerance [1–3]. In this process, some of the immune checkpoints involved are cytotoxic T-lymphocyte-associated antigen 4 (CTLA-4) and programmed cell death protein 1 (PD-1), which work at different stages of the immune response. Medications aimed at both of these checkpoint inhibitors work by enhancing endogenous antitumor activity. BRAF/MEK inhibitors are another group of immunotherapies used as an anticancer treatment, which works by interfering with B-RAF oncogene mutations, slowing down tumor growth. Checkpoint inhibitors and BRAF/MEK inhibitor medications work very well as anticancer medications but are not without side effects.

IntechOpen

Side effects caused by these immunotherapies are known as immune-related adverse events (irAEs). An extensive list of organs can be affected in the myriad of these irAEs. Although with checkpoint inhibitors, only approximately 1% involve the eye [4]. For BRAF/MEK therapies, 25–100% of the patient can have ocular side effects [5]. With the ongoing use of these medications, it is essential to recognize these adverse effects early for adequate management and to prevent further complications. Uveitis associated with immunotherapy can present in multiple anatomic locations and with varying degrees of inflammation. The most accepted form of treatment is the use of topical and or systemic corticosteroids. If the inflammation is severe, enough consideration can be taken to discontinue the anticancer medication. This chapter will review the most common medications associated with immunotherapy-associated uveitis and how to diagnose, monitor, and manage these patients.

2. Immune checkpoint inhibitors (ICIs)

T-cell-mediated immunity has multiple steps for selecting specific antigens, trafficking them to different sites, and executing their functions. These steps are regulated by counterbalancing stimulatory and inhibitory signals to maintain balance. Under normal physiologic conditions, the immune system has a series of modulating responses to control the duration and amplitude of response to minimize organ damage. These modulations are regulated by special stop signals called immune checkpoints. On tumor cells, there is an overexpression of inhibitory ligands and receptors. With this overexpression, cancer cells can evade T-cell detection of the host immune system.

The soluble and membrane-bound receptor–ligand immune checkpoints are the most targeted for cancer therapy. Antibodies that block immune checkpoints do not target tumor cells directly. Instead, they target lymphocyte receptors or their ligands in order to enhance endogenous antitumor activity [6]. The two immune checkpoints that have been most actively studied in the context of clinical cancer immunotherapy are cytotoxic T-lymphocyte-associated antigen 4 (CTLA-4, also known as CD152) and programmed cell death protein 1 (PD1, also known as CD279) [6]. Checkpoint inhibitors work by blocking the interaction of tumor cells with these ligands leading to increased antitumor response. Inhibition of the immune checkpoint pathways has led to the United States Food and Drug Administration's (FDA) approval of seven drugs in the United States [7]. **Table 1** shows a list of all seven drugs. There are key similarities and differences in these pathways.

2.1 Cytotoxic T-lymphocyte-associated antigen 4 (CTLA-4) inhibitors

CTLA-4 was the first immune checkpoint receptor to be clinically targeted [6]. It is exclusively expressed on T-cells, where it primarily downregulates cellular activation [6, 8, 9]. CTLA-4 is a membrane-bound receptor expressed in the plasma membrane of activated T-cells. During an active immune state, antigen-presenting cells (APCs) bind to CTLA-4 to attenuate T-cell activity, diminishing host organ damage.

2.1.1 Ipilimumab

Currently, only one FDA-approved ICI targets CTLA-4. The generic name is Ipilimumab and the trade name is Yervoy (Bristol-Meyers Squib). It is an intravenous

Name	Target checkpoint
Ipilimumab (Yervoy)	CTLA-4-blocking antibody
Nivolumab (Opdivo)	PD-1-blocking antibody
Pembrolizumab (Keytruda)	PD-1-blocking antibody
Cemiplimab (Libtayo)	PD-1-blocking antibody
Avelumab (Bavencio)	PD-L1-blocking antibody
Durvalumab (Imfinzi)	PD-L1-blocking antibody
Atezolizumab (Tecentriq)	PD-L1-blocking antibody

Table 1.
FDA-approved immune checkpoint inhibitors.

infusion currently approved to treat metastatic or unresectable melanoma and melanoma recurrence. It is also approved for renal cell carcinoma, non-small cell lung cancer, malignant pleural mesothelioma, and esophageal cancer, but only if used as a combination therapy with nivolumab, PD-1 receptor antibody. In a study by Dow ER et al., they found that in patients with immunotherapy-associated uveitis, 96% of all cases with Ipilimumab were associated with metastatic melanoma [10]. This could be due to the restrictive indications the FDA has approved this medication use as monotherapy.

2.2 Programmed cell death protein 1 (PD-1) and programmed cell death ligand 1 (PD-L1) inhibitor

PD-1 is also an immune receptor involved in downregulating T-cell response. PD-1 regulates T-cell activation by binding to two ligands (PD-L1 and PD-L2). Cancer tumor cells can block antitumor host responses by upregulating PD-1 ligands. PD-1 has similar effects on T-cells as CTLA-4 but differs in its timing of downregulation and the anatomic location of immune inhibition [3]. PD-1 is more expressed on activated T-cells, B-cells, and myeloid cells compared to CTLA-4 [2, 3, 11]. While CTLA-4 functions during the priming phase of T-cell activation, PD-1 functions during the effector phase, predominantly within peripheral tissues [3, 6]. Chronic antigen exposure, as it occurs in cancer, can lead to an excess PD-1 expression on T-cells, leading to a state of "exhaustion" that can be partially reversible by PD-1 pathway blockade [6]. By inhibiting PD-1 pathway with either antibody to the receptor or its ligands, we can increase antitumor activity. There are currently three PD-1 inhibitor medications approved by the FDA (Nivolumab, Pembrolizumab, and Cemiplimab) and three anti-PD-L1 (Avelumab, Durvalumab, and Atezolizumab).

2.2.1 Nivolumab

Trade name Opdivo (Bristol-Meyers Squib) is a PD-1-blocking antibody. It is administered via intravenous infusion, currently approved for metastatic melanoma, non-small-cell lung cancer, metastatic small-cell lung cancer, metastatic squamous cell carcinoma of the head and neck, urothelial cancer, hepatocellular carcinoma, Hodgkin lymphoma, and metastatic colorectal cancer. Nivolumab has numerous approved indications to be used in combination with other therapies, including anti-CTLA-4

Ipilimumab. Nivolumab + Ipilimumab combination is approved for metastatic melanoma and renal cell carcinoma.

2.2.2 Pembrolizumab

Trade name Keytruda (Merck) is a PD-1-blocking antibody. It is administered via intravenous infusion, currently approved for melanoma, non-small cell lung cancer, head and neck squamous cell cancer, classical Hodgkin lymphoma, primary mediastinal B-cell lymphoma, urothelial carcinoma, metastatic colon and rectal cancer, unresectable or metastatic solid tumors with high microsatellite instability, PD-L1 positive cervical cancer, hepatocellular carcinoma, Merkel cell carcinoma, renal cell carcinoma, and advanced endometrial carcinoma. Pembrolizumab is the only approved ICI to demonstrate objective tumor regression [12].

2.2.3 Cemiplimab

Trade name Libtayo (Regeneron/Sanofi Genzyme) is a PD-1-blocking antibody. It is administered via intravenous infusion, currently approved for metastatic or advanced cutaneous squamous cell carcinoma and non-small cell lung cancer.

2.2.4 Avelumab

Trade name Bavencio (EMD Serono & Pfizer) is a PD-L1-blocking antibody. It is administered via intravenous infusion and is currently approved for urothelial and renal cell carcinoma.

2.2.5 Durvalumab

Trade name Imfinzi (AstraZeneca) is a PD-L1-blocking antibody. It is administered via intravenous infusion and approved for the treatment of unresectable stage III non-small cell lung cancer, extensive-stage small cell lung cancer and for bile duct and gallbladder cancer.

2.2.6 Atezolizumab

Trade name Tecentriq (Genentech) is a PD-L1-blocking antibody. It is administered via intravenous infusion. It is approved for the treatment of non-small cell lung cancer, small cell lung cancer, hepatocellular carcinoma, and melanoma.

3. Immune-related adverse events (irAEs)

With the increasing use of ICIs as novel therapies for cancer treatment, it is expected to observe more side effects and adverse events secondary to these medications. The use of ICIs is rising exponentially, with approximately 40% of patients with cancer in the United States in 2019 eligible for treatment [13]. ICIs are not the only medication class to cause adverse effects, as other types of immunotherapies can cause this. With more immunotherapies currently being investigated, the number of available treatments could exponentially increase over time. Despite the observed clinical advantages these medications demonstrate, they produce a myriad of side effects that can involve several body systems. These side effects are called irAEs. The incidence and onset of irAEs vary depending on the class and dose of ICIs, the type of cancer, and factors related to patients [13]. More than two-thirds of reported cases of cancer immunotherapy-related irAEs are related to ICIs, and three drugs (Ipilimumab, Nivolumab, and Pembrolizumab) are responsible for almost 60% of reported cases [14]. It is believed that CTLA-4 might be more closely related to causing irAEs since its mechanism of action is less specific compared to PD-1/PD-L1 medications [10]. The onset of irAEs has been described as occurring as early as within a few days of ICI initiation and ≥ 1 year after completion of therapy. The median onset is within 2–16 weeks from the commencement of therapy [14–16]. Patients treated with combined therapy, anti-PD-1/PD-L1 + anti-CTLA-4 have an increased incidence, severity, and earlier onset of irAEs [13, 14].

The exact mechanism as to why irAEs occur due to ICIs is not entirely understood. It is important to note that there are differences in the clinical presentation and frequency of specific irAEs and the organs most commonly involved [17]. The most frequent irAEs include gastrointestinal, endocrine, and dermatological [18]. **Table 2** shows a full list of all reported irAEs. Uveitis only accounts for approximately 1% of

Cardiac	o Autoimmune hepatitis	o Panuveitis
• Myocarditis[a]	o Eosinophilic hepatitis	o Posterior uveitis
o Autoimmune myocarditis	• Lymphocytic gastritis	• Vogt–Koyanagi–Harada syndrome
o Myocardial fibrosis	• Pancreatitis	**Pulmonary**
• Pericarditis	**Hematological**	• Interstitial lung disease[a]
o Autoimmune pericarditis	• Aplastic anemia/pure red cell aplasia	o Alveolitis
o Pericardial effusion	• Autoimmune hemolytic anemia	o Organizing pneumonitis
o Pericardial tamponade	• Autoimmune neutropenia	o Pneumonitis
Dermatological	• Hemophagocytic lymphohistiocytosis	o Pulmonary fibrosis
• Alopecia areata/universalis	• Immune thrombocytopenic purpura	o Pulmonary hemorrhage
• Dermatitis herpetiformis	**Muscular**	**Renal**
• Erythema multiforme	• Myalgias[a]	• Acute tubulointerstitial nephritis/renal tubular acidosis
• Granuloma annulare	• Myositis[a]	• Glomerulonephritis
• Lichen planopilaris/planus/lichenoid dermatitis	o Anti-synthetase syndrome	**Skeletal**
• Panniculitis/erythema nodosum	o Bulbar myopathy	• Arthralgia[a]/polyarthralgia
• Pemphigoid/pemphigus	o Dermatomyositis	• Arthritis[a]
• Psoriasis	o Diaphragmatic lymphocytic polymyositis	o Monoarthritis
• Pyoderma gangrenosum	o Necrotizing myopathy	o Oligoarthritis
• Sweet syndrome	o Orbital myositis	o Polyarthritis
• Vitiligo[a]	**Neurological**	• Enthesitis

Endocrine	• Aseptic meningitis	• Fasciitis/eosinophilic fasciitis
• Adrenitis[a]	• Encephalitis	• Jaccoud arthropathy
o Adrenal insufficiency	• Cranial nerve involvement	• Polymyalgia rheumatica
o Cortisol deficiency	o Bilateral hearing loss	• Psoriatic arthritis
o Hypercortisolism	o Facial palsy	• Rheumatoid arthritis
o Hypoadrenalism	o Oculomotor paresis	• Spondyloarthropathy
o Isolated adrenocorticotropic hormone deficiency	• Motor neuropathy	• Tenosynovitis
• Autoimmune diabetes mellitus	o Acute generalized motor neuropathy	**Systemic**
• Hyperparathyroidism	o Multifocal motor block neuropathy	• Antiphospholipid syndrome
• Hypogonadism	• Myasthenia gravis	• Lupus
• Hypophysitis[a]	• Neuromyelitis optica spectrum disorders	o Lupus nephropathy
o Autoimmune hypophysitis	o Optic neuritis	o Subacute cutaneous lupus erythematosus
o Hypopituitarism	o Transverse myelitis	o Systemic lupus erythematosus
o Pan-hypopituitarism	• Polyneuropathies[a]	• Sarcoidosis
• Thyroiditis[a]	o Axonal sensory-motor polyneuropathy	o Cutaneous sarcoidosis
o Autoimmune thyroiditis	o Multiplex mononeuritis	o Pulmonary sarcoidosis
o Hyperthyroidism	o Peripheral sensory neuropathy	o Renal sarcoidosis
o Hypothyroidism	• Polyradiculopathies	• Sicca syndrome[a]/Sjögren syndrome
o Graves' disease	o Chronic inflammatory demyelinating polyneuropathy	• Systemic sclerosis
o Thyrotoxicosis	o Guillain–Barré syndrome	• Vasculitis[a]
Gastrointestinal	**Ocular**	o Cerebral vasculitis
• Enterocolitis[a]	• Conjunctivitis	o Cryoglobulinaemia
o Ileitis	• Episcleritis/scleritis	o Cutaneous vasculitis
o Ileocolitis	• Orbital inflammation	o Eosinophilic granulomatosis with polyangiitis
o Ischemic colitis	• Uveitis[a]	o Giant cell arteritis
o Microscopic colitis	o Anterior uveitis	o Pulmonary vasculitis
o Ulcerative colitis	o Chorioretinopathy	o Henoch–Schönlein purpura
• Hepatitis[a]	o Iridocyclitis/iritis	[a]More than 100 cases reported.

Obtained from Ramos-Casals M, Brahmer JR, Callahan MK, et al. Immune-related adverse events of checkpoint inhibitors. Nat Rev. Dis Prim. 2020;6 (1). doi:10.1038/s41572-020-0160-6.

Table 2.
Organ-based reported irAEs.

patients with irAEs. However, it is of utmost importance to be aware of it since delay in diagnosis and treatment could lead to detrimental irreversible visual consequences.

Treatment depends on the organ system affected and the grade of toxicity according to the Common Terminology Criteria for Adverse Events (CTCAE) classification. Specific treatments for irAEs beyond uveitis are out of the scope of this chapter. However, some of the treatments used are glucocorticoids, hormone replacement, immunosuppressive agents, IV immunoglobulin, plasma exchange, and monoclonal antibodies.

4. Target therapies of proto-oncogene B-RAF and mitogen-activated protein kinase BRAF/MEK

ICIs are not the only immunomodulatory medication associated with uveitis. Approximately 25–100% of patients treated with BRAF/MEK inhibitors develop ocular adverse effects [5]. These medications are primarily used in the treatment of melanoma. Nearly 50% of the patients with advanced melanoma have BRAF (V600E) mutations [19]. The MEK gene is closely connected to the BRAF gene, so drugs that target MEK also help with BRAF mutation melanomas. BRAF inhibitor drugs as monotherapy have shown high rapid response rates not previously seen in melanoma patients. However, the duration of responses is limited in most patients. The same occurs in MEK monotherapy. The combination of BRAF/MEK inhibitors has shown significant improvement in response rates [19]. BRAF inhibitors include vemurafenib (Zelboraf), dabrafenib (Tafinlar), and encorafenib (Braftovi). MEK inhibitors approved are trametinib (Mekinist), cobimetinib (Cotellic), and binimetinib (Mektovi).

A cohort study by F. Dimitriou et al., published in 2021, investigated if the occurrence of uveitis under treatment with BRAF/MEK and ICI is more frequent than in a general population of patients without treatment for cutaneous melanoma and found that patients treated with BRAF/MEK inhibitors had a two-fold higher hazard of developing uveitis. Clinical findings were similar in patients treated with ICI and BRAF/MEK inhibitors. They do not specify treatments but state that the course was complicated in four of eleven patients requiring systemic steroids. No patients had to discontinue their cancer treatment due to the uveitis. There are minimal reports of BRAF/MEK clinical trials, which could account for an underreporting of rare adverse events, such as uveitis [5]. But as we gather more data, more information can be gathered, and more accurate treatment and diagnostic recommendations can be made.

5. Immunotherapy-associated uveitis

The medical term for intraocular inflammation is uveitis. Uveitis is an inflammation involving uveal tissue, consisting of its three main components: iris, ciliary body, and choroid. The etiology can be of infectious or non-infectious inflammatory origin. This difference is essential to establish when diagnosing patients with intraocular inflammation since the treatments will differ vastly. Immunotherapy-associated uveitis is the term given to patients who develop intraocular inflammation while taking immune-modulating medications. The novel immunotherapies being used to treat cancer have been linked to causing uveitis. The overall reported incidence is 1%, although patients with a combination of ICIs might have a higher incidence [4, 10, 13]. The median onset is 5–9 weeks, depending on various reports [10, 13]. But it can range from 1 to 72 weeks [13]. There is a difference in the onset and severity of uveitis depending on the type of ICI used. Some reports have stated an incident of uveitis in 64% of patients taking the anti-CTLA-4 Ipilimumab [20]. It is important to note that most PD-1 and PD-L1 medications have been approved by the FDA for less time and have fewer indications than Ipilimumab, which could also be a reason for the decreased reported incidence.

A comprehensive literature review of 126 cases of immune checkpoint-associated uveitis in 2020 by E.R Dow et al. showed that 93.5% of patients had bilateral inflammation. The most common anatomic location was anterior with 37.7%, followed by panuveitis at 34.0%, posterior at 25.7%, and intermediate at 0.01% [10]. They also noted that five of their eight unilateral cases were from single case series, suggesting a possible disconnect between the descriptions and interpretations of laterality. Comparing the ICIs, Ipilimumab had the highest anterior uveitis percentage, while atezolizumab had the highest percentage of posterior uveitis. Interestingly the posterior findings of atezolizumab resembled deep capillary ischemic pathologies such as acute macular neuroretinopathy and paracentral acute middle maculopathy with retinal vasculitis or venulitis, while 0% of anterior uveitis. Another common posterior uveitis finding was a Vogt–Koyanagi–Harada (VKH)-like syndrome. This VKH-like presentation gives us more insight into the pathophysiology associated with immune-associated uveitis, which may represent a spectrum of autoimmune diseases within the eye due to a loss of tolerance in an immune-privileged organ and the subsequent development of T-cell- driven inflammation [8].

Presenting symptoms may include blurred vision, change in color vision, photophobia, visual distortion, scotomas, visual field changes, double vision, tenderness, pain with eye movement, eyelid swelling, proptosis, redness, and dryness [13]. Symptoms may not always correlate with the severity of inflammation. Unfortunately, no standardized controlled trials are available, and there is no information regarding whether the onset is acute or insidious in these immunotherapy-associated uveitis cases. Below we will discuss grading systems used as well as monitor and treatment recommendations.

5.1 Grading

Uveitis grading is based on the terminology proposed by the Standardization of Uveitis Nomenclature for disease classification criteria (SUN Criteria) [21]. It assigns a name based on the predominant anatomical location of active intraocular inflammation. The SUN criteria subdivide the eye into anatomic compartments; anterior, which refers to inflammation in the anterior chamber, intermediate = inflammation located in the vitreous cavity, anterior/intermediate = inflammation equally located in the anterior chamber and vitreous cavity, and posterior = inflammation located in the retina and/or choroid. Panuveitis is termed when all compartments of the eye are equally inflamed. As part of the SUN Criteria classification, they also established a grading system to quantify intraocular inflammation. This consists of grades 0.5+ to 4 + cells. Refer to **Table 3** for grading classification.

The CTCAE is used to grade ocular, and other irAEs secondary to immunotherapies used to treat cancer. The most recent version grades uveitis as follows: grade 1 refers to anterior uveitis with trace cells (0.5+), grade 2 refers to anterior uveitis with 1 to 2+ cells, grade 3 to anterior uveitis with 3+ or greater cells or intermediate/posterior/panuveitis, and grade 4 to 20/200 vision or worse in the affected eye [22]. Though a helpful guideline, the CTCAE has limitations since it does not consider

0	<1
1+	1–5
2+	6–15
3+	16–25
4+	26–50
5+	>50

Table 3.
SUN criteria grading for anterior chamber cells.

prior/baseline ophthalmological conditions that could affect visual acuity. The CTCAE cannot be accurately applied to patients with decreased baseline visual acuity.

5.2 Treatment options

Immunotherapy-associated uveitis is a phenomenon that has been rising with the increased use of ICIs. Currently, no randomized controlled trials are available to provide specific treatment algorithm recommendations since most cases have been reported through case reports and small case series. The most common treatment for immunotherapy-associated uveitis is topical corticosteroids. The main goal is to keep patients on glucocorticoids for as little time as possible and maintain them on their possible life-saving anticancer medication without interruption. General recommendations are to slowly taper the corticosteroids over 4–6 weeks after clinical improvement is confirmed.

In recognition of an increasing need for guidance, The American Society of Clinical Oncology (ASCO) and the National Comprehensive Cancer Network (NCCN) partnered to develop guidelines on the management of irAEs, which are resumed in **Table 4** [13, 23, 24]. These guidelines agree in general with the treatment recommendations. For grade 1, both guidelines agree to continue ICI treatment and only use topical corticosteroids. Grade 2 can be treated with topical and/or systemic corticosteroids, but patients can resume ICI therapy once inflammation improves to grade ≤ 1. Grades 3–4 ICI therapy should be permanently discontinued, and treatment should be with high-dose systemic steroids. The decision of suspending or discontinuing ICI is a very complex one. There should be good and clear communication between ophthalmologists and oncology specialists for better assessment and decision-making since there are potentially devastating consequences of stopping potentially life-saving treatments.

When and how to reinstate ICI therapy after a uveitis episode is not standardized due to the low amount of data. The NCCN provides the following recommendations: for grade 2, if ICI were stopped, may consider resumption of immunotherapy in consultation with ophthalmologists if inflammation improves to grade ≤ 1. Permanent discontinuation of immunotherapy is warranted in the setting of severe intraocular inflammation (grade 3–4) and episcleritis symptomatic episcleritis with visual acuity worse than 20/40 [24, 25].

5.3 Monitoring

Patients on ICI should undergo prompt ophthalmic evaluation if they develop worsening vision, floaters, or conjunctival injection [8]. Patients with any ocular

Grade	Definition CTCAE	ASCO	SITC
1	Anterior uveitis with trace cells	o Continue ICI o Refer to ophthalmology within 1 week o Artificial tears	• Continue ICI • Refer to ophthalmology within 1 week • Artificial tears
2	Anterior uveitis with 1+ or 2+ cells	o Hold ICI temporarily until after ophthalmology consult. o Topical (e.g., 1% prednisolone) and systemic steroids o Resume ICI treatment once off systemic corticosteroids or once corticosteroids for other concurrent systemic irAEs are reduced to 10 mg; continued topical corticosteroids are permitted when resuming therapy to manage and minimize local toxicity.	o Hold ICI o Ophthalmology referral within 2 days, prior to initiating uveitis treatment o Topical corticosteroids, and/ or systemic corticosteroids
3	Anterior uveitis with 3+ or greater cells; intermediate posterior or panuveitis	o Permanently discontinue ICI o Systemic corticosteroids and intravitreal or periocular/ or topical corticosteroids. o Methotrexate may be used in patients who respond poorly to systemic corticosteroids or those with severe sight-threatening inflammation.	o Permanently discontinue ICI o Systemic corticosteroids in addition to intravitreal/ periocular corticosteroids/ topical corticosteroid.
4	Best corrected visual acuity of 20/200 or worse in the affected eye	o Permanently discontinue ICI. o Systemic corticosteroids—prednisone 1–2 mg/kg/day or methylprednisolone 0.8–1.6 mg/ kg/day o Intravitreal or periocular or topical corticosteroids	o Permanently discontinue ICI o Same as grade 3

Table 4.
Grading and treatment recommendations of ocular irAEs.

symptoms should be referred to ophthalmology. Based on the most current cancer association guidelines for grade 1, ophthalmology referral should be within one week of symptoms. For Grades 2–3, an urgent referral is recommended; based on SITC, it should be within two days [24]. For grade 4, an emergent evaluation is recommended.

An initial ophthalmologic evaluation must include visual acuity measurement of each eye separately, color vision assessment, pupil evaluation, eye pressure, slit lamp, and dilated funduscopic evaluation. Current guidelines recommended by cancer associations do not include how to manage or monitor patients with baseline ophthalmologic conditions, making the management and monitoring of this patient population a complex one. Patients with metastatic or unresectable cancers are also in a delicate state of health which predisposes them to a series of infectious pathologies, and therefore if there is suspicion, it is always recommended to rule-out infectious uveitis processes prior to commencing high-dose systemic steroids.

Close follow-up is recommended while inflammation is active and should continue after the inflammation resolves due to the risk of possible reactivation. In the case series by E.R Dow et al. [10], in most cases, the ICI was stopped, and in more than half of the patients whose ICI was restarted, there was a recurrence of uveitis that was sometimes more severe than the initial episode. We can create more standardized monitoring guidelines as we continue to monitor patients with ICI.

6. Conclusion

Immunotherapy-associated uveitis is an increasing occurrence that has become more apparent with the increased use of immunologic cancer treatments. Both ICI and BRAF/MEK therapies help improve survival in cancer patients by improving the patient's ability to attack cancer cells. Due to the positive effects these medications provide to metastatic and unresectable cancer patients, we hypothesize that more patients would continue to benefit from their use. With ongoing approvals and combinations of new medications, we may continue to foresee new information about ocular irAEs. Generally, most patients can be treated successfully with topical or systemic steroids without needing to hold or completely discontinue their cancer treatment. The way we treat and monitor these uveitis patients is based on limited literature, for which more controlled and standardized studies are needed to help have better treatment and monitoring algorithms. It remains unclear when to stop or discontinue cancer immunotherapies in patients with immunotherapy-associated uveitis. However, it is of utmost importance for oncologists, ophthalmologists, and all physicians involved in the care of cancer patients to be aware of the complications of these medications for prompt diagnosis and referral to improve patient care. Although relatively rare, the most crucial aspect of immunotherapy-associated uveitis is that it requires prompt recognition and treatment to avoid irreversible ocular damage. Any decision to hold or permanently discontinue these potentially lifesaving cancer medications should be thoroughly evaluated and discussed between the oncologists and ophthalmologists.

Conflict of interest

Erick Rivera-Grana has no conflict of interests to disclose. Stephanie M. Llop has no conflict of interests to disclose.

Author details

Erick Rivera-Grana[1] and Stephanie M. Llop[2*]

1 Ophthalmology Department, University of Puerto Rico, San Juan, Puerto Rico, USA

2 Bascom Palmer Eye Institute, University of Miami Miller School of Medicine, Miami FL, USA

*Address all correspondence to: sxl1789@med.miami.edu

References

[1] Goldrath AW, Bevan MJ. Selecting and maintaining a diverse T-cell repertoire. Nature. 1999;**402**(6759): 255-262. DOI: 10.1038/46218

[2] Fife BT, Bluestone JA. Control of peripheral T-cell tolerance and autoimmunity via the CTLA-4 and PD-1 pathways. Immunological Reviews. 2008;**224**:166-182. DOI: 10.1111/ j.1600-065X.2008.00662.x

[3] Buchbinder EI, Desai A. CTLA-4 and PD-1 pathways similarities, differences, and implications of their inhibition. Am J Clin Oncol Cancer Clin Trials. 2016; **39**(1):98-106. DOI: 10.1097/ COC.0000000000000239

[4] Venkat AG, Arepalli S, Sharma S, et al. Local therapy for cancer therapy-associated uveitis: A case series and review of the literature. The British Journal of Ophthalmology. 2020;**104**(5): 703-711. DOI: 10.1136/bjophthalmol-2019-314403

[5] Dimitriou F, Urner-Bloch U, Eggenschwiler C, et al. The association between immune checkpoint or BRAF/ MEK inhibitor therapy and uveitis in patients with advanced cutaneous melanoma. European Journal of Cancer. 2021;**144**:215-223. DOI: 10.1016/j. ejca.2020.11.027

[6] Pardoll DM. The blockade of immune checkpoints in cancer immunotherapy. Nature Reviews. Cancer. 2012;**12**(4): 252-264. DOI: 10.1038/nrc3239

[7] Vaddepally RK, Kharel P, Pandey R, Garje R, Chandra AB. Review of indications of FDA-approved immune checkpoint inhibitors per NCCN guidelines with the level of evidence. Cancers (Basel). 2020;**12**(3):738. DOI: 10.3390/cancers12030738

[8] Conrady CD, Larochelle M, Pecen P, Palestine A, Shakoor A, Singh A. Checkpoint inhibitor-induced uveitis: A case series. Graefe's Archive for Clinical and Experimental Ophthalmology. 2017; **256**(1):187-191. DOI: 10.1007/s00417-017-3835-2

[9] Lee K, Chuang E, Griffin M, et al. Molecular basis of T cell inactivation by CTLA-4. Science. 1998;**282**(December): 2263-2266

[10] Dow ER, Yung M, Tsui E. Immune checkpoint inhibitor-associated uveitis: Review of treatments and outcomes. Ocular Immunology and Inflammation. 2021;**29**(1):203-211. DOI: 10.1080/ 09273948.2020.1781902

[11] Keir ME, Butte MJ, Freeman GJ, Sharpe AH. PD-1 and its ligands in tolerance and immunity. Annual Review of Immunology. 2008;**26**:677-704. DOI: 10.1146/annurev.immunol.26. 021607.090331

[12] Chan IS, Bhatia S, Kaufman HL, Lipson EJ. Immunotherapy for Merkel cell carcinoma: A turning point in patient care. Journal for Immunotherapy of Cancer. 2018;**6**(1):23. DOI: 10.1186/ s40425-018-0335-9

[13] Schneider BJ, Naidoo J, Santomasso BD, et al. Management of Immune-Related Adverse Events in patients treated with immune checkpoint inhibitor therapy: ASCO guideline update. Journal of Clinical Oncology. 2021;**39**(36):4073-4126. DOI: 10.1200/JCO.21.01440

[14] Ramos-Casals M, Brahmer JR, Callahan MK, et al. Immune-related adverse events of checkpoint inhibitors. Nature Reviews Disease Primers. 2020; **6**(1):38. DOI: 10.1038/s41572-020-0160-6

[15] Yoest JM. Clinical features, predictive correlates, and pathophysiology of immune-related adverse events in immune checkpoint inhibitor treatments in cancer: A short review. ImmunoTargets Ther. 2017;**6**: 73-82. DOI: 10.2147/ITT.S126227

[16] Weber JS, D'Angelo SP, Minor D, et al. Nivolumab versus chemotherapy in patients with advanced melanoma who progressed after anti-CTLA-4 treatment (CheckMate 037): A randomised, controlled, open-label, phase 3 trial. The Lancet Oncology. 2015;**16**(4):375-384. DOI: 10.1016/S1470-2045(15)70076-8

[17] Khoja L, Day D, Wei-Wu Chen T, Siu LL, Hansen AR. Tumour- and class-specific patterns of immune-related adverse events of immune checkpoint inhibitors: A systematic review. Annals of Oncology. 2017;**28**(10):2377-2385. DOI: 10.1093/annonc/mdx286

[18] Choi J, Lee SY. Clinical characteristics and treatment of immune-related adverse events of immune checkpoint inhibitors. Immune Netw. 2020;**20**(1):e9. DOI: 10.4110/in.2020.20.e9

[19] Eroglu Z, Ribas A. Combination therapy with BRAF and MEK inhibitors for melanoma: Latest evidence and place in therapy. Ther Adv Med Oncol. 2016; **8**(1):48-56. DOI: 10.1177/1758834015616934

[20] Voskens CJ, Goldinger SM, Loquai C, et al. The price of tumor control: An analysis of rare side effects of anti-CTLA-4 therapy in metastatic melanoma from the ipilimumab network. PLoS One. 2013;**8**(1):e53745. DOI: 10.1371/journal.pone.0053745

[21] Jabs DA, Nussenblatt RB, Rosenbaum JT, et al. Standardization of uveitis nomenclature for reporting clinical data. Results of the first international workshop. American Journal of Ophthalmology. 2005;**140**(3): 509-516. DOI: 10.1016/j.ajo.2005.03.057

[22] National Cancer Institute. Common Terminology Criteria for Adverse Events (CTCAE V. 5.0). U.S. Department of Health and Human Services; Maryland, USA. 2019. Available from: https://ctep.cancer.gov/protocoldevelopment/electronic_applications/ctc.htm#ctc_60

[23] Brahmer JR, Lacchetti C, Schneider BJ, et al. Management of immune-related adverse events in patients treated with immune checkpoint inhibitor therapy: American society of clinical oncology clinical practice guideline. Journal of Clinical Oncology. 2018;**36**(17):1714-1768. DOI: 10.1200/JCO.2017.77.6385

[24] Puzanov I, Diab A, Abdallah K, et al. Managing toxicities associated with immune checkpoint inhibitors: Consensus recommendations from the Society for Immunotherapy of cancer (SITC) toxicity management working group. Journal for Immunotherapy of Cancer. 2017;**5**(1):1-28. DOI: 10.1186/s40425-017-0300-z

[25] Thompson JA, Schneider BJ, Brahmer J, et al. Management of immunotherapy-related toxicities, version 1.2019. JNCCN J Natl Compr Cancer Netw. 2019;**17**(3):255-289. DOI: 10.6004/jnccn.2019.0013

Chapter 9

Nutraceutical Approach for the Treatment of Retinal Inflammation after Infections

Ilaria Piano, Francesca Corsi and Claudia Gargini

Abstract

This chapter described the ability of Zika virus, a hemostat-borne flavivirus, to infect retinal pigment epithelium cells and to generate chronic inflammation capable of generating permanent damage in the host that can progress eventually to the onset of pathology related to retinal degeneration. In addition, given the lack of an effective vaccine against ZIRK, the possibility of using as a therapeutic strategy the reduction of inflammatory processes that are established as a result of viral infection through the use of bioactive phytonutrients was analyzed.

Keywords: retinal degeneration, RPE cells, Zika virus, inflammation, phytonutrients

1. Introduction

Age-related macular degeneration (AMD) is an idiopathic degenerative disease of the retina and the cause of irreversible and profound vision loss in people older than 60 years [1]. Because of the rapidly aging population, it is easy to predict a worldwide increase in the incidence of AMD, resulting in increased costs on healthcare services. AMD presents in two main forms: Dry-AMD and Wet-AMD. Dry-AMD is characterized by atrophy of retinal pigment epithelial (RPE) cells and degeneration of adjacent photoreceptors. This form of the disease accounts for approximately 25% of cases, and patients experience severe loss of central vision. In contrast, wet-AMD is characterized by the formation at the level of the choroid of new vessels (CNVs) that branch out to the outer layers of Bruch's membrane, located beneath the basal membrane of the RPE, or across the RPE into the subretinal space. These vessels are usually constituted by a fragile endothelium and therefore subject to injury with subsequent hemorrhage and macular neuroretinal detachment. This form accounts for 75% of cases with severe central vision loss [2]. Despite their different pathophysiology and symptomatology, the two forms of AMD share similar risk factors for their development.

AMD is an aging-related syndrome caused by multiple factors including environmental, nutritional, and behavioral [3, 4] as well as genetic background can make an individual more or less susceptible to these factors [4, 5]. As in most diseases affecting the outer retina, loss of visual function in AMD results from degeneration and death of photoreceptors in the central retina, but in the initial pathogenesis of dry

AMD, the involvement of RPE cells [6] has been studied. The specific genetic and biochemical mechanisms responsible for RPE degeneration in AMD are still under investigation, but recent advances in understanding dry AMD suggest that oxidative stress and inflammation may be two of the cellular mechanisms underlying RPE cell death with an important role in drusen biogenesis and perhaps in the etiology of AMD in general [7, 8].

The RPE is a monolayer of cuboidal cells subjacent to the neural retina [9]. The basal cell membrane of the RPE is in contact with Bruch's membrane, a multilayered matrix that separates the RPE from the underlying choroidal vasculature. The apical membrane of the RPE is intimately interdigitated to the outer segments of the underlying photoreceptors. The main function of the RPE, which forms a part of the blood-retinal barrier, is to support the survival and normal function of the photoreceptors, in fact it controls the exchange of nutrients, waste products, ions, and gases between the choroidal blood vessels and the photoreceptors [10]; RPE is involved in the transport of retinol necessary for the synthesis of the visual pigment of photoreceptors [11] and in the phagocytosis of photoreceptor outer segment membrane disks (POS) [12]. In addition, RPE cells produce trophic and immunological factors necessary for the survival and protection of photoreceptors and the entire eye [13].

In addition to oxidative stress and inflammation, triggered by multifactorial events, infection by pathogens may also be a cause of damage and degeneration of RPE cells [14] and eventually lead to the onset of AMD.

2. Viral infections that induce eye damage

In the last decade, the World Health Organization (WHO) has identified a list of infectious diseases that have the potential to evolve into epidemics resulting in health emergencies and increased economic pressure on healthcare systems worldwide. Moreover, for the viral infections included in the list, there are no effective preventive or curative countermeasures to date. Among the diseases included in the list were coronaviruses, responsible for the pandemic that exploded in 2020, Crimean-Congo hemorrhagic fever, Filovirus diseases (Marburg hemorrhagic fever and EVD), Lassa Fever, Nipah virus infection, Rift Valley fever, and Zika virus [15].

2.1 Ocular complications from coronavirus infections

Coronaviruses include a family of viruses capable of infecting humans discovered for the first time in 1969; the transmission of the virus occurs mainly through respiratory droplets that in contact with the mucous membranes allow the virus to penetrate in the cells. There are seven coronaviruses that infect humans, and in 2002, the virus, named SARS-CoV-1, was isolated that mainly caused benign and mild infections of the upper respiratory tract [https://www.who.int]. Then in 2012, another virus causing respiratory syndrome named MERS-CoV was isolated in the Middle East [16]. The recent pandemic of Coronavirus-19 (COVID-19) due to SARS-CoV-2, which began in December 2019, has resulted in over 108 million cases and 2.3 million deaths. These highly transmissible pathogens cause lower respiratory tract infections that can rapidly progress to severe pneumonia with an estimated mortality rate of <1% for those aged 20–54 years, 1–5% in those aged 55–64 years, and 3–11% in individuals aged 65–84 years [17]. Unlike the other two diseases, COVID-19 symptomatology varies significantly between individuals. Indeed, while many patients develop respiratory distress and fever, cough, and fatigue, some patients may have no respiratory symptoms at onset and present with extra pulmonary manifestations, including headache, diarrhea, and vomiting.

Ocular complications have not been reported in association with SARS-CoV-1 or MERS-CoV. However, a study of healthcare workers with SARS-CoV showed that three of 36 patients (8%) had traces of SARS-CoV RNA in their tear fluid [18]. Ocular involvement was reported to a greater extent in association with COVID-19. The most common ocular manifestation is conjunctivitis with disease prevalence ranging from 2% to 32% [19]. In addition, several studies have found the presence of viral RNA in lachrymal fluid such that there is a risk of transmission through the tear film [20]. Retinal manifestations have been described through imaging studies. In a study of retinal changes in 12 adults with COVID-19, all patients showed hyperreflective lesions at the level of ganglion cells and inner plexiform layers on OCT, and four had cotton wool and microhemorrhages [21]. Another study showed that six of 27 (22%) of the COVID-19 positive patients with bilateral pneumonia showed cotton wool at an average of 43 days after the onset of COVID-19 symptoms [22].

In addition, the development of optic neuritis, disc edema, vascular tortuosity, acute macular neuroretinopathy (AMN), retinal occlusive vasculopathy (RVO), retinal artery occlusion, intraretinal hemorrhages, cotton wool, uveitis, and endogenous endophthalmitis has been reported in patients who tested positive and had moderate to severe COVID-19 symptoms. Often these diseases affecting the retina and retinal vasculature are the subject of single-case studies so it is necessary to expand these investigations in order to test the incidence of ocular complications of COVID-19 on a large scale [23].

2.2 Zika virus

The Zika virus is a flavivirus transmitted by Aedes mosquitoes and is related to yellow fever virus, dengue virus, and West Nile virus. Flaviviruses are single-stranded RNA viruses contained in capsid and coated with pericapsid. The genome encodes for a total of 10 proteins of which seven are nonstructural and three structural including: glycoprotein E (responsible for host cell infection and antigenic determinant of antibody response), capsid protein C, and membrane protein M (**Figure 1**) [24]. Zika virus was first identified in Uganda in 1947 in macaques and then in humans as early

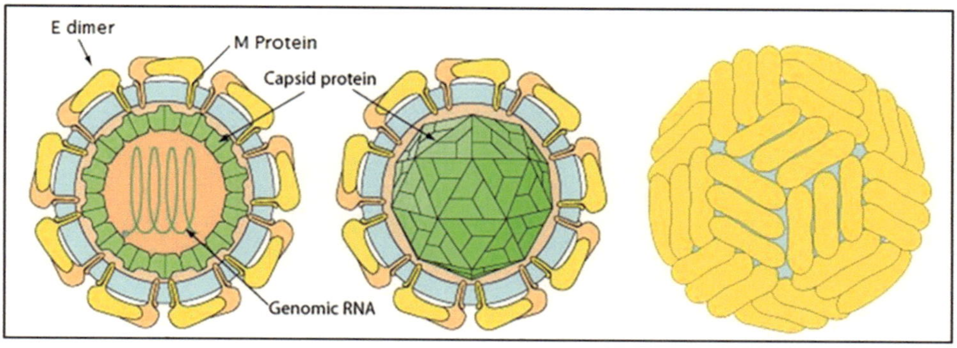

Figure 1.
Zika virus 3-D structure (Font: modified https://www.socialnews.xyz/2016/04/01/scientists-reveal-zika-virus-structure/).

as 1968. It has also been identified in French Polynesia, where an outbreak has been associated with perinatal transmission and fetal abnormalities. The virus currently present in Brazil appears to have originated from Polynesia. The clinical findings of the primary infection mimic both the dengue virus and the chikungunya virus, also present in Brazil and carried by the same mosquito. Testing for Zika virus is not readily available, making diagnosis challenging; however, serologic testing (IgM quantification) can be performed, and polymerase chain reaction (PCR) is available [25].

In adults, Zika virus infection induces symptoms such as: fever, headache, skin rash, muscle aches, diarrhea, and eye redness (**Figure 2**); but the most serious complications occur if the virus is contracted during pregnancy and especially within the first trimester. Zika virus infection, contracted in the first or second trimester of pregnancy, results in the development of microcephaly and retinal lesions in the fetus. In a study of 29 infants born to mothers who had experienced symptomalogy attributable to Zika virus, ocular abnormalities were present in 35% of the infants examined, and in seven of 10 cases they were bilateral. Characteristic lesions included posterior pole pigment deposits and areas of chorioretinal atrophy [26].

2.2.1 Ocular complications from Zika virus infections

The endemic emergence of Zika virus (ZIKV in various regions of the planet) has been accompanied by an unprecedented increase in the spectrum of ZIKV-associated diseases. It is becoming increasingly clear that ZIKV infection has implications that go beyond microcephaly, as infants born with congenital ZIKV have pathologies that also affect the eyes, ears, limbs, and possibly other organs [27]. Consequently, there has been a growing interest in understanding the pathogenesis of ZIKV in neurological diseases.

Since clinical studies have linked ZIKV to ocular abnormalities, mainly in the retina of infants and adults [28, 29] and to uveitis in children [30, 31]; for these reasons, it is important to study the pathogenesis of ZIKV in the eye to identify potential targets for therapeutic intervention since this virus currently has no effective vaccine.

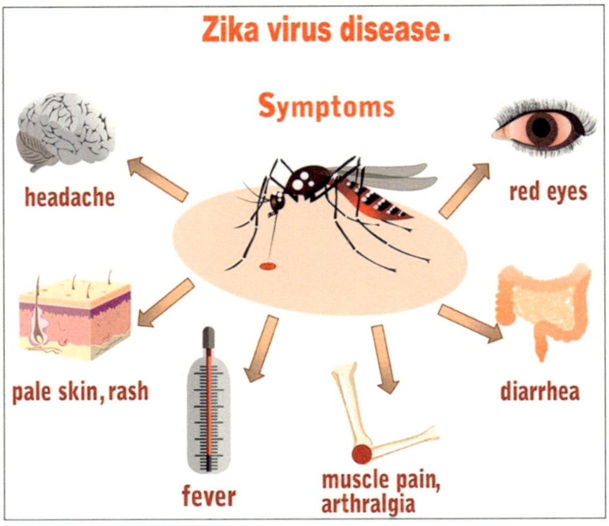

Figure 2.
Symptomatology attributable to Zika virus infection.

It has been shown that direct inoculation of ZIKV into the eye of an adult mouse causes retinal lesions with signs (chorioretinal atrophy and mottling of the RPE) that resemble of the ZIKV-associated ocular pathology described in humans. It has also been observed that ZIKV infects different retinal cell types and stimulates an innate antiviral response in the retina.

The main protective mechanism that controls the influx of innate immune cells and pathogens into the posterior segment of the eye is the presence of the blood-retinal barrier (BRB), consisting internally of retinal vascular endothelial cells and externally of RPE cells [32]. BRB dysfunction is known to allow infectious agents to enter the retina and cause inflammation and tissue damage [33].

The study by Kumar Singh and coworkers [34] shows that ZIKV has the ability to induce the expression of TLR3, RIGI, and MDA5 in RPE, HRvECs, and in the retina, suggesting that these PRRs might be involved in ZIKV recognition in the eye. Activation of PRRs leads to the production of various inflammatory mediators, including cytokines, chemokines, and IFNs both in vitro and in vivo. In this study, it was also shown that direct inoculation of ZIKV has the ability to create retinal lesions in adult WT mice, with evidence of choroidal inflammation, activation of antiviral innate immune response, and damage with atrophy and death of the RPE. The limitation of this study, in the in vivo experiments, was the intravitreal inoculation method, which itself bypasses the BRB and directly infects retinal cell types (**Figure 3**).

A further study investigated the potential mechanisms of ZIKV-induced degeneration by going to analyze retinal inflammation and endoplasmic reticulum (ER) stress in retinas at p8, a stage when the retinal tissue is still developing. The authors of this study [35] demonstrate how ZIKV-infected retinas are morphologically damaged compared with control retinas (**Figure 4**) and found that the levels of several key inflammatory molecules including chemokines (CCL2 and CXCL10), pro-inflammatory cytokines (TNFα, IL-1β, and IL-6), adhesion molecules (ICAM-1 and VCL-1), and iNOS were increased by 1.6–1300-fold in ZIKV-infected retinas. Similarly, key

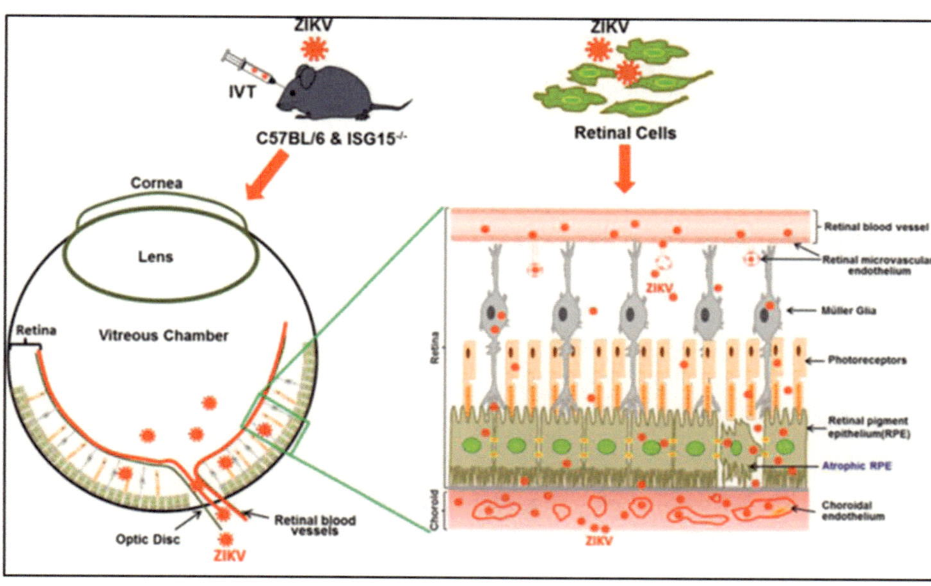

Figure 3.
Zika virus eye infection and related retinal damage. Image modified from Kumar Singh et al. [34].

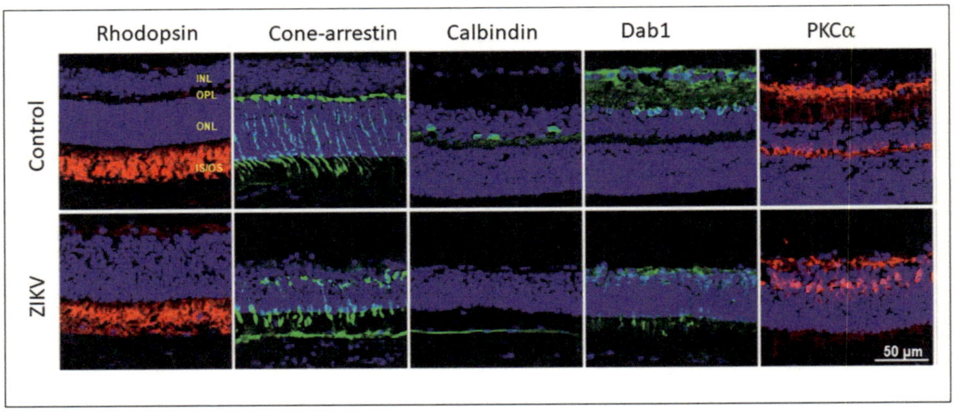

Figure 4.
Retinal degeneration induced by ZIKV infection. The image was modified from Li et al. [35].

molecules involved in ER stress, including XBP1s, GRP78, and CHOP, were significantly increased. Furthermore, in association with the increase in inflammation and ER stress, levels of cleaved caspase 3, a marker of apoptosis, and phosphorylated receptor-interacting protein 3 (pRIP3), a marker of necroptosis, were also increased in ZIKV-infected retinas. The cells most affected by this infection appeared to be localized mainly in the INL, where cleaved caspase 3-positive cells were visible, and in the IPL and GCL where pRIP3-positive cells were localized (**Figure 5**). These results

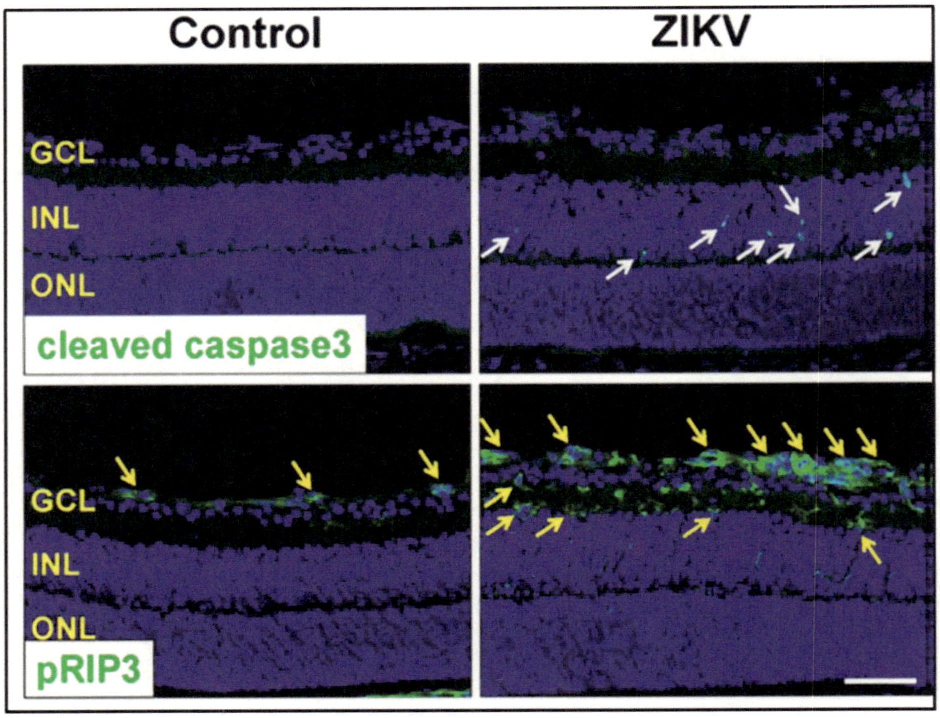

Figure 5.
Localization of key markers of apoptosis (green, cleaved caspase 3) and necroptosis (green, pRIP3) in ZIKV-infected retinas. The image was modified from Li et al. [35].

suggest that ZIKV-induced retinal degeneration may involve inflammation and ER stress by mediating cell apoptosis and necroptosis.

All of the evidence reported in the various studies concurs in suggesting that ZIKV infection leads to degeneration that can be likened to AMD-like degeneration where processes of chronic inflammation drive the progression of the disease. To date, however, it is not possible to permanently prevents this type of infection because there is no effective vaccine available, so one of the possible strategies to counteract ZIKV-induced chronic inflammation could be to use anti-inflammatory molecules. To this end, possible anti-inflammatory approaches through the use of nutraceutical molecules will be reported in the next section.

3. Phytonutrients and their applications

Natural products and their derivatives have played a significant role in medicine, generating many of the first new molecular entities (NMEs) and nearly half of all approved NMEs [36].

Scientific research is more and more focused on identifying biologically active food components that can optimize physical and mental well-being and reduce the risk of disease onset. Nutraceuticals or phytonutrients are products of natural origin, foods, or parts of them, that promote good health, longevity, and quality of life and, what is more, they can be used, in some cases, for the prevention and even treatment of chronic diseases.

Phytonutrients include the polyphenols. Polyphenols and their derivatives are widely distributed bioactive compounds in plant-derived foods (fruits, vegetables, legumes, cereals, seeds, spices, wine, tea, coffee, cocoa, and herbs) [37]. These bioactive compounds have received considerable interest over the past decade because of their wide range of biological activities. They are a broad group of compounds organic, plant secondary metabolites. The polyphenolic composition of plants is highly variable, both qualitatively and quantitatively; some of them are ubiquitous, while others are restricted to specific families or species [38]. From a structural point of view, polyphenols are compounds with one or more hydroxyl groups, associated with the aromatic ring, which can be present either in the oxidized form (quinone) or in the reduced form (phenol). Depending on the number of phenolic rings (hence the name "polyphenols") and the structural elements attached to them, polyphenols can be distinguished into flavonoids and non-flavonoids (phenolic acids, stilbenes, and lignans) [39]. Currently, about 8000 different structures of plant phenols are found. Flavonoids, in turn, are divided into six main subclasses: isoflavones, flavones, flavonols, anthocyanins, flavanones, flavanols. They are usually associated with a sugar, forming glycosides [40].

Here, in detail, we will review the activity of two polyphenols in neurodegenerative retinal diseases related to Zika virus infection.

3.1 Resveratrol

Resveratrol (3,5,4′-trihydroxy-trans-stilbene) is a plant-derived substance that is a member of the stilbenes group, non-flavonoid compounds belonging to the polyphenol family (**Figure 6**). Stilbenes are produced by the combination of the acetate and shikimate pathway.

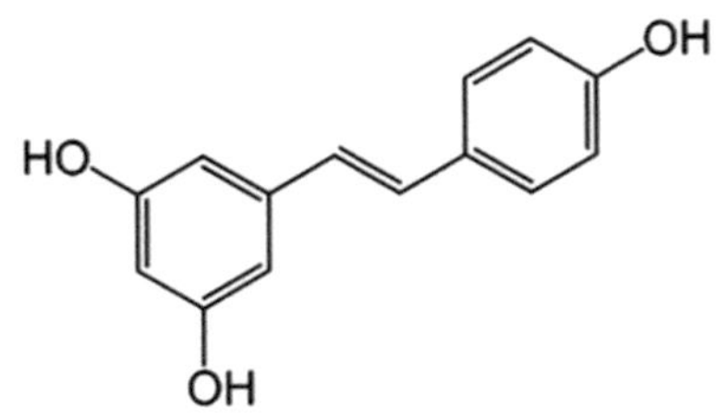

Figure 6.
Resveratrol structure.

Resveratrol is naturally found in the two isomeric forms cis and especially in the trans, which shows greater activity biological activity [41].

The most abundant dietary source of resveratrol is red grapes. Discrete amounts are also found in blueberries, berries, and the polygonum cuspidatum plant.

Resveratrol has been shown to have a powerful antioxidant action. In fact, the presence of this substance in red wine is associated with the benefits obtained by populations that habitually consume it in their diets. The cardioprotective properties of resveratrol are well known, and the presence of this compound in red wine is partly responsible for the phenomenon known as the "French Paradox". In France, habitual consumption of red wine reduces the incidence of mortality from cardiovascular disease. It is also known to have anti-inflammatory, anticancer, protective properties on nerve cells, antiaggregant, immunomodulatory, antibacterial, and antifungal properties of resveratrol. All these activities are due to the interaction of this molecule with several cellular synthetic pathways involving enzymes such as cyclooxygenase, lipoxygenase, and tyrosine kinase.

3.2 Hesperidin

Hesperidin (4′-methoxy-7-O-rutinosyl-3′,5-dihydroxyflavanone; hesperetin 7-O-rutinoside) is a naturally occurring flavanone glycoside found in citrus fruits (most notoriously oranges) and is a sugar-bound form of the flavonoid hesperitin (**Figure** 7) [42].

Flavanones, also called dihydroflavones, have a saturated C ring and can be multi-hydroxylated; in addition, several hydroxyl groups can be methylated and/or glycosylated [43].

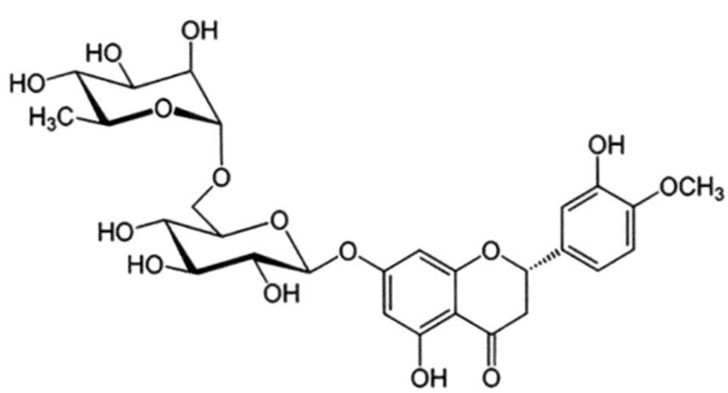

Figure 7.
Hesperidin structure.

Hesperitin is known to mediate the actions of hesperidin in the body, and since hesperidin needs to progress to the colon to be "released" by intestinal bacteria, it acts as a time release for hesperitin; one serving of hesperidin seems to increase blood levels for over the course of a day or so when consumed in this manner.

Various biological and pharmacological effects have been reported for hesperidin. It possesses the antioxidant, anti-inflammatory, and anti-carcinogenic activities [44]. Hesperidin possesses also considerable neuroprotective property in various neurodegenerative diseases, such as Alzheimer's, Parkinson's, stroke, and Huntington's [45].

4. Phytonutrients as a therapeutic perspective in the treatment of Zika-virus-induced ocular inflammation

It is well known that retinal degeneration can be induced by several factors, including genetic mutations, oxidative stress, and inflammation. Several treatments employing natural molecules, with antioxidant and/or anti-inflammatory actions, have shown efficacy in slowing the progression of retinal degeneration (e.g., AMD) [46].

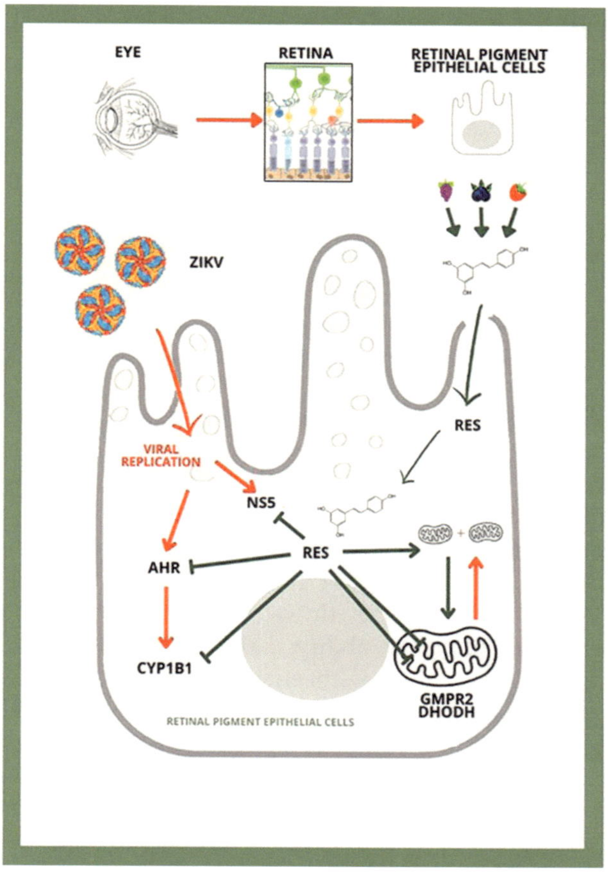

Figure 8.
Mechanism of action of resveratrol in the treatment of Zika virus retinal infection. Zika virus takes advantage of host mitochondrial enzymes for viral replication; resveratrol is able to inhibit these enzymes (GMPR2 and DHODH), effectively blocking virus replication.

Moreover, recent studies have demonstrated the antioxidant activity of Saffron, Naringenin, and Quercetin, the last are two polyphenols with known antioxidant and anti-inflammatory activities, in slowing the progression of retinal degeneration in several animal models [47, 48].

There is also a study that illustrates the efficacy of Hesperidin in protecting a retinal pigmented epithelium cell line (ARPE-19) from H_2O_2-induced damage, by inhibiting both apoptosis and ROS hyperproduction. Showing, once again, the efficacy of a polyphenol in the treatment of a retinal degeneration, such as AMD [49].

Regarding the Zika virus specifically, although the clinical manifestations at the ocular level are known, to date there is still a lack of research on the stages of the virus and consequently on potential treatments with natural molecules.

There is only one study on the efficacy of resveratrol treatment in the Zika-virus-infected ARPE-19 cell line with a focus on mitochondrial morphology.

Russo et al first showed how Zika virus infection altered the balance of mitochondrial dynamics toward the fission process in RPE cell and how these organelles lose their typical tubular shape during infection. Through a docking analysis, they study how resveratrol treatment restores the typical mitochondrial shape by acting as an inhibitor on enzymes critical for viral RNA replication (e.g., GMPR2 and DHODH). Indeed, viruses use host-specific factors to complete their multiplication cycles, and inhibition of mitochondrial enzymes involved in nucleoside biosynthesis has been shown to be an effective antiviral strategy. In conclusion, they demonstrated the efficacy of resveratrol as an antiviral agent in the treatment of Zika-virus-induced eye diseases [50]. A schematic representation of the mechanism of action of resveratrol, proposed by the authors [50], is shown in **Figure 8**.

5. Conclusion

In this chapter, we described how inflammation triggered by virus infection can lead to ocular complications capable of progressing to degenerative diseases such as AMD.

In particular, ocular complications due to COVID-19 and Zika virus have been analyzed, unfortunately this area of research is not yet well explored; especially in the former case given the recent appearance of the new virus responsible for Sars-Cov2 that is constantly evolving.

As for Zika virus, although the etiology at the level of the central nervous system and at the ocular level is known, effective therapies capable of blocking viral replication are not yet available; in fact, a specific vaccine is not yet developed.

Studies on the anti-inflammatory ability, at the ocular level and on retinal degeneration, of natural molecules have been widely resonant in the last decade; this strategy has also received interest in the treatment of Zika-virus-induced inflammation, and promising studies indicate the ability of molecules such as resveratrol and hesperetin to block the viral cell cycle. These notions, while in need of further study, open new perspectives for phytonutrient treatment of virus-induced ocular complications.

Acknowledgements

Thanks to Giulia Corsi for graphic support in the creation of some images.

Author details

Ilaria Piano*, Francesca Corsi and Claudia Gargini
Department of Pharmacy, University of Pisa, Pisa, Italy

*Address all correspondence to: ilaria.piano@unipi.it

References

[1] Evans J, Wormald R. Is the incidence of registrable age-related macular degeneration increasing? The British Journal of Ophthalmology. 1996;**80**(1):9-14

[2] Klein R, Klein BEK, Jensen SC, Meuer SM. The five-year incidence and progression of age-related maculopathy. Ophthalmology. 1997;**104**(1):7-21

[3] Snodderly DM. Evidence for protection against age-related macular degeneration by carotenoids and antioxidant vitamins. The American Journal of Clinical Nutrition. 1995;**62**(6):1448S-1461S

[4] Seddon JM, Ajani UA, Mitchell BD. Familial aggregation of age-related maculopathy. American Journal of Ophthalmology. 1997;**123**(2):199-206

[5] Heiba IM, Elston RC, Klein BEK, Klein R. Sibling correlations and segregation analysis of age-related maculopathy: The beaver dam eye study: Genetic analysis of age-related maculopathy. Genetic Epidemiology. 1994;**11**(1):51-67

[6] Cai J, Nelson KC, Wu M, Sternberg P, Jones DP. Oxidative damage and protection of the RPE. Progress in Retinal and Eye Research. 2000;**19**(2):205-221

[7] Hageman G. An integrated hypothesis that considers drusen as biomarkers of immune-mediated processes at the RPE-Bruch's membrane interface in aging and age-related macular degeneration. Progress in Retinal and Eye Research. 2001;**20**(6):705-732

[8] Rodrigues EB. Inflammation in dry age-related macular degeneration. Ophthalmologica. 2007;**221**(3):143-152

[9] Strauss O. The retinal pigment epithelium in visual function. Physiological Reviews. 2005;**85**(3): 845-881

[10] McBee JK, Palczewski K, Baehr W, Pepperberg DR. Confronting complexity: The interlink of phototransduction and retinoid metabolism in the vertebrate retina. Progress in Retinal and Eye Research. 2001;**20**(4):469-529

[11] Thompson DA, Gal A. Vitamin A metabolism in the retinal pigment epithelium: Genes, mutations, and diseases. Progress in Retinal and Eye Research. 2003;**22**(5):683-703

[12] Nguyen-Legros J, Hicks D. Renewal of photoreceptor outer segments and their phagocytosis by the retinal pigment epithelium. In: International Review of Cytology. Academic Press; 2000;**196**:245-313. DOI: 10.1016/S0074-7696(00)96006-6. ISSN: 0074-7696. ISBN: 9780123646002

[13] Streilein JW, Ma N, Wenkel H, Fong Ng T, Zamiri P. Immunobiology and privilege of neuronal retina and pigment epithelium transplants. Vision Research. 2002;**42**(4):487-495

[14] Qin S, Rodrigues GA. Progress and perspectives on the role of RPE cell inflammatory responses in the development of age-related macular degeneration. Journal of Inflammation Research. 2008;**1**:49-65. DOI: 10.2147/jir.s4354. [Epub 2 Dec 2008]. PMID: 22096347; PMCID: PMC3218720

[15] Kuthyar S, Anthony CL, Fashina T, Yeh S, Shantha JG. World Health Organization High Priority Pathogens: Ophthalmic disease findings and vision health perspectives. Pathogens. 2021;**10**(4):442

[16] Killerby ME, Biggs HM, Midgley CM, Gerber SI, Watson JT. Middle East respiratory syndrome coronavirus transmission. Emerging Infectious Diseases. 2020;**26**(2):191-198

[17] Petersen E, Koopmans M, Go U, Hamer DH, Petrosillo N, Castelli F, et al. Comparing SARS-CoV-2 with SARS-CoV and influenza pandemics. The Lancet Infectious Diseases. 2020;**20**(9):e238-e244

[18] Loon SC. The severe acute respiratory syndrome coronavirus in tears. The British Journal of Ophthalmology. 2004;**88**(7):861-863

[19] Zhang X, Chen X, Chen L, Deng C, Zou X, Liu W, et al. The evidence of SARS-CoV-2 infection on ocular surface. The Ocular Surface. 2020;**18**(3):360-362

[20] Chen L, Liu M, Zhang Z, Qiao K, Huang T, Chen M, et al. Ocular manifestations of a hospitalised patient with confirmed 2019 novel coronavirus disease. The British Journal of Ophthalmology. 2020;**104**(6):748-751

[21] Landecho MF, Yuste JR, Gándara E, Sunsundegui P, Quiroga J, Alcaide AB, et al. COVID-19 retinal microangiopathy as an in vivo biomarker of systemic vascular disease? Journal of Internal Medicine. 2021;**289**(1):116-120

[22] Marinho PM, Marcos AAA, Romano AC, Nascimento H, Belfort R. Retinal findings in patients with COVID-19. The Lancet. 2020;**395**(10237):1610

[23] Al-Namaeh M. Ocular manifestations of COVID-19. Ophthalmological Eye Diseases. 2022;**14**:2515

[24] Firth AE, Atkins JF. A conserved predicted pseudoknot in the NS2A-encoding sequence of West Nile and Japanese encephalitis flaviviruses suggests NS1' may derive from ribosomal frameshifting. Virology Journal. 2009;**6**(1):14

[25] Jampol LM, Goldstein DA. Zika Virus infection and the eye. JAMA Ophthalmology. 2016;**134**(5):535

[26] de Paula FB, de Oliveira Dias JR, Prazeres J, Sacramento GA, Ko AI, Maia M, et al. Ocular findings in infants with microcephaly associated with presumed Zika Virus Congenital Infection in Salvador, Brazil. JAMA Ophthalmology. 2016;**134**(5):529

[27] Vogel G. Experts fear Zika's effects may be even worse than thought. Science. 2016;**352**(6292):1375-1376

[28] de Miranda HA, Costa MC, Frazão MAM, Simão N, Franchischini S, Moshfeghi DM. Expanded spectrum of congenital ocular findings in microcephaly with presumed Zika infection. Ophthalmology. 2016;**123**(8):1788-1794

[29] Ventura CV, Maia M, Travassos SB, Martins TT, Patriota F, Nunes ME, et al. Risk factors associated with the ophthalmoscopic findings identified in infants with presumed Zika Virus congenital infection. JAMA Ophthalmology. 2016;**134**(8):912

[30] Furtado JM, Espósito DL, Klein TM, Teixeira-Pinto T, da Fonseca BA. Uveitis associated with Zika Virus infection. The New England Journal of Medicine. 2016;**375**(4):394-396

[31] Parke DW, Almeida DRP, Albini TA, Ventura CV, Berrocal AM, Mittra RA. Serologically confirmed Zika-related unilateral acute maculopathy in an adult. Ophthalmology. 2016;**123**(11):2432-2433

[32] Kumar A, Pandey RK, Miller LJ, Singh PK, Kanwar M. Muller glia in

retinal innate immunity: A perspective on their roles in endophthalmitis. Critical Reviews in Immunology. 2013;**33**(2):119-135

[33] Coburn PS, Wiskur BJ, Miller FC, LaGrow AL, Astley RA, Elliott MH, et al. Bloodstream-to-eye infections are facilitated by outer blood-retinal barrier dysfunction. PLoS One. 2016;**11**(5):e0154560

[34] Singh PK, Guest JM, Kanwar M, Boss J, Gao N, Juzych MS, et al. Zika virus infects cells lining the blood-retinal barrier and causes chorioretinal atrophy in mouse eyes. JCI Insight. 2017;**2**(4):e92340. DOI: 10.1172/jci.insight.92340. PMID: 28239662; PMCID: PMC5313066

[35] Li Y, Shi S, Xia F, Shan C, Ha Y, Zou J, et al. Zika virus induces neuronal and vascular degeneration in developing mouse retina. Acta Neuropathology Communication. 2021;**9**(1):97

[36] Patridge E, Gareiss P, Kinch MS, Hoyer D. An analysis of FDA-approved drugs: Natural products and their derivatives. Drug Discovery Today. 2016;**21**(2):204-207

[37] Manach C, Scalbert A, Morand C, Rémésy C, Jiménez L. Polyphenols: Food sources and bioavailability. The American Journal of Clinical Nutrition. 2004;**79**(5):727-747

[38] Velderrain-Rodríguez GR, Palafox-Carlos H, Wall-Medrano A, Ayala-Zavala JF, Chen CYO, Robles-Sánchez M, et al. Phenolic compounds: Their journey after intake. Food & Function. 2014;**5**(2):189-197

[39] Del Rio D, Rodriguez-Mateos A, Spencer JPE, Tognolini M, Borges G, Crozier A. Dietary (Poly)phenolics in human health: Structures, bioavailability, and evidence of protective effects against chronic diseases. Antioxidants & Redox Signaling. 2013;**18**(14):1818-1892

[40] Kumar S, Pandey AK. Chemistry and biological activities of flavonoids: An overview. The Scientific World Journal. 2013;**2013**:1-16

[41] Souto AA, Carneiro MC, Seferin M, Senna MJH, Conz A, Gobbi K. Determination of trans-resveratrol concentrations in Brazilian Red Wines by HPLC. Journal of Food Composition and Analysis. 2001;**14**(4):441-445

[42] Kim J, Wie MB, Ahn M, Tanaka A, Matsuda H, Shin T. Benefits of hesperidin in central nervous system disorders: A review. Analytical Cell Biology. 2019;**52**(4):369

[43] Marella S. Flavonoids-the most potent poly-phenols as antidiabetic agents: An overview. MADD. 2017;**1**(3)

[44] Roohbakhsh A, Parhiz H, Soltani F, Rezaee R, Iranshahi M. Molecular mechanisms behind the biological effects of hesperidin and hesperetin for the prevention of cancer and cardiovascular diseases. Life Sciences. 2015;**124**:64-74

[45] Hajialyani M, Hosein Farzaei M, Echeverría J, Nabavi S, Uriarte E, Sobarzo-Sánchez E. Hesperidin as a neuroprotective agent: A review of animal and clinical evidence. Molecules. 2019;**24**(3):648

[46] Dziedziak J, Kasarełło K, Cudnoch-Jędrzejewska A. Dietary antioxidants in age-related macular degeneration and glaucoma. Antioxidants. 2021;**10**(11):1743

[47] Piano I, Di Paolo M, Corsi F, Piragine E, Bisti S, Gargini C, et al. Retinal neurodegeneration: Correlation

between nutraceutical treatment and animal model. Nutrients. 2021;**13**(3):770

[48] Piano I, Corsi F, Polini B, Gargini C. Nutraceutical molecules slow down retinal degeneration, in Tvrm4 mice a model of retinitis pigmentosa, by genetic modulation of anti-oxidant pathway. Frontiers in Neuroscience. 2022;**16**:868750. DOI: 10.3389/fnins.2022.868750. [Published: 19 Apr 2022]

[49] Zhu C, Dong Y, Liu H, Ren H, Cui Z. Hesperetin protects against H_2O_2-triggered oxidative damage via upregulation of the Keap1-Nrf2/HO-1 signal pathway in ARPE-19 cells. Biomedicine & Pharmacotherapy. 2017;**88**:124-133

[50] Russo CA, Torti MF, Marquez AB, Sepúlveda CS, Alaimo A, García CC. Antiviral bioactivity of resveratrol against Zika virus infection in human retinal pigment epithelial cells. Molecular Biology Reports. 2021;**48**(7):5379-5392

Section 3

Ocular Surface

Chapter 10

Advances in Biomaterials for Corneal Regeneration

Kamal Malhotra and May Griffith

Abstract

The human cornea acts as a protective covering for the eye and plays an important role in light transmission into the eye for vision. Corneal defects due to trauma, infection, or disease can have detrimental effects on the vision, and severe cases lead to vision loss. Twenty-three million people are estimated to be affected by corneal blindness worldwide. Treatment involves corneal transplantation surgery, but there is a severe shortage of donor corneas worldwide. Furthermore, patients with severe pathologies risk rejecting conventional corneal transplantation, thus leaving them untreated. Therefore, there is an urgent need to develop new therapies to replace traditional corneal transplant surgery. This review focuses on recent potential biomaterials development for corneal regeneration and repair. It includes cell-based therapies, cell-free regeneration-inducing biomaterials, and injectable or in-situ gelation-based biomaterials for patients with a high risk of graft failure. It also consists of the emerging role of exosomes and extracellular vesicles in corneal infections and regeneration.

Keywords: corneal regeneration, biomaterials, corneal repair, transplantation, hydrogel, cell-free regeneration

1. Introduction

The cornea is an avascular, transparent, and multilayered tissue whose primary function is to act as a lens to direct light entering the eye toward the retina. It consists of three cellular layers, an epithelium, stroma, and endothelium, and two acellular layers, the Bowman's and Descemet's membrane [1]. A third acellular layer, the Dua membrane, has also been described. The epithelium forms the cornea's outermost layer and comprises stratified epithelial cells. These cells act as a barrier to protect the eye from pathogens and allow the diffusion of essential nutrients and oxygen. The stroma constitutes 90% of the cornea's total thickness and contains keratocyte cells interspersed in lamellae but forming a connected network. The cornea is responsible for focusing approximately 75% of light into the eye for vision. It also protects the eye while preserving its transparency by self-renewal of its epithelium in particular [2]. However, injury, aging, or disease could lead to irreversible loss of clarity and corneal blindness.

Corneal blindness is one of the significant causes of vision loss leading to 23 million patients who have unilateral blindness and 4.9 million patients who have bilateral blindness globally [3]. Although corneal transplant is the most common

IntechOpen

transplanted tissue worldwide, corneal blindness is still rising, with 2 million cases yearly [4]. Due to the increasing demand, eye banks cannot provide the cornea to all the patients, leaving an estimated 12.7 million people on the waiting list for corneal transplantation [5]. Corneal transplant with a human donor cornea has been the go-to treatment for corneal blindness since the twentieth century. In penetrating keratoplasty or full-thickness grafts, a full-thickness button of healthy donor corneal tissue replaces excised pathologic corneal tissue. Only the damaged layers are replaced in lamellar keratoplasty or partial thickness grafts. This helps maintain the integrity of the cornea and surrounding tissue, leading to faster healing and vision improvement. Complications of corneal transplantation include graft failure, of which graft rejection is a leading cause. Disease transmission from graft to host is rare but has been reported, e.g., endophthalmitis, due to donor-to-host microbial transmission [6]. Other issues include complications in immune-compromised patients, infectious diseases, and astigmatism associated with corneal transplants. However, proper donor screening and processing may reduce the risk of infection and related post-surgical complications. However, the donor cornea shortage is a major issue, especially in developing nations. It is even difficult to carry out complex surgical procedures in some developing countries due to insufficient resources/facilities. Thus, there is an urgent need to develop new therapies or biomaterials as alternatives to donor transplantation.

In this chapter, we focus on the biomaterials rather than fabrication techniques such as electrospinning or 3D bioprinting. We refer the reader to Patel et al. 2021 for a review of electrospinning in corneal constructs [7] and to Bin et al. 2019 and Fuest et al. 2020 for reviews on bioprinting of corneal implants [8, 9].

2. Cell-based therapies

Several cell-based therapies are already approved for treatment in clinical settings [10–13]. These include resurfacing the cornea with limbal epithelial cells. Cellular therapy of corneal stroma has gained attention in recent years. Studies revealed that mesenchymal stromal (or stem) cells (MSCs) could survive and differentiate into adult human keratocytes in animal models without eliciting an inflammatory response. In addition, they produced new collagen in the host stroma and were able to remodel scars and improve transparency in animal models for corneal dystrophies [14, 15]. Cell-based therapies can be broadly divided into using stem cells to stimulate regeneration with and without scaffolds. This section focuses on stem-cell-based theories with scaffolds or templates.

Bio-fabrication of stem cell supports from silk fibroin/gelatin (SF/G) film and scaffold to make stem-cell-incorporating corneal epithelial and stromal equivalents for canine corneal regeneration. Canine limbal epithelial stem cells (cLESCs) were seeded in SF/G film, and canine corneal stromal stem cells (cCSSCs) were seeded in SF/G scaffold, respectively, which supported cell adhesion, viability, and proliferation along with differentiation of cLESCs and cCSSCs into keratocytes. Studies revealed endogenous ECM production after 14 days, thus mimicking native cornea [16]. Pitarresi and coworkers were the first ones to use hydrogels based on hyaluronic acid (HA) cross-linked with polyaspartamide derivative (PHEA-EDA) as an alternative to amniotic membrane for the delivery of limbal stem cells (LSCs). HA/PHEA-EDA hydrogel showed biocompatibility with immortalized human corneal epithelial cells or primary cells but only moderate to poor cell adhesion capabilities. These features allow the potential for clinical application of HA/PHEA-EDA as a delivery substrate with easy release of transplanted limbal stem cells to treat damaged corneas [17]. HCECs and human adipose stem cells (HASCs) were co-cultured in 3D hyaluronic acid hydrogel with and without collagen. HASCs could proliferate and differentiate within the proper cell density, and the survival of cells was better in the absence of collagen, showing potential for use in ocular surface reconstruction [18]. Hyaluronan hydrogel scaffold was used to expand human corneal epithelial stem cell ex-vivo in the xeno-free environment. The developed hydrogel behaved as native cornea equivalent, which reduced the risk of xeno-contamination and allowed the expansion of limbal stem cells [19].

3. Decellularized corneas repopulated with stem cells

Decellularized corneas comprising intact ECM composition and integrity hold the potential to use as an implant in the same or cross-species. They maintain the native mechanical strength and stromal structure but lack the cellular components, preventing graft rejection, or activating undesirable immune responses. Recently, Polisetti and coworkers explored the use of decellularized human corneas as scaffolds. The decellularized human corneal scaffold preserves the native extracellular matrix proteins, glycosaminoglycans, and tissue structure to allow regeneration of the epithelium and stroma of the host tissue ex-vivo [20]. Decellularized human limbus (DHL) was used as a biomimetic scaffold for transplanting limbal epithelial progenitor cells (LEPCs) in ex-vivo transplantation. The scaffold provided a limbal niche-specific microenvironment where native ECM composition was preserved and showed excellent biocompatibility for LEPCs and limbal melanocytes (LMS). Furthermore, the scaffold allowed complete epithelization with interspersed melanocytes and stromal repopulation from host tissue, thereby showing potential for regeneration of damaged cornea in patients suffering from limbal stem cell deficiency (LSCD) [21].

A rabbit corneal model was used to study the in-vivo biocompatibility of decellularized human corneal stroma with and without recellularization of human adipose-derived adult stem cells (h-ADASC). The decellularized corneal sheets had intact extracellular matrices and an excellent recellularization capacity with h-ADASC. In addition, it revealed good transparency with no clinical sign of rejection. The post-mortem analysis revealed the survival of transplanted stem cells within the graft and the differentiation of stem cells into functional keratocytes [22].

In a human clinical trial, decellularized porcine corneal stromas were transplanted into 47 patients with corneal fungal infection. There was no recurrent disease observed within 3 years of the study. Seventy-two percent of patients showed visual improvement. However, neovascularization was observed in 53% of patients but was suppressed eventually. Thus, the decellularized cornea has demonstrated promising potential in regenerating damaged corneas while preserving the native ECM composition. However, care must be taken to prevent zoonotic pathogenic transmission, as seen in recent years of global transmission of coronavirus from animals to humans.

4. Cell-free regeneration-inducing biomaterials

Recently biomaterials have shown enormous potential in tissue engineering due to their desirable physical, chemical, and mechanical properties, which can guide cells to grow and promote functionality. Biomaterials developed as corneal substitutes should replicate the structure and functionality of the native cornea. They should mimic the in vivo microenvironment, e.g., extracellular matrix, to support resident cell growth, proliferation, and integration within the host tissue for bifunctional regeneration of damaged cornea. Biomaterials should also possess desirable characteristics such as biodegradability, biocompatibility, non-immunogenicity, and seamless integration with host tissues. In addition, biomaterials should possess sufficient mechanical (tensile) strength to support suturing or gluing and to withstand the intraocular pressure to support the fluctuations. Besides this, it is important to have optical transparency and a refractive index like that of a healthy cornea, plus allow the diffusion of nutrients into the scaffold and waste out of it [23]. Thus, it is important to have these considerations in mind for designing corneal construct mimicking native cornea. Griffith and coworkers have provided an extensive guide to consider beforehand while designing biosynthetic alternatives for clinical applications [24].

Natural, synthetic, and composite polymers are the main biomaterials used for corneal tissue engineering. Natural polymers tend to have inherent biocompatibility and bio-integration compatibilities, whereas synthetic polymers allow for customization of desired chemical and mechanical properties. Composite polymers have the advantage of both natural and synthetic polymers, i.e., they are both biocompatible and tunable to allow for desirable mechanical and chemical properties for corneal tissue engineering.

4.1 Naturally derived and synthetic hydrogels

The main advantage of using naturally derived polymers for corneal tissue engineering is their biocompatibility. Commonly used natural polymers for corneal regeneration include collagen, silk fibroin, gelatin, chitosan, cellulose, hyaluronic acid (HA), and decellularized cornea. They are formed by chemical cross-linking and formation of physical bonds and networks.

4.1.1 Collagen and collagen-based hydrogels

One of the most attractive natural polymers is collagen, the most abundant extracellular matrix component in several tissues including the human cornea. Collagen is the main component of corneal tissue. It possesses unique properties such as biocompatibility, bio-adhesiveness, suitable biodegradability, and low immunogenicity, which is to support corneal regeneration. In addition, collagen supports the corneal epithelial growth and cell adhesion without eliciting toxicity. The source of collagen plays important role in its physiochemical properties. Type I and type II collagen possess adequate tensile strength, whereas type III collagen is superior in mechanical strength and optical clarity [25]. Collagen from different sources such as porcine, bovine, rat, recombinant human collagen type I and III are commercially available. On their own, collagen hydrogels are soft and unstable. Attempts to improve the physicochemical properties of collagen-based hydrogels include chemical cross-linking and development of composite hydrogels with synthetic polymers to add mechanical strength. Examples include cross-linking by glutaraldehyde, 1-ethyl-3-(3-dimethyl aminopropyl) carbodiimide hydrochloride (EDC), and multifunctional dendrimers to improve the elastic and mechanical strength of collagen scaffolds [26]. One limitation of using chemical linkers is that they can be cytotoxic and not cell-friendly, limiting their use to fabricating cell-free scaffolds. A naturally derived cross-linker such as genipin was tested to reduce the cytotoxic effect of cross-linker, but the concentration of genipin required to enhance the mechanical strength resulted in dark-blue-colored collagen scaffold [27].

Further, to reduce the heterogenicity of collagen derived from animal source, Fagerholm and team [28] performed the first successful clinical trials where they used the cell-free implant made from recombinant human collagen type III (RHCIII). Trial includes the treatment of 10 patients with keratoconus or central scarring with RHCIII implant, which showed stable regeneration of epithelium, stroma, and nerves after 2 years of implantation. The long-term observation also revealed the immune compatibility of implants. Cell-free implant containing carbodiimide cross-linked recombinant human collagen (RHC) was grafted into patients and revealed stable integration of regenerated neo-corneas without rejection. In addition, nerve and stromal cell regeneration observed over 4 years mimic microarchitecture of healthy corneas without recruiting inflammatory dendritic cells into the implant area [29]. Next, Griffith and coworkers conducted a clinical study in cornea patients with a high risk of implant rejection [30]. 2-methacryloyloxyethyl phosphorylcholine (MPC), a synthetic phosphorylcholine with reported inflammation suppressing properties, was incorporated into RHCIII to form interpenetrating networks. The resulting RHCIII-MPC hydrogels were implanted into the corneas of unilaterally blind seven patients (one dropout) by anterior lamellar keratoplasty after excision of the pathologic tissue. The patients were followed up for an average of 24 months (**Figure 1**). The implants supported the stable regeneration of the epithelium, stroma, and nerves over the observation period [30]. Short collagen-like peptides (CLPs) conjugated to polyethylene glycol (PEG) showed promising functionality equivalent to recombinant human collagen. CLP-PEG hydrogel supported stable regeneration of corneal tissue and nerve in preclinical animal testing [31].

Recently, a cross-linker-free supramolecular gel strategy has been explored to make collagen gel where collagen molecules were intertwined inside a pyrene conjugated dipeptide amphiphile (PyKC) without any functional group modification. The newly developed collagen implant was optically transparent, mechanically stable, and supported the growth of all corneal cells. It also triggered anti-inflammatory differentiation while suppressing the pro-inflammatory differentiation of human monocytes [32]. Plant-derived recombinant human collagen I was used to make hydrogel-based corneal graft to support mechanical stability, biocompatibility, and transparency in mini-pigs. Thus, showed the potential of plant-based RHC1 as an alternative to animal-derived collagen or allografts [33].

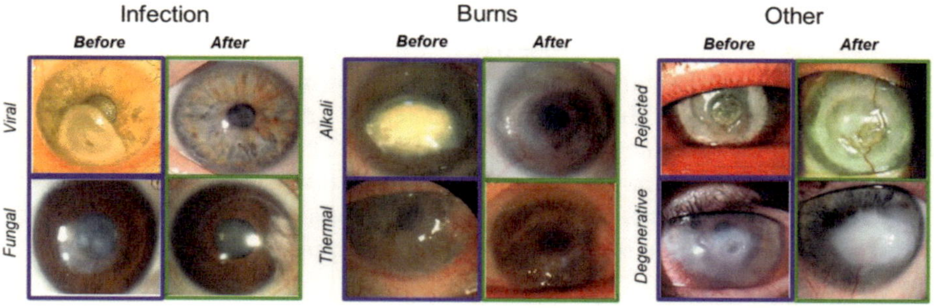

Figure 1.
Clinical trial of RHCIII MPC corneal implant in high-risk patient at the last follow-up showing three groups of patients as per the preoperative diagnosis: Infection (herpes and fungal keratitis), burn (alkali or thermal), and other (failed graft and post-stroke neurotrophic keratitis). Patient with infection showed best recovery with mostly clear regenerative cornea followed by cornea with burns. Reproduced from [30].

4.1.2 Gelatin-based hydrogel

Recently, methacrylated gelatin (GelMA)-based hydrogels have gained attention for corneal tissue engineering because of their appropriate mechanical strength and optical properties. GelMA hydrogels showed good biocompatibility with 98% survival rate of keratocyte after 21 days of culture. In vivo studies of Gel MA in rabbit model showed no signs of ulcer, edema, or infection when hydrogel was implanted in mid-stromal pocket and observed for 8 weeks. Hematoxylin and Eosin staining showed hydrogel integration within the host tissue with negligible foreign body reaction [34]. The efficacy of GelMA in repairing rat corneas compared with lamellar keratoplasty (LKP) showed significant differences between the two groups in terms of inflammatory cell infiltrates, corneal cell thickness, and expression of α-SMA and TGF-β after 3 months of observation. Thus, supporting the ability of Gel MA in alleviating the corneal stroma fibrosis and reducing the loss of corneal refractive power due to fibrosis [35]. Electrospinning was used to make Gel MA fibers that were then complexed with poly (2-hydroxymethyl methacrylate) (p(HEMA)) through UV photo-polymerization to form GelMA-p(HEMA) composite hydrogels. The composite hydrogel showed optical transmittance equivalent to that of the human cornea, highly promising mechanical strength, improved structural integrity, and supported proliferation of BCE C/D¬1b corneal endothelial cells in 3D culture [36].

Gelatin-based hydrogels have also been explored for the drug delivery applications to overcome the poor bioavailability of traditional eye drop method. Dual cross-linking reactions prepared gelatin hydrogel/contact lens composite via in situ free radical polymerization and carboxymethyl cellulose/N-hydroxysulfosuccinimide to encapsulate rutin for corneal wound healing. The composite hydrogel showed sustained release of rutin for 14 days and without eliciting toxicity. In vivo studies in rabbit cornea injury model showed that the rutin-encapsulating composite hydrogel supported faster healing (98.3% ± 0.7%) at 48 h post-operation compared with the composite alone (healing rate, 87.0% ± 4.5%). Results also revealed the role of ERK/MAPK and PI3K/AKT signal pathways in corneal wound healing [37]. Injectable photo-cross-linked gelatin hydrogels were formed using acrylated gelatin and thiolated gelatin with tunable mechanical properties, biocompatibility, and biological properties that support the repair of corneal wound. The hydrogel showed promising cell viability in cell seeding and cell encapsulation studies and supported the regeneration of new tissues under focal corneal wounds in rabbit corneas [38]. Collagen/gelatin/alginate (CGA) hydrogels were used for the sustained delivery of moxifloxacin (MFX) and dexamethasone (DEX) loaded into nanoparticles, for the treatment of infectious ocular keratitis. Lipid nanocarrier loaded with MFX/DEX (Lipo-MFX/DEX) and encapsulated within the hydrogel showed promising cell proliferation ability when co-cultured with ocular epithelial cells. CGA-Lipo-MFX/DEX composite hydrogel showed the sustained release of drug for up to 12 h and exhibit the ability to inhibit bacterial growth to improve corneal wound healing [39]. Thus, gelatin-based hydrogels are not only promising alternatives for stimulating corneal regeneration but could also be a viable option for ocular drug delivery applications.

4.1.3 Silk-fibrion-based hydrogels

Silk fibroin is a structural protein extracted from the silkworm's cocoon, Bombyx mori. Silk represents a unique choice to use as a biomaterial for tissue engineering due to its tunable and robust mechanical properties, controlled degradation, and non-immunogenic properties [40]. Photoactivated, in-situ forming antimicrobial silk-based hydrogels were developed for treating corneal injuries. Gentamicin-loaded methacrylated-silk (SilkMA) hydrogels adopted the corneal injury shape and gelled within a few minutes upon exposure to low-intensity UV. The mechanical strength, transparency, and water content approached those of the human cornea, and hydrogel inhibited the growth of *Staphylococcus aureus* and *Pseudomonas aeruginosa* for up to 72 h [41]. Silk-fibroin-based films (SF) were also complexed with lysophosphatidic acid (LPA) to form a functionalized graft for corneal endothelial cell (CEnCs) regeneration. The functionalized graft supported cell adhesion provided good biocompatibility and expressed CEnCs-specific genes and protein when tested in rabbit corneas [42]. A hybrid transparent fibrillar film made from SF/GelMA could be tuned as needed to form matrices with different properties by modifying the volume ratio of SNF to GelMA. The SNF/GelMA ratio of 30/70 was optimal and showed mechanical strength, transparency, and stability (reduction in degradation rate) that approximated the properties of the human cornea. The SNF/GelMA film supported cell attachment, spreading, and proliferation of stromal cells, making it an ideal candidate for corneal regeneration [43].

Recently, a study reported the upregulation of cytokine IL-1β, which induces undesirable phenotypic changes in keratocytes by downregulating the gene and protein expression of keratocyte corneal stromal markers: Keratocan, Lumican, Aldh3a1, and CD34. These markers play important role in maintaining corneal epithelial homeostasis and corneal transparency during normal conditions [44, 45]. The selective IKKβ inhibitor, TPCA-1, can reverse the phenotypic change and preserve the keratocyte phenotype in diseased corneas. Zhang and coworkers developed silk fibroin hydrogels with sustained release of TPCA-1, which accelerated in vivo wound healing, and increased keratocyte expression marker while supporting the regeneration of epithelium and stroma [46]. Thus, showing the promising potential of silk-fibroin-based hydrogel for corneal regeneration and drug delivery applications in vivo (**Table 1**).

Biomaterial	Target tissue	Novelty	Developmental status	Refs.
Natural and Biosynthetic hydrogels				
Collagen	Stroma	Collagen-based porous hydrogel with good transparency and mechanical strength; showed sustained release drug delivery in-vitro, developed new Flap-ALK surgical implantation model inspired from LASIK surgery	Animal model: rabbit	[47]
Gelatin	Corneal surface: Epithelium	Glycidyl methacrylate grafted on gelatin to form elastic protein-based, adhesive hydrogel that showed 4 times better stretchability, biocompatibility, and higher tensile strength	In-vitro studies	[48]
Gelatin	Stroma	Visible-light-based stereolithography (SLA) 3D bioprinting methodology developed to make gelatin methacrylate (GelMA) hydrogels that can be molded into dome shaped corneal implants	In-vitro studies	[49]

Biomaterial	Target tissue	Novelty	Developmental status	Refs.
Recombinant human collagen type III	Epithelium and stroma	Biosynthetic recombinant human collagen implant can be fabricated using chemical or photochemical cross-linking. The former cross-linking methodology results in hydrogels promoting in situ tissue regeneration; of sufficient toughness to allow handling but requires overlying sutures for retention	Animal model: mini pigs, rabbits	[25]
o-nitroso benzaldehyde group (NB)-modified gelatin (GelNB)	Corneal surface: Epithelium	Developed molecular coating to attach covalently to corneal surface, enhanced corneal epithelial cell migration in-vitro, promoted self-healing, and inhibit disorder of regeneration	Animal model: rabbit	[50]
Recombinant human collagen	Epithelium and stroma	RHC hydrogel tested in 10 patients with significant vision loss and results showed stable integration, supported corneal reepithelization, nerve regeneration and restore touch sensitivity:	Pilot clinical trial	[28]
Composite hydrogels				
Collagen (Col) and polycaprolactone (PCL)	Epithelium	Corneal graft made from Col-PCL membrane, comprising transparent central part made from Col and mechanically robust edge from Col-PCL with high tensile strength (1.1 ± 0.3 MPa)	In-vitro and ex-vivo studies	[51]
Gelatin methacrylate (GelMA) and long-chain poly (ethylene glycol) diacrylate (PEGDA)	Epithelium and stroma	3 D printing of bi-layer dome shaped cell laden scaffold made from GelMA and PEGDA, demonstrated high transmission, swelling, nutrient permeation and appropriate degradation rate	Animal model: rabbit	[52]
methacrylated gelatin (GelMA) and poly(2-hydroxyethyl methacrylate) (pHEMA)	Stroma	Developed novel cell loaded IPN hydrogel made from GelMA-HEMA for corneal stroma model, appropriate mechanical strength, and high transparency	In-vitro	[53]
Collagen and glycol polymer	Full thickness cornea	Interpenetrating polymer network (IPN) hydrogel made from type I collagen and 6-methacryloyl-a-D-galactopyranose (MG) slow biodegradation	In-vitro	[54]
Collagen and phosphorylcholine	Full thickness cornea	Improved mechanical strength and enzymatic stability from collagenase, promising optical clarity	Animal model: mini pigs	[55]

Biomaterial	Target tissue	Novelty	Developmental status	Refs.
Collagen (Col) and pyrene conjugated dipeptide amphiphile (PyKC)	Epithelial, stroma and endothelium	Developed cross-linker-free collagen hydrogel, optically transparent, mechanically, and enzymatically stable, restrict human adenovirus propagation	In-vitro	[32]
Gelatin and poly (ε-caprolactone)-polyethylene glycol)	Stroma	Poly (ε-caprolactone)-poly (ethylene glycol) micro-fibrous scaffold was infused with gelatin methacrylate (GelMA) to make 3D fiber hydrogel, supported differentiation of limbal stromal stem cells to keratocytes or fibroblasts	Animal model: rat	[56]
Recombinant human collagen type III (RHC III) and 2 methacryloyl oxyethylphosphoryl-choline (MPC)	Full thickness cornea	Optimized RHC-III MPC hydrogel to enhance mechanical strength and make it suitable for post-fabrication modification that included micro-contact printing and laser re-shaping	In-vitro studies	[57]
Recombinant human collagen type III (RHC III) and 2 methacryloyl oxyethylphosphoryl-choline (MPC)	Epithelium and stroma	Optimized RHCIII-MPC hydrogel, where the incorporation of the MPC polymer network with reported inflammation suppression properties allowed stable regeneration in corneas of patients with active ulcers and infectious keratitis scarring	Pilot clinical study	[30]
In-situ forming, injectable hydrogels				
Gelatin	Stroma	Visible light crosslinking was used in conjunction with the bioadhesive in-situ GelCORE hydrogel. This hydrogel showed higher tissue adhesiveness than commercially available adhesives	Animal model: rabbit	[58]
Hyaluronate and collagen	Stroma	In-situ forming bio-orthogonally linked hydrogel, highly transparent and good mechanical strength	Animal model: rabbit	[59]
Short collagen-like peptides (CLPs) and polyethylene glycol (PEG)	Epithelium and stroma	In-situ forming, self-assembled liquid hydrogel (LiQD cornea) which gelled spontaneously at body temperature, stimulated regeneration of corneal epithelium, stroma, and nerves for over 1 year, acts as an effective glue filler for patching perforated corneas	Animal model: rabbit and cat	[60]

Table 1.
Advances in the use of natural, biosynthetic, composite, and in-situ forming biomaterials for corneal reconstruction.

5. In-situ gelation-based biomaterials

Recently, in-situ gelation-based, injectable hydrogels have gained attention in corneal tissue engineering because of several advantages over conventional solid implants. Injectable hydrogels can be delivered in a doctor's or ophthalmologist's clinic instead of an operating theater, since there is no need for surgical intervention. The risk of parasurgical infection, patient discomfort, or scar formation is reduced. The in-situ forming hydrogel can adapt to complex tissue cavities, mold, or irregular wounds with better integration [61]. It is easy to encapsulate therapeutic molecules such as peptides, drugs, or exosomes into the hydrogel for synergistic effect. The clinical potential of in-situ forming hydrogels for corneal regeneration has been reviewed by Poudel et al. [61].

In-situ composite hydrogels made from hydroxypropyl chitosan (HPCTS) and sodium alginate dialdehyde via Schiff's base chemistry showed histocompatibility, nontoxicity, and biodegradability. The composite hydrogel incorporating corneal endothelial cells was tested in a rabbit cornea injury model and showed its ability to support the reconstruction of corneal endothelium [62]. An Avastin® containing in-situ forming PEG hydrogel was explored for sustained release of the drug to treat corneal neovascularization. The transparent PEG hydrogel was nontoxic to L-929 cells after 1 week of incubation. The in-situ forming hydrogel showed sustained release of Avastin for up to 14 days without any apparent hydrolysis of the drug molecule [63].

To improve the drug efficacy and increase ocular drug availability, another in-situ forming, thermoresponsive chitosan-gelatin-based hydrogel was developed. The fast-gelling hydrogel was fabricated using β-glycerophosphate disodium salt hydrate (β-GD) and genipin to encapsulate timolol maleate for sustained release. The chitosan gelatin solution was instilled into the lower conjunctival sac of rabbits' eyes to form a hydrogel that provided sustained release of timolol maleate for up to 24 h [64]. Chun et al. developed injectable in-situ forming hydrogel comprising collagen type I that was cross-linked using a multifunctional polyethylene glycol (PEG)-N-hydroxysuccinimide (NHS). When tested for its ability to heal corneal defects, the hydrogel allowed the migration of epithelial cells to form multilayer at the site of corneal stromal defects without inflammation [65].

The GelCORE bioadhesive hydrogel was developed for the sutureless repair of corneal injuries. The highly biocompatible, transparent hydrogel is cured in-situ by visible light cross-linking. In-vivo studies in rabbit corneas showed regeneration of the stroma and epithelium after excision of rabbit corneal tissues [58]. Bio-orthogonally cross-linked hydrogels comprising hyaluronan and collagen showed improved mechanical strength for corneal repair. The in-situ forming hydrogel possesses low refractive index than the native cornea, showed excellent biocompatibility and epithelization in in-vitro and in-vivo studies of partial thickness defects [59].

Griffith and coworkers have recently explored the clinical potential of a fully synthetic hydrogel made from CLP-PEG that incorporated fibrinogen. The "LiQD Cornea" gelled spontaneously in situ at body temperature without the need for light exposure. The hydrogel stimulated the stable (over 1 year) regeneration of corneal epithelium, stroma, and nerves, serving as an alternative to a partial thickness anterior lamellar allografts (**Figure 2C**) [56]. For patients who have corneal perforations (**Figure 2A**), these are emergencies that require patching. The LiQD Cornea was tested and found to also be effective glue-fillers for patching perforated corneas in rabbits, mini-pigs (**Figure 2B** and **C**) [60], and in a cat model [66].

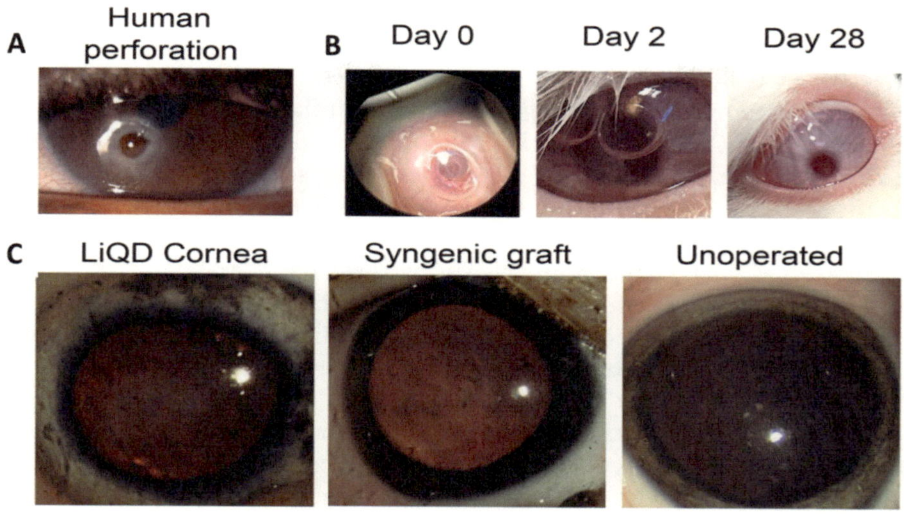

Figure 2.
LiQD hydrogel evaluation in rabbit and mini-pigs (A) Human cornea perforation. (B) Postsurgical perforated rabbit cornea containing LiQD cornea hydrogel at Day 0, 2, and 28. Perforation can be easily seen at Day 0. At Day 2, the air bubble introduced during surgery was prominent, indicating the perforation was sealed. Perforation was healed after 28 days of injecting LiQD cornea hydrogel. (C) Mini pig corneas showing presence of LiQD cornea, syngeneic graft, and unoperated cornea after 12 months of surgery. Reproduced from [60].

6. Role of exosomes in corneal infection and regeneration

Exosomes are membrane-bound extracellular vesicles (EVs) secreted from most cell types into the extracellular space, ranging from 30 to 150 nm in size. The role of exosomes in corneal diseases and their biogenesis during pathological or physiological immune responses has been documented in several studies [67–69]. Secreted exosomes could regulate immune responses as they have the potential for transferring and presenting antigenic peptides, regulating gene expression, and inducing various immune signaling pathways. Furthermore, their detection in a biological fluid can offer a window to the altered cellular or tissue states, and cell-to-cell communication in healthy and disease patients could lead to early diagnosis and potential treatment [70].

Exosomes are natural nanovesicles and are superior to synthetic nanovesicles like liposomes in terms of their stability, biocompatibility, plasma half-life, ability to enter non-accessible tissue regions, and their role in immunomodulation. Exosomes are potentially effective drug delivery vehicles, but their nonspecific targeting feature limits their use in drug delivery applications [71]. However, engineered exosomes secreted by specific cell types could overcome this problem.

Exosomes have recently shown potential in regulating therapeutic functions via cell-to-cell communications. Induced pluripotent stem cells derived exosomes (iPSCs-Exos) are being examined as a natural therapeutic nanoparticle for treating corneal epithelial defects. iPSCs-Exos have induced cell proliferation, migration, cell cycling, and apoptosis inhibition of human corneal epithelial cells (HCECs) in-vitro. Studies also showed the upregulation of cyclin A and CDK2 that induce the HCECs to enter the S phase of the cell cycle for potential regeneration. In vivo studies also revealed the accelerated healing potential of iPSCs-Exos in treating corneal epithelial defects [72]. Zhong and coworkers showed that when exosomes derived from human umbilical cord mesenchymal stem cells (HucMSC-Exos) were combined with an autophagy activator, they positively affected the repair of a corneal injury (CI). The repair process was regulated by accelerated cell proliferation and migration while inhibiting apoptosis and inflammation by activating the AMPKmTOR-ULK1 autophagy pathway [73]. Han et al. [74] examined the possible role of exosomes in corneal wound healing and neovascularization. They showed exosomes between epithelium and stroma after epithelium debridement during the wound healing process. Exosome-like vesicles were also observed in the stroma after anterior stromal keratectomy. They were fused with keratocytes to induce myofibroblast transformation in vitro. These epithelial-derived exosomes also helped induce endothelial cell proliferation, indicating the ability of exosomes to communicate among corneal epithelial cells, keratocytes, and vascular endothelial cells [74].

As these naturally derived nanotherapeutics show emerging potential in treating corneal infection and regeneration, it would be interesting to encapsulate these particles into scaffold/hydrogel for sustained release in clinical applications. In this context, chitosan-based thermoresponsive hydrogels encapsulating exosomes derived from induced pluripotent stem cell–derived mesenchymal stem cells (iPSC-MSCs) were reported to reduce corneal scar formation and accelerated wound healing [75]. In addition, the sustained release of miRNA-containing exosomes helped regenerate the corneal epithelium and stromal layer. The exosomes prevented ECM deposition by downregulating the translocation-associated membrane protein 2 (TRAM2) gene, providing a new strategy for the clinical treatment of fibrotic corneal diseases [75]. Exosomes are paving a new path with their potential utility for early diagnosis and treatment of corneal diseases. Their incorporation into biomaterial-based hydrogels could facilitate their use as therapeutic particles for sustained release in clinical applications.

7. Conclusion and perspective

Corneal transplantation is the only widely accepted treatment for corneal blindness. However, the shortfall of high-quality donor cornea worldwide has made it very challenging. Several approaches have been explored to replace donor corneas, ranging from incorporation of stem cells and decellularized extracellular matrix scaffold to cell-free approaches. Cell-free biomaterial approaches have shown promising potential in promoting in situ corneal regeneration without aggravating the risk of rejection. In-situ gelation of biomaterials opens a new path in corneal regeneration as it does not require extensive surgical intervention, and could reduce the risk of infection, scar formation, and patient discomfort. However, this technique is ineffective in patients with depleted stem or progenitor cells.

More research focusing on developing of biomaterials for high-risk patients is needed. Exosomes derived from cells have recently shown potential in early diagnosis and capabilities to modulate pathological disease state. Future studies should focus on understanding the role of exosomes in corneal pathologies and combining biomaterials with exosomes to explore the additive effect of both strategies.

Finally, it is essential to consider regulatory pathway beforehand while designing and developing corneal implants for clinical applications for effective translation from bench-to-bench side.

Acknowledgements

MG holds a Canada Research Chair Tier 1 in Biomaterials and Stem Cells in Ophthalmology and the Caroline Durand Foundation Chair for Stem Cell Therapy in the Eye. Work done in the Griffith lab has been supported by grants from FRQS, CIHR, NSERC, and the Stem Cell network in Canada, and previous funding from the Swedish Research Council and Vinnova in Sweden.

Conflict of interest

MG's previous university has filed patents that cover RHCIII and RCIII-MPC implants. She has IP disclosures filed for the LiQD Cornea and fully synthetic pro-regeneration corneal implants.

Nomenclature

ALDH3A1	aldehyde dehydrogenase 3A1 (ALDH3A1)
β-GD	β-glycerophosphate disodium salt hydrate
CD34	Cluster of differentiation 34
CEnCs	Corneal endothelial cells
CI	Corneal injury
cLESCs	Canine limbal epithelial stem cells
CLPs	Collagen-like peptides
Col	Collagen
DEX	Dexamethasone
DHL	Decellularized human limbus
ECM	Extra cellular matrix
EDC	1-ethyl-3-(3-dimethyl aminopropyl) carbodiimide hydrochloride
EVs	Extracellular vesicles
Gel MA	Methacrylated gelatin
HA	Hyaluronic acid
HASCs	Human adipose stem cells
HPCTS	Hydroxypropyl chitosan
HucMSC	Human umbilical cord mesenchymal stem cells
iPSCs-Exos	Induced pluripotent stem cells derived exosomes
iPSC-MSCs	Induced pluripotent stem cell-derived mesenchymal stem cells
LEPCs	Limbal epithelial progenitor cells
LKP	Lamellar keratoplasty
LMs	Limbal melanocytes
LSCs	Limbal stem cells
LSCD	Limbal stem cell deficiency
MFX	Moxifloxacin
MPC	2-methacryloyloxyethyl phosphorylcholine
MSCs	Mesenchymal stem cells
NHS	N-hydroxysuccinimide
PCL	Polycaprolactone
PEG	Polyethylene glycol

PEGDA	Poly (ethylene glycol) diacrylate
p(HEMA)	Poly (2-hydroxymethyl methacrylate)
RHC	Recombinant human collagen
RHC III	Recombinant human collagen type III
SF/G	Silk fibroin/gelatin
Silk MA	Methacrylated-silk

Author details

Kamal Malhotra[1,2*] and May Griffith[1,2,3]

1 Department of Ophthalmology, Université de Montréal and Maisonneuve-Rosemont Hospital Research Centre Montreal, Quebec, Canada

2 Centre de recherche du Centre hospitalier de l'Université de Montréal, Montreal, Quebec, Canada

3 Institute of Biomedical Engineering, Université de Montréal, Quebec, Canada

*Address all correspondence to: malhotrakamal.kavi@gmail.com

References

[1] Mobaraki M, Abbasi R, Omidian Vandchali S, Ghaffari M, Moztarzadeh F, Mozafari M. Corneal repair and regeneration: Current concepts and future directions. Frontiers in Bioengineering and Biotechnology. 2019;**7**:135

[2] Mahdavi SS, Abdekhodaie MJ, Mashayekhan S, Baradaran-Rafii A, Djalilian AR. Bioengineering approaches for corneal regenerative medicine. Tissue Engineering and Regeneration Medicine. 2020;**17**(5):567-593

[3] Oliva M, Schottman T, Gulati M. Turning the tide of corneal blindness. Indian Journal of Ophthalmology. 2012;**60**(5):423

[4] Ong JA, Auvinet E, Forget KJ, Lagali N, Fagerholm P, Griffith M, et al. 3D corneal shape after implantation of a biosynthetic corneal stromal substitute. Investigative Ophthalmology & Visual Science. 2016;**57**(6):2355

[5] Gain P, Jullienne R, He Z, Aldossary M, Acquart S, Cognasse F, et al. Global survey of corneal transplantation and eye banking. JAMA Ophthalmology. 2016;**134**(2):167

[6] Hassan SS, Wilhelmus KR, Dahl P, Davis GC, Roberts RT, Ross KW, et al. Infectious disease risk factors of corneal graft donors. Archieves of Ophthamology. 2008;**126**(2):235-239

[7] Patel G, Na KS, Lee HJ, et al. Electrospun fibers for corneal regeneration. Current Ophthalmological Report. 2021;**9**:146-157

[8] Zhang B, Xue Q, Li J, Ma L, Yao Y, Ye H, et al. 3D bioprinting for artificial cornea: Challenges and perspectives. Medical Engineering & Physics. 2019;**71**:68-78

[9] Fuest M, Yam GHF, Mehta JS, Duarte Campos DF. Prospects and challenges of translational corneal bioprinting. Bioengineering. 2020;**7**(3):71

[10] Hsu CC, Peng CH, Hung KH, Lee YY, Lin TC, Jang SF, et al. Stem cell therapy for corneal regeneration medicine and contemporary nanomedicine for corneal disorders. Cell Transplantation. 2015;**24**(10):1915-1930

[11] Sacchetti M, Rama P, Bruscolini A, Lambiase A. Limbal stem cell transplantation: Clinical results, limits, and perspectives. Stem Cells International. 2018;**2018**:8086269

[12] Calonge M, Nieto-Miguel T, de la Mata A, Galindo S, Herreras JM, López-Paniagua M. Goals and challenges of stem cell-based therapy for corneal blindness due to limbal deficiency. Pharmaceutics. 2021;**13**(9):1483

[13] Baylis O, Figueiredo F, Henein C, Lako M, Ahmad S. 13 years of cultured limbal epithelial cell therapy: A review of the outcomes. Journal of Cellular Biochemistry. 2011;**112**(4):993-1002

[14] Demirayak B, Yüksel N, Çelik OS, Subaşı C, Duruksu G, Unal ZS, et al. Effect of bone marrow and adipose tissue-derived mesenchymal stem cells on the natural course of corneal scarring after penetrating injury. Experimental Eye Research. 2016;**151**:227-235

[15] Yan D, Yan C, Yu F, Zhang S, Chen L, Wu N, et al. Exploitation of human mesenchymal stromal cell derived matrix towards the structural and functional restoration of the

ocular surface. Biomaterials Science. 2020;**8**(17):4712-4727

[16] Torsahakul C et al. Bio-fabrication of stem cell incorporated corneal epithelial and stromal equivalents from silk fibroin and gelatin-based biomaterial for canine corneal regeneration. PLoS One. 2022;**17**(2):e0263141

[17] Fiorica C, Senior RA, Pitarresi G, Palumbo FS, Giammona G, Deshpande P, et al. Biocompatible hydrogels based on hyaluronic acid cross-linked with a polyaspartamide derivative as delivery systems for epithelial limbal cells. International Journal of Pharmaceutics. 2011;**414**(1-2):104-111

[18] Kiiskinen J. Co-culture of corneal epithelial cells and adipose stem cells – toward the use of hydrogels in ocular surface reconstruction. University of Tampere: Tampere, Finland. 2016:58

[19] Chen D, Qu Y, Hua X, Zhang L, Liu Z, Pflugfelder S, et al. A hyaluronan hydrogel scaffold-based xeno-free culture system for ex vivo expansion of human corneal epithelial stem cells. Eye. 2017;**31**:962

[20] Polisetti N, Schmid A, Schlötzer-Schrehardt U, Maier P, Lang SJ, Steinberg T, et al. A decellularized human corneal scaffold foranterior corneal surface reconstruction. Scientific Reports. 2021;**11**(1):2992

[21] Polisetti N, Roschinski B, Schlötzer-Schrehardt U, Maier P, Schlunck G, Reinhard T. A decellularized human limbal scaffold for limbal stem cell Niche reconstruction. IJMS. 2021;**22**(18):10067

[22] Alio del Barrio JL, Chiesa M, Garagorri N, Garcia-Urquia N, Fernandez Delgado J, Bataille L, et al. Acellular human corneal matrix sheets seeded with human adipose-derived mesenchymal stem cells integrate functionally in an experimental animal model. Experimental Eye Research. 2015;**132**:91-100

[23] Chen Z, You J, Liu X, Cooper S, Hodge C, Sutton G, et al. Biomaterials for corneal bioengineering. Biomedical Materials. 2018;**13**(3):032002

[24] Griffith M, Poudel BK, MalhotraK, AklaN, González-AndradesM, Courtman D, et al. Biosynthetic alternatives for corneal transplant surgery. Expert Review of Ophthalmology. 2020;**15**(3):129-143

[25] Liu W, Merrett K, Griffith M, Fagerholm P, Dravida S, Heyne B, et al. Recombinant human collagen for tissue engineered corneal substitutes. Biomaterials. 2008;**29**(9):1147

[26] Nong LM, Zhou D, Zheng D, Jiang YQ, Xu NW, Zhao GY, et al. The effect of different cross-linking conditions of EDC/NHS on type II collagen scaffolds: An in vitro evaluation. Cell and Tissue Banking. 2019;**20**(4):557-568

[27] Avila MY, Gerena VA, Navia JL. Corneal crosslinking with genipin, comparison with UV-Riboflavin in ex-vivo model. Molecular Vision. 2012;**18**:1068-1073

[28] Fagerholm P, Lagali NS, Merrett K, Jackson WB, Munger R, Liu Y, et al. Biosynthetic alternative to human donor tissue for inducing corneal regeneration: 24-month follow-up of a phase 1 clinical study. Science Translational Medicine. 2010;**2**(46):46ra61

[29] Fagerholm P, Lagali NS, Ong JA, Merrett K, Jackson WB, Polarek JW, et al. Stable corneal regeneration four years after implantation of a cell-free recombinant human collagen scaffold. Biomaterials. 2014;**35**(8):2420-2427

[30] Islam MM, Buznyk O, Reddy JC, Pasyechnikova N, Alarcon EI, Hayes S, et al. Biomaterials-enabled cornea regeneration in patients at high risk for rejection of donor tissue transplantation. NPJ Regeneration Medicine. 2018;**3**(1):2

[31] Jangamreddy JR, Haagdorens MKC, Mirazul Islam M, Lewis P, Samanta A, Fagerholm P, et al. Short peptide analogs as alternatives to collagen in pro-regenerative corneal implants. Acta Biomaterialia. 2018;**69**:120-130

[32] Islam MM, Chivu A, AbuSamra DB, et al. Crosslinker-free collagen gelation for corneal regeneration. Scientific Reports. 2022;**12**:9108

[33] Haagdorens M, Edin E, Fagerholm P, Groleau M, Shtein Z, Ulčinas A, et al. Plant recombinant human collagen Type I hydrogels for corneal regeneration. Regeneration and Engineering Translational Medicine. 2022;**8**(2):269-283

[34] Kilic Bektas C, Burcu A, Gedikoglu G, Telek HH, Ornek F, Hasirci V. Methacrylated gelatin hydrogels as corneal stroma substitutes: In vivo study. Journal of Biomaterials Science. 2019;**30**(18):1803-1821

[35] Chen Y, Dong L, Kong B, Huang Y, Zhong S, Connon C, et al. Effects of gelatin methacrylate hydrogel on corneal repair and regeneration in rats. Translational Vision Science & Technology. 2021;**10**(14):25

[36] Arica TA, Guzelgulgen M, Yildiz AA, Demir MM. Electrospun GelMA fibers and p(HEMA) matrix composite for corneal tissue engineering. Materials Science and Engineering: C. 2021;**120**:111720

[37] Zhao L, Qi X, Cai T, Fan Z, Wang H, Du X. Gelatin hydrogel/contact lens composites as rutin delivery systems for promoting corneal wound healing. Drug Delivery. 2021;**28**(1):1951-1961

[38] Li L, Lu C, Wang L, Chen M, White J, Hao X, et al. Gelatin-based photocurable hydrogels for corneal wound repair. ACS Applied Materials & Interfaces. 2018;**10**(16):13283-13292

[39] Chang MC, Kuo YJ, Hung KH, Peng CL, Chen KY, Yeh LK. Liposomal dexamethasone–moxifloxacin nanoparticle combinations with collagen/gelatin/alginate hydrogel for corneal infection treatment and wound healing. Biomedical Materials. 2020;**15**(5):055022

[40] Lawrence BD, Marchant JK, Pindrus MA, Omenetto FG, Kaplan DL. Silk film biomaterials for cornea tissue engineering. Biomaterials. 2009;**30**(7):1299-1308

[41] Barroso IA, Man K, Hall TJ, Robinson TE, Louth SET, Cox SC, et al. Photocurable antimicrobial silk-based hydrogels for corneal repair. Journal of Biomedical Materials Research. 2022;**110**(7):1401-1415

[42] Choi J, Jeon H, Song J, Oliveira J, Reis R, Khang G. Biofunctionalized lysophosphatidic acid/silk fibroin film for cornea endothelial cell regeneration. Nanomaterials. 2018;**8**(5):290

[43] Farasatkia A, Kharaziha M, Ashrafizadeh F, Salehi S. Transparent silk/gelatin methacrylate (GelMA) fibrillar film for corneal regeneration. Materials Science and Engineering: C. 2021;**120**:111744

[44] Kao R, Liu CY. Roles of lumican and keratocan on corneal transparency. Glycoconjugate Journal. 2002;**19**(4-5):275-285

[45] Koppaka V, Chen Y, Mehta G, Orlicky DJ, Thompson DC, Jester JV,

et al. ALDH3A1 plays a functional role in maintenance of corneal epithelial homeostasis. PLoS ONE. 2016;**11**(1):e014

[46] Zhang W, Chen J, Qu M, Backman LJ, Zhang A, Liu H, et al. Sustained release of TPCA-1 from silk fibroin hydrogels preserves keratocyte phenotype and promotes corneal regeneration by inhibiting interleukin-1β signaling. Advanced Healthcare Materials. 2020;**9**(17):e2000591

[47] Xeroudaki M, Thangavelu M, Lennikov A, et al. A porous collagen-based hydrogel and implantation method for corneal stromal regeneration and sustained local drug delivery. Scientific Reports. 2020;**10**:16936

[48] Sharifi S, Islam MM, Sharifi H, Islam R, Koza D, Reyes-Ortega F, et al. Tuning gelatin-based hydrogel towards bioadhesive ocular tissue engineering applications. Bioactive Materials. 2021;**6**(11):3947-3961

[49] Mahdavi SS, Abdekhodaie MJ, Kumar H, Mashayekhan S, Baradaran-Rafii A, Kim K. Stereolithography 3D bioprinting method for fabrication of human corneal stroma equivalent. Annals of Biomedical Engineering. 2020;**48**(7):1955-1970

[50] Zhang Y, Li C, Zhu Q, Liang R, Xie C, Zhang S, et al. A long-term retaining molecular coating for corneal regeneration. Bioactive Materials. 2021;**6**(12):4447-4454

[51] Sun X, Yang X, Song W, Ren L. Construction and evaluation of collagen-based corneal grafts using polycaprolactone to improve tension stress. ACS Omega. 2020;**5**(1):674-682

[52] He B, Wang J, Xie M, Xu M, Zhang Y, Hao H, et al. 3D printed biomimetic epithelium/stroma bilayer hydrogel implant for corneal regeneration. Bioactive Materials. 2022;**17**:234-247

[53] Kilic Bektas C, Hasirci V. Cell loaded GelMA:HEMA IPN hydrogels for corneal stroma engineering. Journal of Materials Science: Materials in Medicine. 2020;**31**(1):2

[54] Deng C, Li F, Hackett JM, Chaudhry SH, Toll FN, Toye B, et al. Collagen and glycopolymer based hydrogel for potential corneal application. Acta Biomaterialia. 2010;**6**(1):187-194

[55] Liu W, Deng C, McLaughlin CR, Fagerholm P, Lagali NS, Heyne B, et al. Collagen–phosphorylcholine interpenetrating network hydrogels as corneal substitutes. Biomaterials. 2009;**30**(8):1551-1559

[56] Kong B, Chen Y, Liu R, Liu X, Liu C, Shao Z, et al. Fiber reinforced GelMA hydrogel to induce the regeneration of corneal stroma. Nature Communications. 2020;**11**(1):1435

[57] Mirazul Islam M, Cėpla V, He C, Edin J, Rakickas T, Kobuch K, et al. Functional fabrication of recombinant human collagen–phosphorylcholine hydrogels for regenerative medicine applications. Acta Biomaterialia. 2015;**12**:70-80

[58] Shirzaei Sani E, Kheirkhah A, Rana D, Sun Z, Foulsham W, Sheikhi A, et al. Sutureless repair of corneal injuries using naturally derived bioadhesive hydrogels. Science Advances. 2019;**5**:eaav1281

[59] Chen F, Le P, Fernandes-Cunha GM, Heilshorn SC, Myung D. Bio-orthogonally crosslinked hyaluronate-collagen hydrogel for suture-free corneal defect repair. Biomaterials. 2020;**255**:120176

[60] McTiernan CD, Simpson FC, Haagdorens M, Samarawickrama C,

Hunter D, Buznyk O, et al. LiQD Cornea: Pro-regeneration collagen mimetics as patches and alternatives to corneal transplantation. Science Advances. 2020;**6**:eaba2187

[61] Poudel B, Robert M, Simpson F, Malhotra K, Jacques L, Labarre P, et al. In situ tissue regeneration in the cornea from bench to bedside. Cells, Tissues, Organs. 2022;**211**:506-526

[62] Liang Y, Liu W, Han B, Yang C, Ma Q, Song F, et al. An in situ formed biodegradable hydrogel for reconstruction of the corneal endothelium. Colloids and Surfaces. B, Biointerfaces. 2011;**82**(1):1-7

[63] Yu J, Xu X, Yao F, Luo Z, Jin L, Xie B, et al. In situ covalently cross-linked PEG hydrogel for ocular drug delivery applications. International Journal of Pharmaceutics. 2014;**470**(1-2):151-157

[64] Song Y, Nagai N, Saijo S, Kaji H, Nishizawa M, Abe T. In situ formation of injectable chitosan-gelatin hydrogels through double crosslinking for sustained intraocular drug delivery. Materials Science and Engineering: C. 2018;**88**:1-12

[65] Chun YH, Park SK, Kim EJ, Lee HJ, Kim H, Koh WG, et al. In vivo biocompatibility evaluation of in situ-forming polyethylene glycol-collagen hydrogels in corneal defects. Scientific Reports. 2021;**11**(1):23913

[66] Juarez A, Djallali M, Piché M, Thériault M, Groleau M, Beroual S, et al. A liquid hydrogel to restore long term corneal integrity after perforating and non-perforating trauma in feline eyes. Frontiers in Bioengineering and Biotechnology. 2021;**9**:773294

[67] Robbins PD, Morelli AE. Regulation of immune responses by extracellular vesicles. Nature Reviews. Immunology. 2014;**14**(3):195-208

[68] Liu J, Jiang F, Jiang Y, Wang Y, Li Z, Shi X, et al. Roles of exosomes in ocular diseases. International Journal of Nanomedicine. 2020;**15**:10519-10538

[69] Li N, Zhao L, Wei Y, et al. Recent advances of exosomes in immune-mediated eye diseases. Stem Cell Research & Therapy. 2019;**10**:278

[70] Kalluri R, LeBleu VS. The biology, function, and biomedical applications of exosomes. Science. 2020;**367**(6478): eaau 6977

[71] Li X, Corbett AL, Taatizadeh E, Tasnim N, Little JP, Garnis C, et al. Challenges and opportunities in exosome research-perspectives from biology, engineering, and cancer therapy. APL Bioengineering. 2019b;**3**(1)

[72] Wang S, Hou Y, Li X, Song Z, Sun B, Li X, et al. Comparison of exosomes derived from induced pluripotent stem cells and mesenchymal stem cells as therapeutic nanoparticles for treatment of corneal epithelial defects. Aging. 2020;**12**(19): 19546-19562

[73] Ma S, Yin J, Hao L, Liu X, Shi Q, Diao Y, et al. Exosomes from human umbilical cord mesenchymal stem cells treat corneal injury via autophagy activation. Frontiers in Bioengineering and Biotechnology. 2022;**10**:879192

[74] Han KY, Tran JA, Chang JH, Azar DT, Zieske JD. Potential role of corneal epithelial cell-derived exosomes in corneal wound healing and neovascularization. Scientific Reports. 2017;**7**(1):40548

[75] Tang Q, Lu B, He J, Chen X, Fu Q, Han H, et al. Exosomes-loaded thermosensitive hydrogels for corneal epithelium and stroma regeneration. Biomaterials. 2022;**280**:121320

Chapter 11

Current Diagnostic Tests for Dry Eye Disease in Sjögren's Syndrome

María del Rosario Sánchez Valerio

Abstract

Sjogren's syndrome (Sicca Syndrome) is mainly characterized by the presence of dry eye disease (DED). The diagnosis of DED in patients with Sjogren's syndrome has been limited to tests such as the Schirmer test, tear breakup time (TBUT), and corneal stains; however, currently we can evaluate the functional unit in detail lacrimal, which is affected in patients with dry eye and Sjögren's syndrome; thanks to technology that provides objective details for this difficult diagnostic. The newer evaluations that provide the greatest diagnostic value for Sjogren's syndrome are: noninvasive keratograph tear rupture time (NIKBUT), tear meniscus height (TMH), Schirmer's test, meibography, ocular surface disease index (OSDI), Vital stains of the ocular surface, Matrix Metalloproteinase 9 (MMP-9), Tear osmolarity (TearLab); all of these are important complements to the existing tests, which, although less objective, are not substitutable.

Keywords: NIKBUT (noninvasive keratograph tear rupture time), TMH (tear meniscus height), Schirmer's test, meibography, ocular surface disease index (OSDI), vital stains of the ocular surface, matrix metalloproteinase 9 (MMP-9), tear osmolarity (TearLab)

1. Introduction

Sjögren's syndrome (SS) is a chronic inflammatory disorder characterized by immune-mediated exocrinopathy (inflammation and lymphoplasmacytic infiltration of the lacrimal and salivary glands) with resulting dysfunction. It can occur primarily or in association with a second well-defined rheumatic disease (secondary form). Both ways, they produce inflammation of the exocrine glands with subsequent dry eye and dry mouth [1, 2].

Patients with Sjögren's syndrome (SS) may present with symptoms suggestive of dry eyes. Dry eye typically manifests itself in up to 95% of SS patients; whose complaints are inability to tear, foreign body sensation, conjunctival inflammation, eye fatigue, and decreased visual acuity [3]. Dry eye disease (DED) can be complicated by keratoconjunctivitis sicca, blepharitis, bacterial keratitis, or corneal ulcer [4]. Uveitis, episcleritis, and orbital pseudotumor are systemic manifestations that rarely occur in patients with Sjogren's syndrome [5].

2. Dry eye disease (DED)

"Dry eye disease (DED) is a multifactorial disease of the ocular surface characterized by a loss of homeostasis of the tear film, and accompanied by ocular symptoms, in which tear film instability and hyperosmolarity, ocular surface inflammation and damage, and neurosensory abnormalities play etiological roles." [6]. The description to understand this definition implies the term "multifactorial disease" recognizes DED as a significant and complex functional disorder that cannot be characterized by a single process, sign, or symptom. The term "ocular surface" encompasses structures including the tear film, the lacrimal and meibomian glands, the cornea, the conjunctiva, and the eyelids. "Homeostasis" describes a state of dynamic equilibrium in the body with respect to its various functions and the chemical composition of fluids and tissues. The key elements that contribute to the pathophysiological process, including tear film instability, hyperosmolarity, inflammation, and damage, recognized as etiological triggers of the vicious cycle, were considered important, along with neurosensory abnormalities, which have appeared more and more in recent literature, for inclusion in the definition [6].

2.1 Classification

The DED classification is based on its pathophysiology, acuodeficiency dry eye (ADDE), and evaporative dry eye (EDE). The limit in these categories is extremely diffuse [6]. The Sjogren's syndrome–related ADDE is a secondary phenomenon to immune-mediated exocrinopathy affecting the lacrimal and salivary glands [6]. Findings include decreased tear flow, staining of the ocular surface of injured tissue with vital dyes, and increased tear osmolarity. Meibomian gland dysfunction is also common in SS patients, with a resulting increase in tear evaporation, exacerbating decreased tear production [7, 8].

ADDE not associated with Sjogren's syndrome may be due to primary or secondary deficiency of the lacrimal gland, obstruction of the ducts of the lacrimal gland, and reflex hyposecretion [6]. EDE is due to an excessive loss of water from the exposed ocular surface, in the presence of a normal secretory function, the causes can be extrinsic due to harmful exposure of the ocular surface or intrinsic affecting internal structures or dynamics of the eyelid, may be due to causes related to the eyelid (e.g., Meibomian gland dysfunction [MGD] or decreased blinking) [6].

2.2 Pathophysiology

Tear hyperosmolarity stimulates a cascade of events in ocular surface epithelial cells involving the signaling pathways of MAP and NFkB kinases and the generation of inflammatory cytokines (interleukin 1 [IL-1α; IL-1β]; tumor necrosis factor α [TNF-α]) and proteases, such as MMP-9. This stimulates and readies inflammatory cells on the ocular surface, which become a reservoir for inflammatory mediators. These mediators, in an environment of tear hyperosmolarity, cause a decrease in the expression of mucin in the glycocalyx, the apoptotic death of the superficial epithelial cells, and the loss of goblet cells. However, hyperosmolarity also causes corneal epithelial cell death through nonapoptotic processes. Goblet cell loss is a feature of all types of DED, which is reflected in the reduction of tear levels of MUC5AC. The alteration of mucin expression in the glycocalyx is probably one of the reasons why ocular surface staining occurs in DED and, since it affects the ocular surface wetting, leads to an early breakdown of the film tear. This amplifies or triggers hyperosmolarity on the ocular surface, with which the vicious circle is closed and the mechanism that perpetuates the disease is established [6]. In ADDE, tear hyperosmolarity occurs when tear secretion is reduced due to lack of production, under normal conditions of evaporation from the eye. In EDE, tear hyperosmolarity is caused by excessive evaporation of the tear film with a normally functioning tear gland [6].

2.3 Eye manifestations

Patients with dry eye present with eye irritation, foreign body sensation, burning, tearing, photophobia, stinging, or sharp intermittent pain. They may also complain of blurred vision that improves with blinking or the instillation of artificial tears; and they may have all, some, or none of these symptoms. A well-conducted medical history contributes greatly to a correct diagnosis and guides a more focused slit lamp examination; therefore, a thorough slit lamp examination should be performed prior to performing any other tests, which may alter or mask relevant examination data, resulting in a misdiagnosis. Signs of dry eye identified on slit lamp examination include superficial corneal erosions, inadequate tear lake volume, early tear film breakdown time, conjunctival hyperemia, conjunctival surface irregularities, and meibomian gland dysfunction [7].

2.4 Diagnosis of DED

The evaluation of the tear function is carried out by means of different tests that translate into the presence or absence of DED; however, there is no gold standard for the diagnosis of dry eye disease; therefore, they must frequently be associated with each other for a reliable diagnosis; The most used in the basic ophthalmology office are mentioned in order to compare them with the new technologies for the diagnosis of dry eye and the sequence of how they should be applied; according to diagnosis report methodology subcommittee of the international dry eye workshop (2007) [8]. This is summarized in **Table 1**.

2.5 Current methods of diagnosis

Symptoms and signs found during history and slit lamp examination may suggest dry eye due to water deficiency, evaporation, or both. Additional tests should be performed because the ophthalmologist may be the one who detects SS in a patient with no previous medical history or who debuts with ocular symptoms. Therefore,

Clinic history
Symptom questionnaire (OSDI)
Tear breakup time (TBUT)
Ocular surface by fluorescein staining
Tear secretion (Schirmer test with or without anesthesia)
Other tests according to your availability
Bron et al. [8].

Table 1.
Test sequence basic.

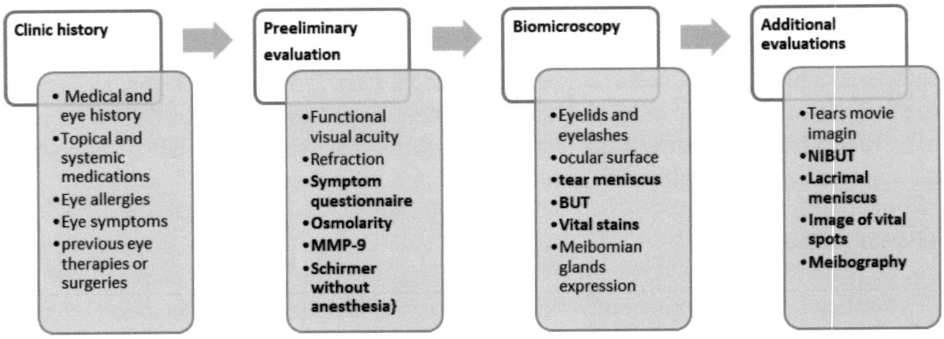

Figure 1.
Sequence of evaluations and tests in dry eye.

the choice of complementary diagnostic methods plays a very important role in the diagnosis, in the same way the sequence to carry out the tests and its correctly applied methodology will be a key point for a successful diagnosis, preventing the tests from overlapping and reporting false negatives or positives [9]. The suggested sequence of evaluations and tests is shown in **Figure 1**.

2.5.1 Symptom questionnaire

The ocular surface disease index (OSDI) was developed to provide a rapid assessment of the symptoms of eye irritation caused by dry eye disease and its impact on vision-related functioning. It is a 12-item questionnaire to evaluate ocular symptoms, functional limitations, and environmental factors related to the environment. Each item has five categories with three subscales with their own type of question; emphasis is placed on symptoms such as photophobia, grit, eye pain, blurred vision, in a period of 2–4 weeks before the visit. The OSDI is a self-administered questionnaire, it contains 12 items to evaluate the symptoms of the ocular surface; that implies little burden and little time for the patient. The OSDI has an overall score and three subscale scores: (A) ocular symptoms [three items], (B) vision-related function [six items], and (C) environmental triggers [three items]. Each OSDI item is scored on a Likert-type scale ranging from 0 to 4 points, where 0 indicates none of the time and 4 all of the time.

The total OSDI score was then calculated based on the following formula; OSDI = [(Sum of the scores of all answered questions) × 100]/[(Total number of answered questions) × 4].

Overall and subscale OSDI scores range from 0 to 100. Based on their OSDI scores, patients can be classified as normal (0–12 points) or mild (13–22 points), moderate (23–32 points) or severe ocular surface disease (33–100 points) [10]. The reliability indices of the OSDI recently reported indicate that it is adequate, the Pearson correlation was higher than 0.8, and the ICC range was from 0.827 to 0.982; In addition, it was evaluated that it has a parallel reliability between the written and web versions [11].

2.5.2 Tear osmolarity

Tear osmolarity in normal subject ranges from 308 to 312 mOsm/l [12]. In individuals with DED associated with SS, osmolarity is significantly higher than in subjects with DED not associated with SS and even more than in healthy controls [13]. Also some studies have shown positive correlations between tear osmolarity and disease activity in patients with SS [14]. Dry eye can be due to both increased evaporation, deficiency in its production, and alteration of the composition, in all cases the pathophysiological sequence culminates with an increase in the osmolarity of the tear film (hyperosmolarity) [15].

The evaporation of a smaller volume for the same surface increases osmolarity during the first 24 h from the beginning of the volumetric decrease [16]. Hyperosmolarity causes epithelial damage directly as it causes cell desquamation, complete disappearance of the superficial epithelial cell layers, decrease in cytoplasmic density, and accumulation of rows of mucus product of osmotically altered goblet cells. This phenomenon is generally evident between 15 and 30 days after the osmolar change of the tear film [17]. The epithelium of the cornea and conjunctiva must be completely moistened for complete wettability; the ocular surface conditions warrant that the surface tension of the aqueous layer at the interface with the epithelium is lower than the surface tension of the epithelium that is exposed to the medium [18]. In the mucous layer, mucopolysaccharides are directly responsible for maintaining surface tension stability. Under hyperosmolar conditions, there is accumulation of mucus and destruction of mucin-secreting cells, which causes an increase in surface tension with the consequent decrease in the wettability of the corneoconjunctival epithelium. The principle of osmosis is characterized by the flow of a solvent through a semipermeable membrane, which is generated when there is a difference in concentrations on one side of the membrane; this movement tends to equalize the solute concentrations on both sides, and there the flow stops. The corneoconjunctival epithelium and the mucous layer are a semipermeable barrier on the ocular surface, by increasing osmolarity in the aqueous layer; the aqueous gradient through the water protein channels present in the stroma and toward the aqueous humor; they change in the opposite direction. This directional fluid change produced by hyperosmolarity can cause dehydration of Sulfated Glycosaminoglycan (GAGS) that occupies the spaces between the collagen fibers of the stroma [19, 20]. When these glycoprotein structures are dehydrated, the correct water balance of the stroma will be affected, which will affect the normal maintenance of corneal transparency [21].

The osmolarity of the tear film in dry eye triggers inflammation, immunological processes, and the presence of autoantigens that enhance the inflammatory process. As an example of this, inflammatory markers such as NF-Kβ that migrates from the nucleus to the cytoplasm in the inflammatory process are directly related to the phenomenon of hyperosmolarity of the tear film. Nuclear translocation of NF-Kβ has been shown to be directly proportional to increased tear film osmolarity [22].

Hyperosmolarity is so important in the pathophysiology of dry eye disease that increased osmolarity of the tear film has been suggested to induce functional and structural damage to the corneal nerves and neurotoxicity [23].

The TFOS Dry Eye Workshop II (DEWS II) subcommittee report concluded: "Tear hyperosmolarity is considered to be the trigger for a cascade of signaling events within surface epithelial cells, leading to the release of inflammatory mediators and proteases. These mediators and tear hyperosmolarity cause the loss of goblet cells, epithelial cells and damage to the epithelial glycocalyx. The inflammatory mediators of activated T cells, recruited on the ocular surface, reinforce the damage; resulting in punctiform epitheliopathy characteristic of DED and tear film instability leading to early tear film rupture. This rupture increases the hyperosmolarity of the tear and completes the vicious circle events that cause damage to the ocular surface" [24]. While sophisticated equipment is required to measure tear film osmolarity, we can assess the sodium concentration that we obtain from tears by wetting a Whatman 41 paper strip in the usual way for the Schirmer test, then colorimetrically measuring the sodium concentration in that. More specifically, the Tear Lab osmolarity system is designed to measure tear osmolarity and facilitate diagnosis in patients with suspected dry eye syndrome. Tear Lab measures osmolarity in 10 s and integrates seamlessly into clinical workflow. The evaluation of tear osmolarity has been shown to be a superior marker to determine the severity of DED, with respect to TBUT, Schirmer I, corneal and conjunctival staining, Meibomian classification and OSDI, whose specificities are (60%, 79%, 85%, 67%, 76%, and 79%) respectively. The test card in conjunction with the Tear Lab Osmolarity System offers a quick and easy method to determine tear osmolarity using nanoliter (nl) volumes of tear fluid obtained directly from the edge of the eyelid. To perform a test, a new test card must be inserted into the collecting pen; then contact the tip of the pen with the tear meniscus, located on the lower eyelid. Once the collection is complete, the pen is placed in the reader's docking station, which will display a quantitative osmolarity test result on the liquid crystal display (LCD) (**Figure 2**). The Tear Lab osmolarity system simplifies the tear collection process by eliminating the need to move tear fluid samples and reducing the risk of evaporation [25].

2.5.3 Matrix metalloproteinase 9 (MMP-9)

The matrix metalloproteinase test (MMP-9) is a useful technique to complement the diagnosis of DED recently developed. Matrix metalloproteinase 9 is an inflammatory biomarker that has been shown to be elevated in the tears of dry eye patients [26]. In tears, MMP-9 expression is normally less than 40 ng/ml and is secreted from the ocular surface epithelium [27]. MMP-9 maintains epithelial barrier function by

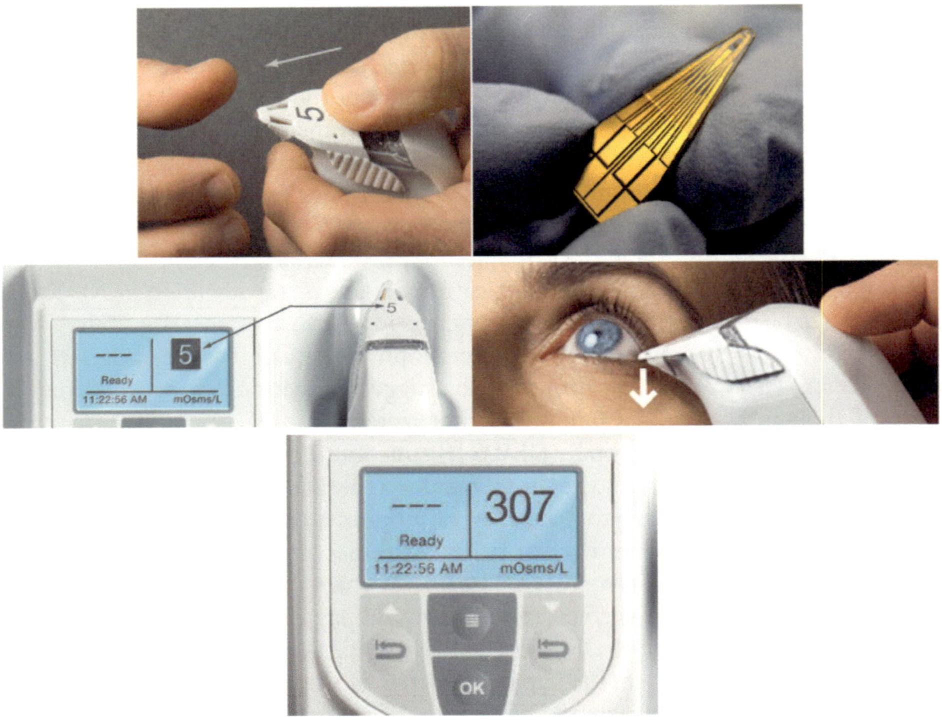

Figure 2.
TearLab.

breaking down components of the epithelial basement membrane and tight junction proteins, such as ZO-1 and occludin [28, 29]. But in addition, MMP-9 is related to the pathogenesis of various diseases, such as sterile ulceration, ocular allergy, keratoconus, conjunctivachalasia, and DED [30–32].

In the pathology of DED, since tear hyperosmolarity begins in the early phase of DED, a vicious circle probably induces inflammatory processes and triggers the release of MMP-9 in a relatively late phase of DED [33]. Detection of elevated MMP-9 in tears could be an ideal tool for the diagnosis and treatment of tear dysfunction [34].

The technique for using the MMP-9 device (InflammaDry test) is as follows: the sampling fleece is contacted three times at each location of the lower eyelid conjunctiva (temporal, middle and nasal; from nasal to temporal direction), and it rests against the temporal conjunctiva of the lower eyelid for an additional 5 s. After the sampling fleece is assembled on a sample collector and pressed, the test strip is immersed in a solution for 20 s; 10 min after taking the sample, the result is read (**Figure 3**).

InflammaDry, this type of device has the advantages of low cost, quick analysis, and ease of device preparation. However, it has been studied that a small sample volume, the reliability of the test result can be significantly affected [35].

It has been studied that the elevation of tear MMP-9 in patients with ED appears to have a good diagnostic yield and a correlation with the clinical severity of DED [26, 27]. The reliability for this test was 85% sensitivity and 94% specificity for the diagnosis of DED [36]. But despite these very promising values, two separate reports showed moderate to low positivity in an immunoassay for MMP-9 in study subjects with DED [36–38]; reporting that there were no differences between subjective symptoms and clinical signs of DED between MMP-9 positive and negative groups [37, 38]. In general, although it is a nonspecific marker for patients with DED [39, 40], various immunoassays have reported its usefulness as an aid in the diagnosis of dry eye; however, there are factors that may influence the results of MMP-9 in tears; one of them was demonstrated in an

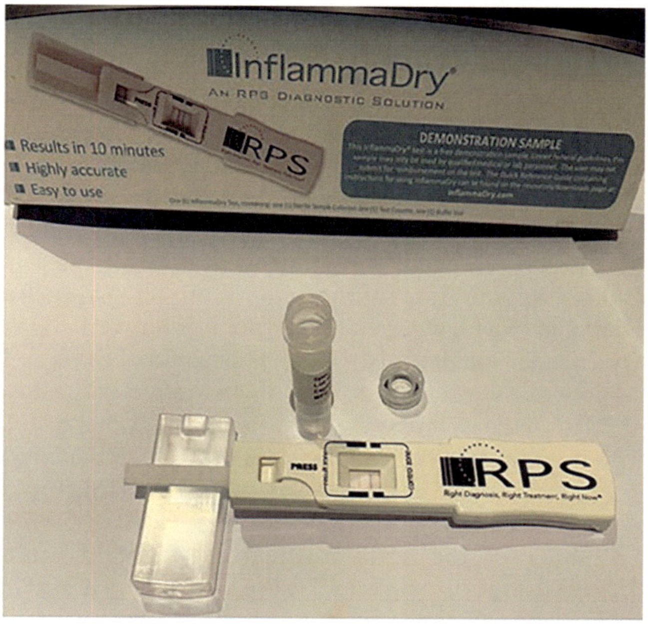

Figure 3.
InflamaDry.

immunoassay where it was concluded that the positivity of the test can depend on the volume of the load and that therefore it can cause false negatives in diseases with aqueous deficiency such as Sjögren's syndrome or graft-versus-host disease [41]. Other useful benefits are the identification of patients with inflammation of the ocular surface and autoimmune disease and can facilitate the decision to establish an anti-inflammatory treatment in these patients [30]. In the same way, its usefulness for the preoperative management of the ocular surface was reported, reducing possible complications when there is an underlying disease. Additionally, this test can also help indicate the need for anti-inflammatory therapies, such as cyclosporine or steroids, and can also predict which patients are most likely to respond [42].

2.5.4 The Schirmer test

The Schirmer test was introduced by Schirmer in 1903, despite the time and disadvantages of performing it, it is still used in most parts of the world, as part of the dry eye test battery. The Schirmer test is a diagnostic method to evaluate the production of watery tears [43, 44]. Topical anesthesia may or may not be used during the procedure, depending on the physician's preference, and may even include nasal stimulation to induce reflex tearing. The Schirmer test allows the study of total tear secretion, that is, it evaluates the sum of the basal secretion plus the reflex secretion if performed without anesthesia; but if performed under anesthesia, it measures the basal secretion produced by the accessory lacrimal glands located in the conjunctiva. The Schirmer test is a diagnostic method to evaluate the production of watery tears [44, 45].

Initially, the method described to perform the Schirmer 1 test is as follows: it should be performed a few minutes after the instillation of topical anesthetic to inhibit the reflex secretion produced by the main lacrimal gland. Whatman No. 1 filter paper 5 mm wide and 35 mm long is used. It is placed in the cul-de-sac at the level of the outer third of the lower eyelid, in a low-light environment, with the patient with his eyes open, and the length of the paper that has absorbed moisture is measured at 5 min [46].

The Schirmer test remains a useful and repeatable test; although over the years several authors have made modifications to their methodology to improve the reliability of the test results; Such studies have been justified by mentioning the lack of practicality for ophthalmologists, especially when performing it routinely due to the 5-min time frame [45]. Therefore, correlations have been evaluated between the different wetting times, the size of the paper strip, or whether it is done with eyes open or closed [45, 47, 48]. The results are controversial. Some authors support the hypothesis that the shorter durations of the 5-min Schirmer test, such as the 1-min test under anesthesia, have a high correlation with the 5-min test and will make this test much more practical for patients [45]. Others affirm that the correlation in this modification was poor and consider it inappropriate to shorten the duration of the Schirmer test [49]. As this controversy has been generated, other tests have been tried with a shorter soak time, such as the Schirmer test of 2 min under anesthesia, and that the 3 mm wide paper strip could be used instead of the standard strip of 5 mm wide; finding results that correlate well with the 5-min test [47]. Then another study was conducted with a 3-min time, the results of which reveal that the 3-min Schirmer test is a reliable alternative for the diagnosis of dry eye and is more useful in daily ophthalmic practice [50]. The position of the eyes (open or closed) when performing the Schirmer test has shown important differences in its results; moisture values in the Schirmer test with eyes open have been reported to show significantly higher results compared with eyes closed [51, 52]; this may be due to the open eyes moving during the blink, stimulating tearing under the influence of the strip.

Other factors that could influence the results of the Schirmer test are head position, lighting, strip position, corneal condition, humidity, and ambient temperature, so it is important to consider these factors to achieve the standardization of this important diagnostic tool [51].

Therefore, the recommendation to perform the Schirmer test under anesthesia is to perform it with the eyes closed; this could reduce humidity variations, evaporation, and especially reflex tearing [51, 52].

The interpretation of the results of the Schirmer test is different depending on whether anesthesia is used or not. In patients with dry eye, there are clinical differences between the ADDE and EDE types, since the presence of ADDE strongly suggests the suspicion of Sjogren's syndrome; however, although they also present differences in the physiology of tears between these types, no significant differences are found in tear osmolarity, volume, or distribution [53]. In the Schirmer test without anesthesia, total secretion (basal and reflex) is evaluated, the cutoff point is between 10 and 15 mm, and in the Schirmer test with anesthesia, reflex secretion is evaluated, and the cutoff point for this test is ≤5.5 mm/5 min; sensitivity is 85% and specificity is 83% [54]. The Schirmer II test is used on special occasions, as it requires stimulation of the nasal surface with a cotton-tipped applicator and subsequent measurement of reflex tear production. The disadvantages of the Schirmer test, in all its variants, are the time required, patient discomfort, and the low reliability of the test [54, 55].

2.5.5 Tear breakup time (TBUT)

The tear breakup time (TBUT) measures the stability of the tear film. With instilled fluorescein, TBUT is the time interval after a patient blinks until the first appearance of dryness in the tear film [56]. TBUT is measured by inoculating fluorescein into the cul-de-sac, asking the patient to hold the eyelids open after 1–2 blinks, and counting the seconds until a dry spot appears. The appearance of dry spots in less than 10 s is considered abnormal (**Figure 4**) [57]. Subsequently, alternative values

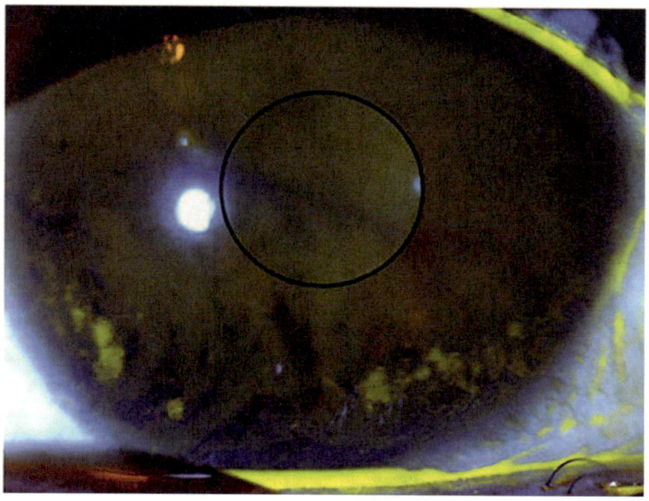

Figure 4.
TBUT.

for BUT are determined by comparing young populations with dry eye and healthy controls, reporting that values less than 5 s occur in subjects with dry eye [58]. The TBUT presents a sensitivity of 72.2% and specificity of 61.6%. The standardization of the method to perform the tear rupture time was carried out by Johnson and Murphy in 2005 [59]. The procedure is summarized in **Table 2**.

Although this test is inexpensive, quick to perform, and uses readily available supplies, it is poorly reproducible and inaccurate [60, 61]. However, the average score of two separate TBUT measurements helps increase their repeatability [62].

2.5.6 Noninvasive keratograph breakup time (NIKBUT)

The tear breakup time (TBUT) was considered one of the most repeatable tear film measurements and although invasive, easy to perform, and interpret [63, 64]. TBUT traditional objective tests are often limited by their invasiveness and low test repeatability and reproducibility [64]. For this reason, new methods of evaluation of the tear film emerged and with the help of the keratograph 5M (K5M) topography, a more objective way of evaluating tear film stability emerged; calling this measurement noninvasive keratograph breakup time (NIKBUT). The time is measured in seconds between the last complete blink and the first alteration of the Placido rings projected on the corneal surface, which the device automatically detects and

1. Instill 1st 5 ul sodium fluorescein 2% in cul-de-sac
2. The patient is asked to blink naturally, loosely so that the fluorescein is naturally distributed.
3. After 10–30 s, the patient is asked to look straight ahead without blinking until instructed.
4. Set the magnification of the biomicroscope to 10×, keep the background illumination constant (cobalt blue light) and use a 12 Wratten yellow filter to improve the observation of the tear film over the entire ocular surface.
5. Use a stopwatch to record the complete blink time and the appearance of a growing micelle.
Tomado de [59].

Table 2.
Evaluation of tear rupture time.

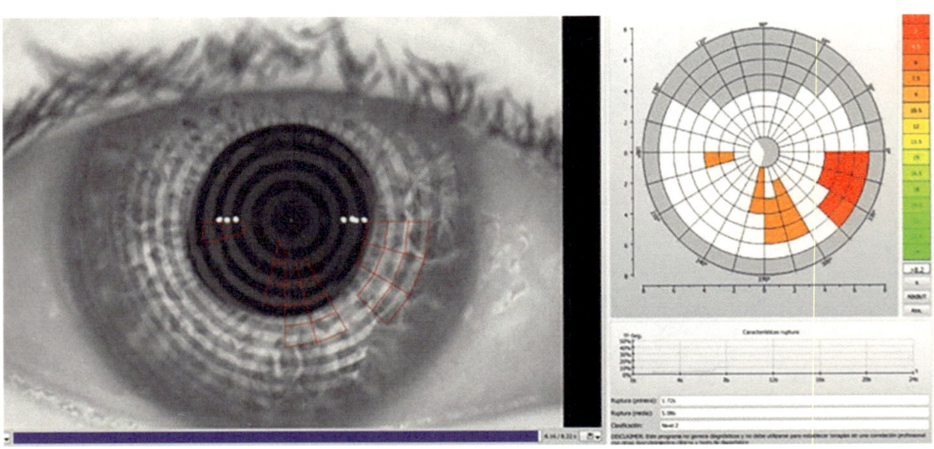

Figure 5.
NIKBUT.

measures. K5M performs two measurements for NIKBUT: the time when the first tear film break occurs (NIKBUT-first) and the average time of all tear incidents (average NIKBUT) (**Figure 5**). Oculus K5M provides noninvasive, objective, and reproducible tear film measurements [65].

2.5.7 Sjögren's international collaborative clinical alliance ocular surface staining (SICA OSS)

Ocular surface staining with various dyes is used to characterize the disease, assess its severity, and monitor the clinical response to therapy. Fluorescein stains macro-ulcerative and punctate epithelial defects (positive staining) and appears orange under cobalt blue light. Classification of ocular surface staining after instillation of vital dyes is a critical diagnostic component of dry eye. These changes in the ocular surface are now documented with various staining scales such as Oxford, Nei-Clek, and SICA OSS [66]. The evaluation of the ocular surface and the qualification of the three scales are carried out with the methodology described in **Table 3**.

To evaluate the SICCA OSS, it gives the same numerical weight to the corneal and conjunctival changes, the staining must be done in two steps. Fluorescein staining is first performed and the cornea is examined with the slit lamp using the cobalt blue filter. Corneal epithelial staining is a dynamic and time-sensitive process; therefore, to ensure that the test is reproducible, the fluorescein evaluation should begin 4–8 min after instillation of the dye. Punctate epithelial erosions (PEE) that stain with fluorescein are counted and scored as follows. If there is no PEE, the score is 0. If 1–5 PEE are seen, the corneal score is 1 (**Figure 1a**). From 6 to 30 PEE they are scored as 2; and >30 PEE are scored as 3. An additional point is added if: (1) PEE occurred in the central 4 mm diameter part of the cornea (**Figure 1b**); (2) one or more filaments are seen anywhere on the cornea; or (3) one or more confluence patches. The spots, including the linear spots, are found anywhere on the cornea (**Figure 1c**). The fluorescein score for the cornea (the PEE grade plus any extra points for modifiers) is noted in the center square of the SICCA eye staining score form (**Figure 2**). The maximum possible score for each cornea is 6 [67].

The second step is the evaluation of the conjunctiva with lysamine green, it is observed in the slit lamp using a 10× magnification but with reduced illumination and using a neutral density filter. It is important to examine and grade the eyes immediately after applying the lysamine green tint because the intensity and spread of the tint in the eye rapidly diminish after the first 2 min. In addition, the patient must blink several times to prevent the dye from accumulating in the conjunctival folds, which can mimic conjunctival staining. If the dye is not properly instilled, a second drop can be administered and the test is performed immediately afterward.

1. Fluorescein is applied
2. The biomicroscope is configured with 10× magnification and use of cobalt blue light in addition to a yellow filter.
3. Cornea: The upper eyelid is lifted to evaluate the total score of the staining or its absence.
4. Conjunctiva: To determine the degree of staining of the nasal and temporal conjunctiva, the subject is asked to look to the opposite side to evaluate said area.
Tomado de [66].

Table 3.
Evaluation of the ocular surface (Oxford, Nei-cleck and Sica OSS).

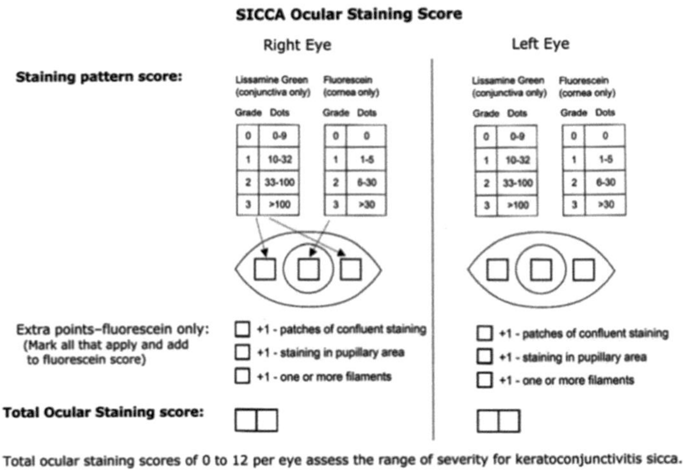

Figure 6.
Sjogren international collaboration clinical Alliance (sicca) ocular staining score form.

The evaluation of this second staining in SICCA OSS, grade 0 (**Figure 3a**) is defined as 0–9 points of lysamine green staining of the interpalpebral bulbar conjunctival (nasal and temporal bulbar conjunctiva classified separately); grade 1 (**Figure 3b**) is defined by the presence of 10–32 points; grade 2 (**Figure 3c**) from 33 to 100; and grade 3 (**Figure 3d**) >100 points. Due to the difficulty of counting individual points in a moving eye in the slit lamp, any area of confluent staining ≥ 4 mm^2 is considered >100 points. The nasal and temporal areas of the conjunctiva are classified separately with a maximum score of 3 for each area or a maximum total score of 6 for each eye (nasal plus temporal). The total SICCA OSS value for each eye is the sum of the fluorescein score for the cornea and the lysamine green scores for the nasal and temporal bulbar conjunctiva. Therefore, the maximum possible score for each eye is 12. The eyes are classified separately and the scores are recorded on the SICCA OSS Eye Staining Scoring Form at each patient visit. Pinguecula stain, pterygium, and Schirmer's strip artifacts should not be included in the evaluation [67].

A value greater than 0 is considered abnormal and can be a sign of KCS. But scores of 1 or 2 can also represent a late staining artifact, if in the corneal fluorescein interpretation the staining pattern is delayed more than 8 min. Since this could lead to a high level of misclassification, an abnormal OSS is defined as a score of 3 or more (**Figure 6**) [67].

In one study, the relationship between serological markers and dry eye severity was investigated in subjects with primary Sjögren's syndrome (SS). The serum markers anti-Ro/SSA, anti-La/SSB, rheumatoid factor (RF) and antinuclear antibody (ANA), ocular surface disease index (OSDI), Schirmer test I values, time to rupture of the tear film, and SICCA ocular staining score (OSS) were determined. Finding what serum RF and ANA levels are associated with conjunctival staining scores and total OSS based on SICCA OSS in primary SS [68].

2.5.8 The tear meniscus height (TMH)

The meniscus, or lacrimal lake, is the amount of tears that rest at the junction of the bulbar conjunctiva and the margin of the lower eyelid. Measurements of the height and curvature of the tear meniscus are used to determine the presence or absence of dry eye [65]. The normal height of the tear meniscus is 0.2–0.5 mm; but in patients with dry eye, it is usually less than 0.2 mm [69, 70]. The evaluation of the tear meniscus should be carried out without having instilled artificial tears or other types of drops; since it can be higher and therefore unreliable; although measurement of the tear meniscus is a good parameter for determining tear production, a low tear lake alone does not necessarily indicate dry eye and should be used as an adjunct to other dry eye tests [69]. The tear meniscus can be reliably assessed using a slit lamp that is capable of micrometer measurements, or it can be done by taking a photograph of the tear meniscus after instilling a small amount of fluorescein. Tear meniscus height (THM) is a noninvasive test for tear quantification and is used as a reliable and repeatable adjunct to the diagnosis of DED [71]. Placido's advanced topography, the keratograph 5M (K5M; Oculus Optikgerate GmbH, Wetzlar, Germany), has additional imaging modalities designed to measure TMH [72, 73]. TMH can also be measured using a corneal adapter, in optical coherence tomography, RTVue-100 FD-OCT system (Optovue, Fremont, AC); reliably and noninvasively. Studies comparing these technologies found that although the tear meniscus height measurements measured with keratography are lower than those taken with OCT, they are closely correlated with each other; therefore, either method could be useful to assess the height of the tear meniscus more objectively [74]. Lacrimal meniscus height (TMH) is an important test because it shows a positive correlation with the value of the Schirmer test [75, 76]. Lacrimal point occlusion in patients with dry eye has been shown to induce increases in the volumes of the upper and lower tear meniscus, but no change in lacrimal menisci of control eyes; this may indicate the presence of a self-regulatory mechanism in the lacrimal system that maintains balance in tear volume (**Figure 7**) [77].

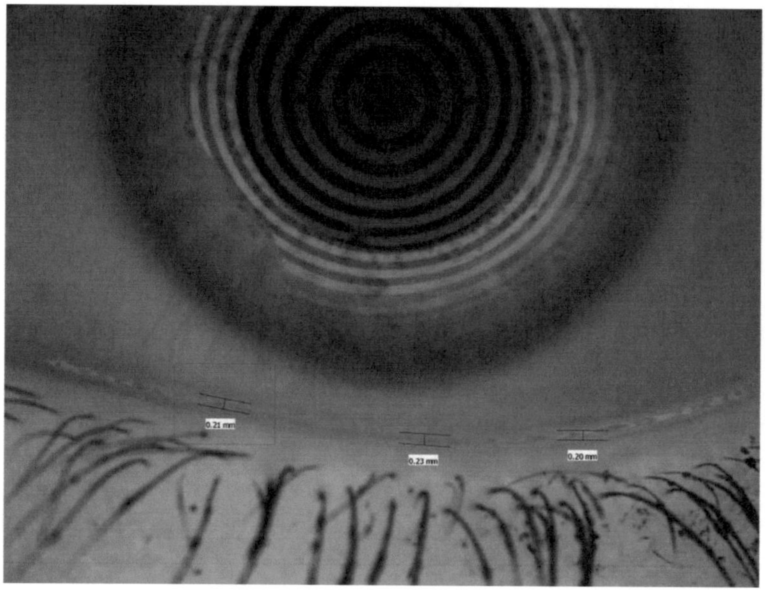

Figure 7.
Tear meniscus height.

2.5.9 Meibography

The meibomian glands are highly specialized sebaceous glands that secrete a lipid compound that is responsible for tear stability. Meibomian gland disease (MGD) is defined as a chronic and diffuse abnormality of the meibomian glands (MG), commonly characterized by terminal duct obstruction and qualitative/quantitative changes in glandular secretion [78]. The prevalence of MGD in published studies ranges from 20% to 70%, depending on diagnostic criteria for evaluating MGD and geographic differences [79, 80]. MGD is considered the main cause of evaporative dry eye [81, 82].

The pathophysiology of MGD is complex and involves several mechanisms and risk factors, including primary obstructive keratinization of the MG orifices, inflammation of the eyelids, abnormal MG secretion, and changes in the microbial flora of the ocular surface or Demodex infestation [24].

Among the main mechanisms of pathophysiology of MGD in patients with SS, the following have been proposed. Women with pSS have been shown to have androgen deficiency similar to that of patients with SLE and RA [83]; in these patients there is a significant decrease in serum levels of androgen precursors (DHEA [dehydroepiandrosterone] and DHEA sulfate), which are the main substrate for androgen synthesis in peripheral tissues. Androgen deficiency in humans has been found to be associated with an increase in eyelid keratinization and the number of occluded and metaplastic orifices of MGs; reduction in the quality of meibum; altered lipid patterns of the meibum; a decrease in the breakup time of the tear film; increased corneal staining with consequent increase in DED symptoms. It has been proposed that the beneficial effect of androgens stimulates the function of this glandular tissue, increasing its lipogenesis and suppressing its keratinization, this may explain why androgen therapy relieves signs and symptoms of DGM and DED in humans [24].

Additionally, it has been proposed that androgen deficiency can lead to a decrease in the influence of insulin-like growth factor 1 (IGF-1) on the meibomian glands. These androgens increase IGF-1 production, positively regulate IGF-1 receptor expression, modulate IGF-1 signaling, and stimulate human meibomian gland epithelial cell function [84]. On the other hand, there is an accumulation of lymphocytes in the conjunctiva of patients with SS and leads to signs of tarsal and periglandular inflammation. Such conjunctival inflammation can create a toxic environment, leading to the release of proinflammatory cytokines that affect the terminal duct of the meibomian gland [85]; as evidence of this, both SSp and SSs subjects and MGD patients showed occluded metaplastic orifices of the MG, as well as decreased quality of the secretions of these glands. These signs are characteristic of obstructive MGD (hyperkeratinization of the terminal duct epithelium, reduced quality of the meibum, and posterior obstruction) [24]. It has been hypothesized that some symptoms in pSS patients, such as sleep disturbances, depressed mood, and fatigue, may also lead to GDM due to decreased blinking, as the above symptoms are already the result of a lower secretion of dopamine, positively with the frequency of blinking. In patients with SS, the lacrimal glands are severely damaged early in the disease; however, the meibomian glands in patients with SSp will undergo further deterioration when the clinical history of dry eye is more than 3 years [85].

Another mechanism contributing to MGD in SS may be that lymphocytic infiltration adjacent to the tarsal conjunctiva in SS could trigger gland destruction.

However, it is possible that conjunctival inflammatory cytokines secreted in the tear film promote hyperkeratinization of the terminal duct epithelium of the meibomian gland [24]. Another process implicated in the pathophysiology of MGD in SSp may be a cytokine-induced alteration in neural-meibomian gland epithelial cell interactions. The meibomian gland is the only sebaceous gland in the human body that has elaborate sensory, sympathetic, and parasympathetic innervation. We found that parasympathetic neurotransmitters and their agonists exert a significant influence on human meibomian gland epithelial cell activity. These cells contain muscarinic acetylcholine and vasoactive intestinal peptide receptors, and the ligands of these receptors stimulate the adenylyl cyclase pathway, enhance intracellular [Ca^{2+}], and can promote cell proliferation [85, 86].

Meibography is a diagnostic technique that allows in vivo evaluation of the morphology of the meibomian glands [87, 88]. For its evaluation, several techniques have been developed, among which are meibography with infrared light. This uses ultraviolet light to produce fluorescence of the gland, the eyelid is everted and through transillumination photographs are obtained to obtain images, which are later graded according to the loss of the meibomian glands. The classification of these images go from 0 to 3; being 0 when there is no loss, 1 when the loss of glands is less than one-third, 2 when the loss is between one-third and two-thirds and 3 when the loss is greater than two-thirds. Meibomian glands are observed differently depending on the method to evaluate them, for example, they appear as dark areas on a lighter background in the contact technique. In contrast, noncontact meibography

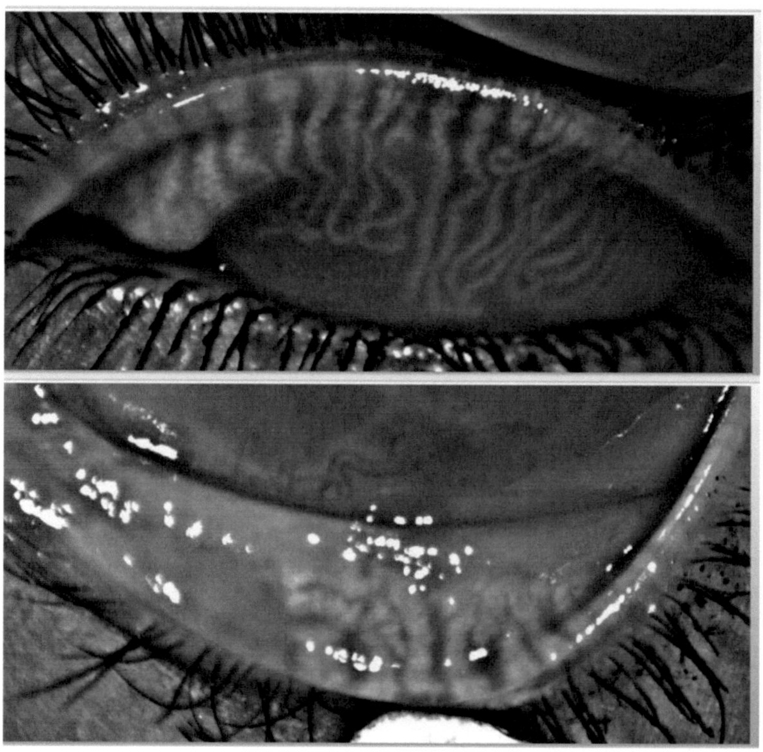

Figure 8.
Meibography.

reveals the meibomian glands as reflected images, and the glands appear as light areas on a darker background [89]. The types of meibography that allow the capture of the morphology of the Meibomian gland in the form of photographs or films are LipiView 2; Tear Science, Cobra, LipiScan, and Tearscope [89]. The meiboscore [87] and the meibo-scale [90] are classification systems to quantify the loss of area of the meibomian gland. The meiboscores of the upper and lower eyelids are summed to obtain a total score of 0–6 for each eye [87]. In contrast, meibo-scale assigns a value from 0 to 4 for each eyelid [90]. The sensitivity and specificity for the diagnosis of MGD by noncontact meibography (cutoff value for meiboscore of +3) as a single test were found to be 49.3% and 64.5%, respectively [91]. The diagnosis of obstructive MGD based on any of the three scores (ocular symptom score, eyelid margin anomaly score, and meiboscore) resulted in a sensitivity of 100% and a specificity of 68.3%; the diagnosis based on two of the three abnormal scores yielded a sensitivity of 84.9% and a specificity of 96.7%; and diagnosis based on the fact that all three scores were abnormal yielded a sensitivity of 66.0% and a specificity of 100% (**Figure 8**) [92].

3. Conclusions

The new emerging technologies for the diagnosis of DED represent a more objective way of talking about this entity that does not have a gold standard for its diagnosis, they facilitate the work and are very useful for research purposes. It is also important to mention that these technologies are of great help to provide an accurate diagnosis and accurate treatment; however, the preexisting tests for the diagnosis of DED are still useful and when applied with adequate methodology and the required sequence, they provide reliable data to make a correct diagnosis of DED; therefore they continue to be valid and must continue to be transmitted to new generations, especially to take advantage of contact with the patient and clinical observation that is not substitutable with anything.

Acknowledgements

My sincere thanks to MD Jose Antonio Alameda Chavez, Laura Ximena Alameda S.; Alondra Alameda S., Angel Antonio Alameda S., for his great collaboration in the elaboration of this manuscript, and in addition to C. Luis Velez, who was involved in its elaboration, was still my source of inspiration.

Conflict of interest

I seriously declare that I have no interest whatsoever, only the academic one, in the elaboration of this chapter.

Notes/thanks/other declarations

I express special thanks for the invitation for the collaboration of this chapter and to the authors of the references included in it.

List of abbreviations

AntiRho/SSA and AntiLa/SSB	Antibodies
ANA	Antinuclear antibodies
DED	Dry eye disease
DEWS II	Dry eye workshop II
ADDE	Acuodeficiency dry eye
EDE	Evaporative dry eye
TMH	Tear meniscus height
RF	Rheumatoid factor
GAGS	Sulfated glycosaminoglycan
IL	Interleukin
K5M	Keratograph 5M
KCS	keratoconjunctivitis sicca
MMP-9	Matrix metalloproteinase 9
MGD	Meibomian gland dysfunction
MUC5A	Mucin 5A
OSDI	Ocular surface disease index
OCT	Optical Coherence Tomography
PEE	Punctate Epithelial Erosions
TBUT	Tear breakup time
TNF	Tumor Necrosis factor
NIKBUT	Noninvasive keratograph breakup time
NFkB	Nuclear factor enhancer of the kappa light chains of activated B cells
SS	Sjögren Syndrome
SICA OSS	Sjögren's International Collaborative Clinical Alliance Ocular Surface Staining

Author details

María del Rosario Sánchez Valerio
Hospital Angeles Puebla, Puebla, México

*Address all correspondence to: rosyoft_@hotmail.com; rosaval79.88@gmail.com

References

[1] Mariette X, Criswell LA. Primary Sjögren's syndrome. The New England Journal of Medicine. 2018;**378**:931

[2] Wang X, Bootsma H, Terpstra J, et al. Progenitor cell niche senescence reflects pathology of the parotid salivary gland in primary Sjögren's syndrome. Rheumatology (Oxford). 2020;**59**:3003

[3] Vivino FB, Bunya VY, Massaro-Giordano G, et al. Sjogren's syndrome: An update on disease pathogenesis, clinical manifestations and treatment. Clinical Immunology. 2019;**203**:81

[4] Kassan SS, Moutsopoulos HM. Clinical manifestations and early diagnosis of Sjögren syndrome. Archives of Internal Medicine. 2004;**164**:1275-1284

[5] Retamozo S, Acar-Denizli N, Rasmussen A, Horváth IF, Baldini C, Priori R, et al. Systemic manifestations of primary Sjögren's syndrome out of the ESSDAI classification: Prevalence and clinical relevance in a large international, multi-ethnic cohort of patients. Clinical and Experimental Rheumatology. 2019;**37**:97-106

[6] Craig J, Nichols K, Akpek E, Caffery B, Dua H, Joo C, et al. TFOS DEWS II definition and classification report. The Ocular Surface. 2017;**15**(3): 276-283

[7] Zeev MS, Miller D, Latkany R. Diagnosis of dry eye disease and emerging technologies. Clinical Ophthalmology. 2014;**8**:581-590

[8] Bron AJ, Abelson MB, Ousler G, Pearce E, Tomlinson A, Yokoi N, et al. Methodologies to diagnose and monitor dry eye disease: Report of the diagnostic methodology subcommittee of the international Dry Eye Workshop (2007). Ocular Surface. 2007;**5**(2):108-152

[9] Milner MS, Beckman KA, Luchs JI, Allen QB, Awdeh RM, Berdahl J, et al. Dysfunctional tear syndrome: Dry eye disease and associated tear film disorders - new strategies for diagnosis and treatment. Current Opinion in Ophthalmology. 2017;**27**(Suppl 1):3-47

[10] Schiffman R. Reliability and validity of the ocular surface disease index. Archives of Ophthalmology. 2000;**118**(5):615

[11] Zhang XM, Yang LT, Zhang Q, Fan QX, Zhang C, You Y, et al. Reliability of Chinese web-based ocular surface disease index questionnaire in dry eye patients: A randomized, crossover study. International Journal of Ophthalmology. 2021;**14**:834-843 10.18240/ijo.2021.06.07

[12] Potvin R, Makari S, Rapuano CJ. Tear film osmolarity and dry eye disease: A review of the literature. Clinical Ophthalmology. 2015;**9**:2039-2047

[13] Méndez GV, Mohamed-Noriega K, Mohamed J, et al. Meibomian gland dysfunction in primary Sjögren's syndrome. ARVO Annual Meeting. 2017;**58**(8)

[14] Schargus M, Wolf F, Tony H-P, Meyer-ter-Vehn T, Geerling G. Correlation between tear film osmolarity, dry eye disease, and rheumatoid arthritis. Cornea. 2014;**33**:1257-1261

[15] Gilbard JP, Farris RL. Tear osmolarity and ocular surface disease in keratoconjunctivitis sicca. Archives of Ophthalmology. 1979;**97**:1642-1646

[16] Holly FJ, Patten JT, Dohlman CH. Surface activity determination of aqueous tear components in dry eye patients and normals. Experimental Eye Research. 1977;**24**:479-491

[17] Gilbard JP, Farris RL, Santamaria J. Osmolarity of tear microvolumes in keratoconjunctivitis sicca. Archives of Ophthalmology. 1978;**96**:677-681

[18] Holly FJ, Lamberts DW. Effect of nonisotonic solutions on tear film osmolarity. Investigative Ophthalmology & Visual Science. 1981;**20**:2336-2345

[19] Fujikawa LS, Foster CS, Gipson IK, Colvin RB. Basement membrane components in healing rabbit corneal epithelial rounds: Immunofluorescence and ultrastructural studies. Journal of Cell Biology. 1984;**98**:128-138

[20] Funderburgh JL, Cintron C, Covington HI, Conrad GW. Immunoanalysis of keratan sulfate proteoglycan from corneal scars. Investigative Ophthalmology & Visual Science. 1988;**29**:116-124

[21] Tseng SCG, Hirst LW, Maumenee AE, Kenyon KR, Sun TT, Green WR. Possible mechanisms for the loss of goblet cells in mucin- deficient disorders. Ophthalmology. 1984;**91**:545-552

[22] Berra A, Berra M. Hyperosmolarity induce nuclear translocation of NF-KB in human conjunctiva epithelial cells. Investigative Ophthalmology & Visual Science. 2005;**46**:4402

[23] Hirata H, Miserska K, Mafurt C, Rosenblatt M. Hyperosmolar tears induce functional and structural alterations of corneal nerves: Electrophysiological and anatomical evidence toward neurotoxicity. Investigative Ophthalmology & Visual Science. 2015;**56**(13):8125-8140

[24] Bron A, de Paiva CS, Chauhan SK, Bonini S, Gabison EE, Jain S, et al. TFOS DEWS II pathophysiology report. The Ocular Surface. 2017;**15**:438-510

[25] Sullivan BD, Whitmer D, Nichols KK, Tomlinson A, Foulks GN, Geerling G, et al. An objective approach to dry eye disease severity. Investigative Ophthalmology & Visual Science. 2010;**51**(12):6125-6130. DOI: 10.1167/iovs.10-5390 Epub 14 July 2010. PMID: 20631232

[26] Yazdani M, Elgstøen KBP, Rootwelt H, Shahdadfar A, Utheim ØA, Utheim TP. Tear metabolomics in dry eye disease: A review. International Journal of Molecular Sciences. 2019;**20**:3755

[27] Korb DR. Survey of preferred tests for diagnosis of the tear film and dry eye. Cornea. 2000;**19**:483-486

[28] Schargus M, Geerling G, Joachim SC. Significance of new methods of examining the tear film in dry eye disease: tear film osmolarity and matrix metalloproteinases (MMP-9). Klinische Monatsblätter für Augenheilkunde. 2018;**235**:597-602

[29] Lemp MA, Bron AJ, Baudouin C, Benítez Del Castillo JM, Geffen D, Tauber J, et al. Tear osmolarity in the diagnosis and management of dry eye disease. American Journal of Ophthalmology. 2011;**151**:792-798

[30] Messmer EM, von Lindenfels V, Garbe A, Kampik A. Matrix metalloproteinase 9 testing in dry eye dis- ease using a commercially available point-of-care immunoassay. Ophthalmology. 2016;**123**:2300-2308

[31] Sambursky R, Davitt WF 3rd, Friedberg M, Tauber S. Prospective, multicenter, clinical evaluation of point-of-care matrix metalloproteinase-9 test for

confirming dry eye disease. Cornea. 2014;**33**:812-818

[32] Asahi M, Wang X, Mori T, Sumii T, Jung JC, Moskowitz MA, et al. Effects of matrix metalloproteinase-9 gene knock-out on the proteolysis of blood-brain barrier and white matter components after cerebral ischemia. The Journal of Neuroscience. 2001;**21**:7724-7732

[33] Sternlicht MD, Werb Z. How matrix metalloproteinases regulate cell behavior. Annual Review of Cell and Developmental Biology. 2001;**17**:463-516

[34] Schargus M, Geerling G, Joachim SC. Significance of new methods of examining the tear film in dry eye disease: tear film osmolarity and matrix metalloproteinases (MMP-9). Klinische Monatsblatter für Augenheilkunde. 2018;**235**:597-602. German. DOI: 10.1055/s-0042-121424 PMID: 28147407

[35] Acera A, Vecino E, Duran JA. Tear MMP-9 levels as a marker of ocular surface inflammation in conjunctivochalasis. Investigative Ophthalmology & Visual Science. 2013;**54**:8285-8291

[36] Sambursky R, Davitt WF, Latkany R, et al. Sensitivity and specificity of a point-of-care matrix metalloproteinase 9 immunoassay for diagnosing inflammation related to dry eye. JAMA Ophthalmology. 2013;**131**(1):24-28

[37] Baudouin C, Messmer EM, Aragona P, Geerling G, Akova YA, Benı'tez-del-Castillo J, et al. Revisiting the vicious circle of dry eye disease: A focus on the pathophysiology of meibomian gland dysfunction. The British Journal of Ophthalmology. 2016;**100**:300-306

[38] Park JY, Kim BG, Kim JS, Hwang JH. Matrix metalloproteinase 9 point-of-care immunoassay result predicts response to topical cyclosporine treatment in dry eye disease. Translational Vision Science & Technology. 2018;**7**:31

[39] Aragona P, Aguennouz M, Rania L, Postorino E, Sommario MS, Roszkowska AM, et al. Matrix metalloproteinase 9 and transglutaminase 2 expression at the ocular surface in patients with different forms of dry eye disease. Ophthalmology. 2015;**122**:62-71

[40] Pinto-Fraga J, Enríquez-de-Salamanca A, Calonge M, González-García MJ, López-Miguel A, López de la Rosa A, et al. Severity, therapeutic, and activity tear biomarkers in dry eye disease: An analysis from a phase III clinical trial. The Ocular Surface. 2018;**16**:368-376

[41] Lanza NL, McClellan AL, Batawi H, Felix ER, Sarantopoulos KD, Levitt RC, et al. Dry eye profiles in patients with a positive elevated surface matrix metalloproteinase 9 point-of-care test versus negative patients. The Ocular Surface. 2016;**14**:216-223

[42] Kaufman HE. The practical detection of mmp-9 diagnoses ocular surface disease and may help prevent its complications. Cornea. 2013;**32**:211-216

[43] Pflugfelder SC, Tseng SC, Sanabria O, et al. Evaluation of subjectiveassessments and objective diagnostic tests for diagnosing tear-film disor-ders known to cause ocular irritation. Cornea. 1998;**17**:38-56

[44] Farris RL, Gilbard JP, Stuchell RN, Mandel ID. Diagnostic tests in kerato-conjunctivitis sicca. The CLAO Journal. 1983;**9**:23-28

[45] Bawazeer AM, Hodge WG. One-minute schirmer test with anesthesia. Cornea. 2003;**22**(4):285-287

[46] Van Bijsterveld OP. Diagnostic tests in the sicca syndrome. Archives of Ophthalmology. 1969;**82**(1):10-14. DOI: 10.1001/archopht.1969.00990020012003

[47] Suphakasem S, Lekskul M, Rangsin R. Assessment of different wetting time and paper strip size of Schirmer test in dry eye patients. Journal of the Medical Association of Thailand. 2012;**95**(Suppl 5):S107-S110 PMID: 22934455

[48] Li N, Deng XG, He MF. Comparison of the Schirmer I test with and without topical anesthesia for diagnosing dry eye. International Journal of Ophthalmology. 2012;**5**(4):478-481. DOI: 10.3980/j.issn.2222-3959.2012.
04.14 Epub 18 August 2012. PMID: 22937509; PMCID: PMC3428545

[49] Recep ÖF. Is it possible to shorten the duration of Schirmer test I? Turk Oftalmoloiji Dergisi. 2012;**42**(5):355-358. DOI: 10.4274/tjo.42.73745 2

[50] Özdemir M, Akçay M. Three-minute Schirmer test. Turkiye Klinikleri Journal of Medical Sciences. 2009;**29**(1):146-149

[51] Rieger G. Schirmer-Test in Lokalanästhesie bei geöffneten oder geschlossenen Augen? [The Schirmer test in local anesthesia in open or closed eyelids]. Fortschr Ophthalmol. German. 1986;**83**(2):79-80. PMID: 3710387

[52] Serruya LG, Nogueira DC, Hida RY. Schirmer test performed with open and closed eyes: Variations in normal individuals. Arquivos Brasileiros de Oftalmologia. Jan-Feb 2009;**72**(1):65-67. DOI: 10.1590/S0004-27492009000100013. PMID: 19347125

[53] Khanal S, Tomlinson A, Diaper CJ. Tear physiology of aqueous deficiency and evaporative dry eye. Optometry and Vision Science. 2009;**86**(11):1235-1240

[54] Methodologies to diagnose and monitor dry eye disease: Report of the diagnostic methodology subcommittee of the International Dry Eye WorkShop (2007). The Ocular Surface. Apr 2007;**5**(2):108-152. DOI: 10.1016/s1542-0124(12)70083-6. PMID: 17508118

[55] Damato BE, Allan D, Murray SB, Lee WR. Senile atrophy of the human lacrimal gland: The contribution of chronic inflammatory disease. The British Journal of Ophthalmology. 1984;**68**:674

[56] Lemp MA. Breakup of the tear film. International Ophthalmology Clinics. 1973;**13**(1):97-102

[57] Vitali C, Moutsopoulos HM, Bombardieri S. The Europen Community Study Group on diagnostic criteria for Sjögren's syndrome. Sensitivity and specificity of tests for ocular and oral involvement in Sjögren's syndrome. Annals of the Rheumatic Diseases. 1994;**5310**:637-647

[58] Abelson M, Ousler G, Nally L. Alternative values for tear film breakup time in normal and dry eye populations. Advances in Experimental Medicine and Biology. 2002;**506**(Part B):1121-1125

[59] Johnson M, Murphy P. The effect of instilled fluorescein solution volume on the values and repeatability of TBUT measurements. Cornea. 2005;**24**(7):811-817

[60] Vanley GT, Leopold IH, Gregg TH. Interpretation of tear film breakup. Archives of Ophthalmology. 1977;**95**(3):445-448

[61] Lin YY, Carrel H, Wang IJ, et al. Effect of tear film break-up on higher order aberrations of the anterior cornea

in normal, dry, and post-LASIK eyes. Journal of Refractive Surgery. 2005;**21**(5):S525-S529

[62] Nichols KK, Mitchell GL, Zadnik K. The repeatability of clinical measurements of dry eye. Cornea. 2004;**23**(3):272-285

[63] Phadatare SP, Momin M, Nighojkar P, Askarkar S, Singh KK. A comprehensive review on dry eye disease: diagnosis, medical management, recent developments, and future challenges. Advances in Pharmaceutics. 2015;**2015** Article ID 704946, 12 pages

[64] Mengher LS, Bron AJ, Tonge SR, Gilbert DJ. A non invasive instrument for clinical assessment of the pre-corneal tear film stability. Current Eye Research. 1985;**4**(1):1-7

[65] Tian L, Qu JH, Zhang XY, Sun XG. Repeatability and reproducibility of noninvasive keratograph 5M measurements in patients with dry eye disease. Journal of Ophthalmology. 2016;**2016**:8013621. DOI: 10.1155/2016/8013621 Epub 12 April 2016. PMID: 27190639; PMCID: PMC4844888

[66] Bron A, Evans V, Smith J. Grading of corneal and conjunctival staining in the context of other dry eye tests. Cornea. 2003;**22**(7):640-650

[67] Whitcher J, Shiboski C, Shiboski S, Heidenreich AM, Kitagawa K, Zhang S, et al. A simplified quantitative method for assessing keratoconjunctivitis sicca from the Sjögren's syndrome international registry. American Journal of Ophthalmology. 2010;**149**(3):405-415

[68] Lim SA, Nam S, Kwok SK, Park SH, Chung SH. Serologic markers are associated with ocular staining score in primary Sjögren syndrome. Cornea. 2015;**34**(11):1466-1470

[69] Mainstone JC, Bruce AS, Golding TR. Tear meniscus measurement in the diagnosis of dry eye. Current Eye Research. 1996;**15**(6):653-661

[70] Guillon JP. Non-invasive tearscope plus routine for contact lens fitting. Contact Lens & Anterior Eye. 1998;**21**(Suppl 1):S31-S40

[71] Holly FJ. Physical chemistry of the normal and disordered tear film. Transactions of the Ophthalmological Societies of the United Kingdom. 1985;**104**(4):374-380

[72] Ibrahim OMA, Dogru M, Takano Y, et al. Application of visante optical coherence tomography tear meniscus height measurement in the diagnosis of dry eye disease. Ophthalmology. 2010;**117**(10):1923-1929

[73] Koh S, Ikeda C, Watanabe S, et al. Effect of non-invasive tear stability assessment on tear meniscus height. Acta Ophthalmologica. 2015;**93**(2): e135-e139

[74] Abdelfattah NS, Dastiridou A, Sadda SR, Lee OL. Noninvasive imaging of tear film dynamics in eyes with ocular surface disease. Cornea. 2015;**34**: S48-S52

[75] Savini G, Barboni P, Zanini M. Tear meniscus evaluation by optical coherence tomography. Ophthalmic Surgery, Lasers & Imaging. 2006;**37**(2):112-118

[76] Chen F, Shen M, Chen W, Wang J, Li M, Yuan Y, et al. Tear MENISCUS VOLUME IN DRY EYE AFTER PUNCTAL occlusion. Investigative Ophthalmology & Visual Science. 2010;**51**(4):1965-1969

[77] Lamberts DW, Foster CS, Perry HD. Schirmer test after topical anesthesia and the tear meniscus height in normal eyes.

Archives of Ophthalmology. 1979;**97**(6):1082-1108

[78] Arita R. Meibography: A Japanese perspective. Investigative Ophthalmology and Visual Science. 2018;**59**(14 Special Issue):DES48-DES55

[79] Geerling G, Baudouin C, Aragona P, et al. Emerging strategies for the diagnosis and treatment of meibomian gland dysfunction: Proceedings of the OCEAN group meeting. The Ocular Surface. 2017;**15**:179-192

[80] Eballe' AO, Ellong A, Wang RE, et al. Meibomian glands dysfunction and ocular surface in black people. Journal Français d'Ophtalmologie. 2019;**42**:127-132

[81] Stapleton F, Alves M, Bunya VY, et al. TFOS DEWS II epidemiology report. The Ocular Surface. 2017;**15**:334-365

[82] Schaumberg DA, Nichols JJ, Papas EB, et al. The international workshop on meibomian gland dysfunction: Report of the subcommittee on the epidemiology of, and associated risk factors for, MGD. Investigative Ophthalmology & Visual Science. 2011;**52**:1994-2005

[83] Sullivan DA, Rocha EM, Aragona P, Clayton JA, Ding J, Golebiowski B, et al. TFOS DEWS II sex, gender, and hormones report. The Ocular Surface. 2017;**15**:284-333

[84] Ding J, Liu Y, Sullivan DA. Effects of insulin and high glucose on human meibomian gland epithelial cells. Investigative Ophthalmology & Visual Science. 2015;**56**:7814-7820

[85] Sullivan DA, Dana R, Sullivan RM, Krenzer KL, Sahin A, Arica B, et al. Meibomian gland dysfunction in primary and secondary sjogren syndrome. Ophthalmic Research. 2018;**59**:193-205. DOI: 10.1159/000487487

[86] Hikichi T, Yoshida A, Tsubota K. Lymphocytic infiltration of the conjunctiva and the salivary gland in Sjögren's syndrome. Archives of Ophthalmology. 1993;**111**:21-22

[87] Arita R, Itoh K, Inoue K, Amano S. Noncontact infrared meibography to document age-related changes of the meibomian glands in a normal population. Ophthalmology. 2008;**115**:911-915

[88] Alsuhaibani AH, Carter KD, Abramoff MD, et al. Utility of meibography in the evaluation of meibomian glands morphology in normal and diseased eyelids. Saudi Journal of Ophthalmology. 2011;**25**:61-66

[89] Robin M, Liang H, Rabut G, Augstburger E, Baudouin C, Labbé A. The role of meibography in the diagnosis of meibomian gland dysfunction in ocular surface diseases. Translational Vision Science and Technology. 2019;**8**(6):14-46

[90] Pult H, Riede-Pult BH. Non-contact meibography: Keep it simple but effective. Contact Lens & Anterior Eye. 2012;**35**:77-80

[91] Finis D, Ackermann P, Pischel N, et al. Evaluation of meibomian gland dysfunction and local distribution of meibomian gland atrophy by non-contact infrared meibography. Current Eye Research. 2015;**40**:982-989

[92] Arita R, Itoh K, Maeda S, et al. Proposed diagnostic criteria for obstructive meibomian gland dysfunction. Ophthalmology. 2009;**116**:2058-2063

Section 4

Retinal Imaging

Chapter 12

Optic Coherence Tomography Angiography in Diabetic Retinopathy

Sara Crespo Millas, Salvatore Di Lauro, David Galarreta Mira and Maria Isabel López Gálvez

Abstract

Diabetic retinopathy (DR) is a progressive microvascular disease considerer as the most important cause of acquired vision loss in the world. OCT angiography (OCT-A) has drastically improved the diagnosis and follow-up of DR showing alterations before changes in the fundus will be visible. With OCT-A, it is possible to quantify several parameters such as the macular vascular density (MVD) and foveal avascular zone (FAZ). This new technique will be important for early detection, follow- up, and monitoring treatment response. OCTA is a very promising image technique that is continually improving and offers numerous advantages over FA in DR management; nevertheless, there are technical limitations that must be improved.

Keywords: diabetic retinopathy, retina, optic coherence tomography

1. Introduction

Diabetic retinopathy (DR) is a progressive microvascular disease considered as the most important cause of acquired vision loss in the world [1]. World Health Organization (WHO) estimated that in 2030 about 366 millions of adults will be affected with diabetes mellitus (DM) and 191 million with DR [2].

DR is characterized by functional and structural alterations on retinal microcirculation. Ischemia is one of the most important factors for progression of DR. Retinal ischemia is responsible of oxygen defect in retinal tissues because retinal neurons need high levels of oxygen, and this supposes an increased production of pro-angiogenic factor such as vascular endothelial growth factor (VEGF) [3, 4].

Histopathological findings show the existence of structural changes in vascular wall that preceded the visible changes on fundus [5, 6].

On the last decade, optical coherence tomography (OCT) and its recent evolution to the OCT angiography (OCT-A) have drastically improved the diagnosis and follow-up of DR [7].

OCT-A is a technic that allows analysis *in vivo*, is painless, and separates the different retinal vascular plexus, something impossible with the traditional techniques. Currently, it has recognized four vascular plexus: superficial capillary plexus (SCP), intermediate capillary plexus(ICP), deep capillary plexus (DCP), and peripapillary radial plexus (PRP) (localized in the peripapilar retinal nervous fiber layer) [8].

The OCT-A shows alterations in these plexus before changes in the fundus will be visible. The earlier stage of DR is defined for the presence of microaneurysm (MA) on the fundus but before that already exist histopathological changes on retinal capillaries. Thus, OCT-A would allow to identify patients affected with DR without fundus changes.

2. Retinal lesions and OCT-A

OCT-A identifies a large number of MA that cannot be detectable on fundus exploration, but less than fluorescein angiography (FA) due to slow hematic flow in the aneurismatic dilatations [9]. Also it is possible to analyze each plexus separately. For that, it has been possible to observe that the majority of MA is located in the DCP [9, 10]. The MA could be classify following its internal reflectivity (hyper or hypo). The hyperreflective ones are associated with high flow and damage in the hemato-retinal barrier and edema. The hyporreflectives has low flow and are more difficult to detect by the OCT-A [11].

Furthermore, OCT-A is capable of detecting other vascular anomalies such as intraretinal vascular anomalies (IRMA) and define its structural characteristics and extension. It is possible to identify the changes in these vascular anomalies after the treatment with anti-VEGF drugs or laser photocoagulation.

Shimouchi et al. studied the characteristics of IRMAs before and after panretinal photocoagulation and identified five types of IRMA: (1) without changes after laser; (2) tuft type; (3) with reperfusion; (4) mix of 2 and 3; (5) worse after the laser. Types 2 and 5 were more related with proliferative diabetic retinopathy (PDR) [12].

IRMAs were identified as dilated and tortuous vessels near ischemia areas [13–15]. Compared with IRMAs, retinal neovascularization (RNV) alters the internal limiting membrane (ILM) [13] and could be identified by observing the flow signal above ILM [13, 16].

With OCT-A it is possible to identify early points of retinal neovascularization, impossible to differentiate from an MA in FA. Furthermore, OCT-A is better than FA in the accuracy identification of lesion limits as the leakage of the FA could blur the RNV border [13].

3. Measure parameters in OCT-A

With OCT-A it is possible to quantify the macular vascular density (MVD), defined as the proportion of vessels related to the total area studied over the base of a binarized image [9]. It is necessary to interpret the images with caution as the values vary according to sex and age, and they are related with image quality. In general, MVD values are progressively minor from healthy people to diabetic patients without DR and PDR [9, 17].

It is especially clear that the visualization of the foveal avascular zone (FAZ) has improved with the introduction of OCT-A. In healthy eyes, FAZ has very well-defined edges without interruptions [8]. FAZ enlargement can result from capillary occlusion with perifoveal arteriole loss easily identified by OCT-A [17]. In addition, there is a clear association between FAZ enlargement and vision loss in patients with DR [18]. OCTA is better than FA for FAZ detection because there is no interference caused by colorant leakage, it is noninvasive and fast, allowing a better imaging comparison over the time. Several studies show that FAZ enlargement already occurs in patients with DM1 and DM2 before any sign of DR can be detected [19–22]. These findings could be useful to identify patients without DR but with higher risk to develop the disease. However, there is a great variability in FAZ size in healthy people (0.071–0.527 mm^2), with higher values in eyes with short axial length [9]. For this reason, FAZ circularity more than size may be useful to identify pathological changes. Some of the quantitative parameters about the ZAF include: ZAF area, acircularity index (AI), axis ratio (AR), and perimeter. AI is the ratio between the ZAF perimeter and the perimeter of a circle with equal area. The AR is the ratio between major and minor axis [13]. AI and AR are greater in patients with DR and greater in patients with PDR versus NPDR [23].

3.1 New parameters

Some of the new parameters that are being studied include: vascular diameter index (VDI), fractal dimension (FD), vascular tortuosity (VT), perfusion density (PD), and skeletonized vascular density (SVD) [9, 13]. VDI is an index of the mean vessel caliper [9]. Increased values are related to rapid increases in blood glucose [9]. FD measures the complexity of the vessels pattern. FD values are lower in diabetic eyes in the SCP and DCP, but it is not related to DR severity [24]. VT is higher in diabetic patients and could be useful for early detection of DR [9]. PD is an index of vessel perfusion in a determinate area, and lower values are related with DR severity and BCVA [25]. SVD vessels longitude eliminating potential confusing factors being more sensible in identifying non-perfusion. SVD in SCP and DCP is inversely related with DR severity [26].

OCTA is also useful to identify and quantify macular ischemia (MI) in the different retinal plexus.

Diabetic macular edema (DME) is the leading cause of vision loss in patients with DR and can be visualized in the OCTA en face as non-flow areas with smooth edges that do not follow surrounding vessels [27].

3.2 The role of OCTA in DR early detection

MVD is reduced in DM1 and DM2 patients in the SCP and DCP in the foveal and perifoveal area without detectable DR [28–31].

FAZ is also affected, being greater in patients without DR [22, 32].

Sun et al. have found an association between FAZ, MVD and FD values in the DCP with the risk of develop DR [33]. Greater FAZ area was related with a risk ratio (RR) of 1.829 for increase of standard deviation (SD), low MVD with a RR of 1.908 for decrease of SD and low FD with a RR of 4.464 for decrease of SD [33]. Furthermore, low values of MDV in the SCP are related with the development of DME [33].

3.3 DR severity

Increased FAZ, reduced FAZ circularity, low MVD, increased VDI, reduced FD, and increased VT are associated with DR severity [25, 34–38]. Basing on these findings, it has been investigated the possibility to automatically detect and grade the severity of DR with the aid of the artificial intelligence and using the MVD, vascular caliper, and FAZ in the SCP and DCP with an accuracy of 94.3% (area under the curve (AUC) = 0.92) and reaching an accuracy of 96% (AUC = 0.96) when OCTA is combined with OCT [39].

3.4 DR progression

Actually, we have very limited knowledge about the predictive value of OCTA in DR progression (most of published studies are transversal). Nevertheless, some recent prospective studies have found a relation between DCP parameters and DR progression with statistical significance [33]. On contrary, SCP parameters do not seem to be associated with DR progression, probably because the DCP is more susceptible to ischemia (higher metabolic requirements of external retina) [40].

3.5 OCTA and DME

DME is still a problem for a correct interpretation of OCTA images. In fact, cystic macular edema affects the automatic segmentation of the software and affects image quality. This is especially evident in the DCP, because signal intensity is lower [41]. Cysts may compress the vessel wall, lowering the flow. OCTA can consider these areas as avascular [42].

According to Coscas et al., three patterns of DME can be identified by OCTA [43]:

- Hypointense intraretinal spaces: rounded structures located near non-perfusion areas in the DCP

- Grayish intraretinal spaces: big grayish cysts, can be confused with intervascular spaces

- Focal hyperintense points: hard exudates

3.6 OCTA and choroid

The choroid is the main source of oxygen and nutrients for external retina to understand DR pathogeny. Increased choriocapillaris (CC) non-perfusion has been described already in patients without signs of DR [37]. OCTA surely represents a significant advance compared with FA for studying the CC, but the deep localization of this complex vascular structure makes it difficult to get high-quality images. The perfusion defect (PD) is the area where it is not possible to identify flow between the OCTA limits of detection [44, 45]. PD could be an interesting parameter to study CC involvement in DR and is significantly higher in DM patients compared with normal eyes [45]. New prospective studies are needed to clarify the importance of the CC in DR.

3.7 OCTA limitations

One of the most important limitations of OCTA is the great variability in the algorithms used by different manufacturers. The immediate consequence is the difficulty of comparing images obtained with different devices [13, 46]. Projection and movement artifacts can be especially frequent in patients with macular lesions and DME, severely affecting image quality (up to 30% of images have to be discarded) [38, 46]. Simple vitreous opacities can affect image quality and interpretation [46]. Furthermore, most of the quantitative and qualitative parameters used in the literature are obtained with an external software after exporting the images, through a slow process and, on many occasions, with manual segmentation. This is absolutely unfeasible in clinical practice, where fast processing systems directly associated with the devices are needed [46]. Without these premises, these OCTA parameters will not be useful in clinical practice.

4. Conclusions

OCTA is a very promising image technique that is continually improving and offers numerous advantages over FA in DR management. Many clinical studies indicate their usefulness in early diagnosis, follow-up, identification of prognostic factors, and treatment of DR and related complications. Nevertheless, OCTA is a relatively new technique and the usefulness of most of the quantitative data it allows to obtain needs to be investigated. Finally, it would be important to have greater interchangeability between data offered by different software and improve image quality by reducing artifacts.

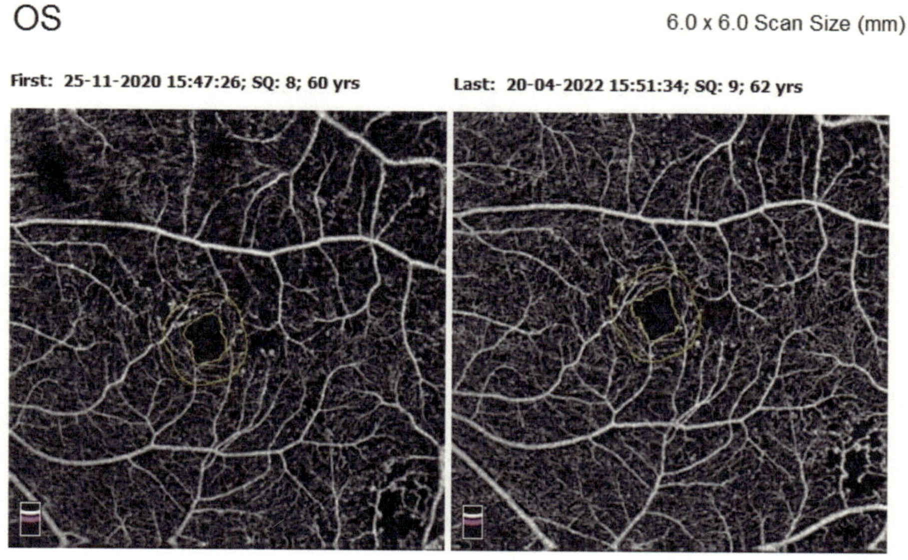

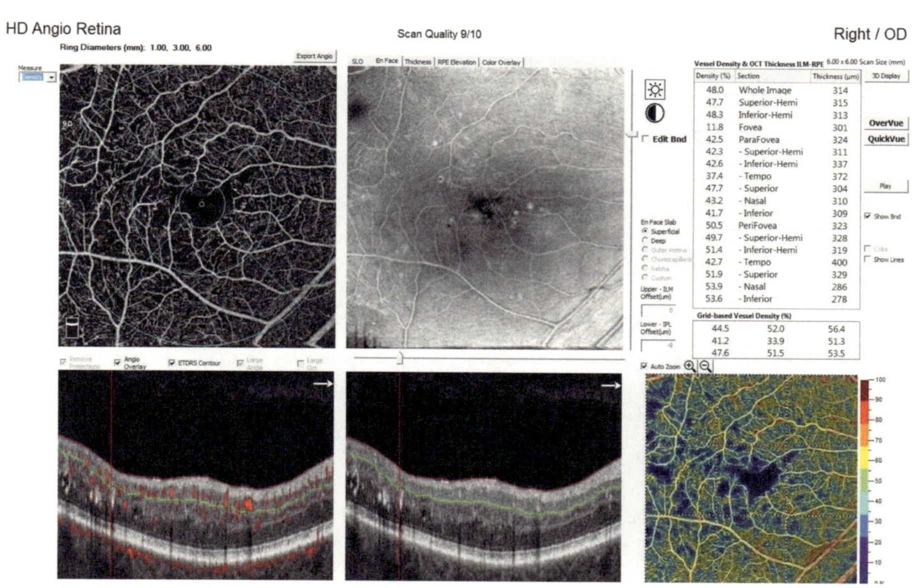

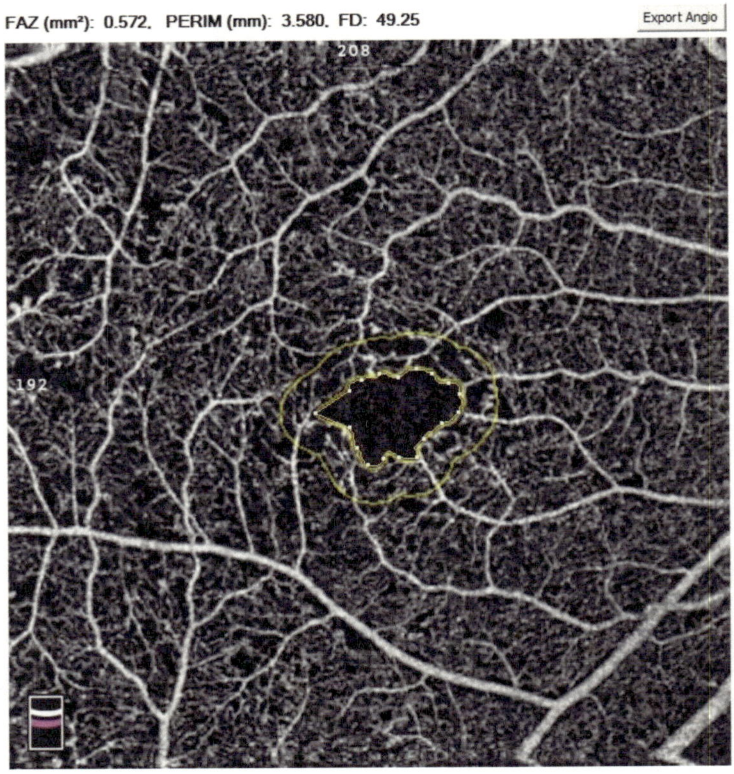
FAZ (mm²): 0.572. PERIM (mm): 3.580. FD: 49.25
Export Angio
208
192

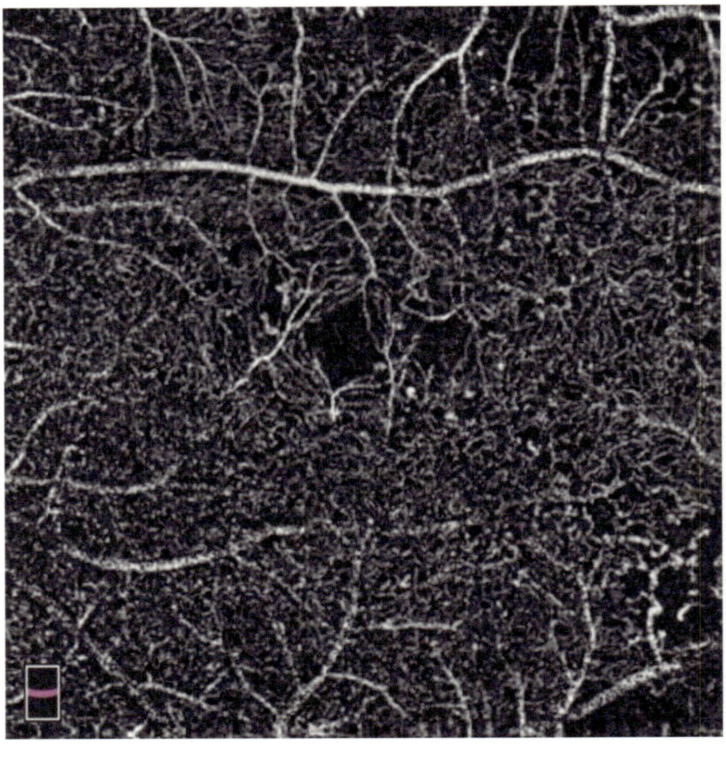

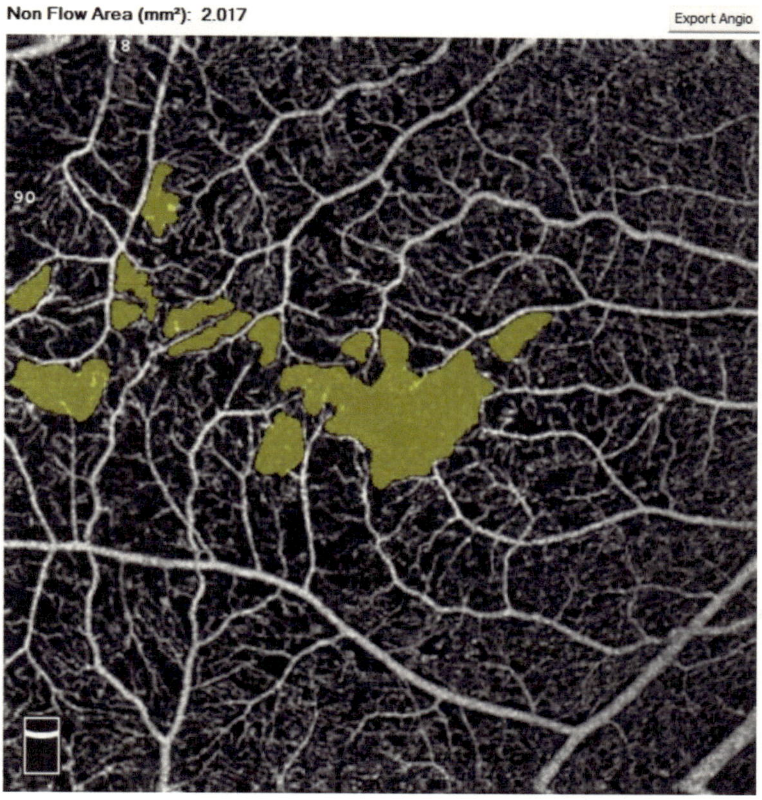

Author details

Sara Crespo Millas[1], Salvatore Di Lauro[1,2]*, David Galarreta Mira[1,2] and Maria Isabel López Gálvez[1]

1 Department of Ophthalmology, Hospital Clinico Universitario de Valladolid, Valladolid, Spain

2 Instituto Oftalmolgico Recoletas (IOR), Valladolid, Spain

*Address all correspondence to: sadilauro@live.it

References

[1] Wild S, Roglic G, Green A, Sicree R, King H. Global prevalence of diabetes: Estimates for the year 2000 and projections for 2030. Diabetes Care. 2004;**27**(5):1047-1053

[2] Ting DS, Cheung GC, Wong TY. Diabetic retinopathy: Global prevalence, major risk factors, screening practices and public health challenges: A review. Clinical & Experimental Ophthalmology. 2016;**44**(4):260-277

[3] Ishibazawa A, De Pretto LR, Alibhai AY, Moult EM, Arya M, Sorour O, et al. Retinal nonperfusion relationship to arteries or veins observed on Widefield optical coherence tomography angiography in diabetic retinopathy. Investigative Ophthalmology & Visual Science. 2019;**60**(13):4310-4318

[4] Duh EJ, Sun JK, Stitt AW. Diabetic retinopathy: Current understanding, mechanisms, and treatment strategies. JCI Insight. 2017;**2**(14):1-13

[5] Blaslov K, Bulum T, Duvnjak L. The role of endothelial dysfunction driven by adipocitokines in the development and progression of microvascular complications in patients with Type 1 and Type 2 diabetes. Medical Hypotheses. 2015;**84**(6):593-595

[6] Tan F, Chen Q, Zhuang X, Wu C, Qian Y, Wang Y, et al. Associated risk factors in the early stage of diabetic retinopathy. Eye and Vision (London, England). 2019;**6**:23

[7] Kwan CC, Fawzi AA. Imaging and biomarkers in diabetic macular edema and diabetic retinopathy. Current Diabetes Reports. 2019;**19**(10):95

[8] Battista M, Borrelli E, Sacconi R, Bandello F, Querques G. Optical coherence tomography angiography in diabetes: A review. European Journal of Ophthalmology. 2020;**30**(3):411-416

[9] Sun Z, Yang D, Tang Z, Ng DS, Cheung CY. Optical coherence tomography angiography in diabetic retinopathy: An updated review. Eye (London, England). 2021;**35**(1):149-161

[10] Ishibazawa A, Nagaoka T, Takahashi A, Omae T, Tani T, Sogawa K, et al. Optical coherence tomography angiography in diabetic retinopathy: A prospective pilot study. American Journal of Ophthalmology. 2015;**160**(1):35-44

[11] Parravano M, De Geronimo D, Scarinci F, Querques L, Virgili G, Simonett JM, et al. Diabetic microaneurysms internal reflectivity on spectral-domain optical coherence tomography and optical coherence tomography angiography detection. American Journal of Ophthalmology. 2017;**179**:90-96

[12] Shimouchi A, Ishibazawa A, Ishiko S, Omae T, Ro-Mase T, Yanagi Y, et al. A proposed classification of Intraretinal microvascular Abnormalities in diabetic retinopathy following Panretinal photocoagulation. Investigative Ophthalmology & Visual Science. 2020;**61**(3):34

[13] Sorour O, Arya M, Waheed N. New findings and challenges in OCT angiography for diabetic retinopathy. Annals of Eye Science. 2018;**3**(8):44

[14] Or C, Sabrosa AS, Sorour O, Arya M, Waheed N. Use of OCTA, FA, and ultra-widefield imaging in quantifying retinal ischemia: A review. The Asia-Pacific Journal of Ophthalmology. 2018;**7**(1):46-51

[15] Schaal KB, Munk MR, Wyssmueller I, Berger LE, Zinkernagel MS, Wolf S. Vascular abnormalities in diabetic retinopathy assessed with swept-source optical coherence tomography angiography widefield imaging. Retina. 2019;**39**(1):79-87

[16] de Carlo TE, Bonini Filho MA, Baumal CR, Reichel E, Rogers A, Witkin AJ, et al. Evaluation of Preretinal neovascularization in proliferative diabetic retinopathy using optical coherence tomography angiography. Ophthalmic Surgery, Lasers & Imaging Retina. 2016;**47**(2):115-119

[17] Nesper PL, Soetikno BT, Zhang HF, Fawzi AA. OCT angiography and visible-light OCT in diabetic retinopathy. Vision Research. 2017;**139**:191-203

[18] Balaratnasingam C, Inoue M, Ahn S, McCann J, Dhrami-Gavazi E, Yannuzzi LA, et al. Visual acuity is correlated with the area of the Foveal avascular zone in diabetic retinopathy and retinal vein occlusion. Ophthalmology. 2016;**123**(11):2352-2367

[19] Park YG, Kim M, Roh YJ. Evaluation of Foveal and Parafoveal microvascular changes using optical coherence tomography angiography in type 2 diabetes patients without clinical diabetic retinopathy in South Korea. Journal of Diabetes Research. 2020;**2020**:6210865

[20] Zhang B, Chou Y, Zhao X, Yang J, Chen Y. Early detection of microvascular impairments with optical coherence tomography angiography in diabetic patients without clinical retinopathy: A Meta-analysis. American Journal Of Ophthalmology. 2020;**222**:226-237

[21] Vujosevic S, Muraca A, Alkabes M, Villani E, Cavarzeran F, Rossetti L, et al. Early microvascular and neural changes in patients with Type 1 and Type 2 diabetes mellitus without clinical signs of diabetic retinopathy. Retina (Philadelphia, PA). 2019;**39**(3):435-445

[22] de Carlo TE, Chin AT, Bonini Filho MA, Adhi M, Branchini L, Salz DA, et al. Detection of microvascular changes in eyes of patients with diabetes but not clinical diabetic retinopathy using optical coherence tomography angiography. Retina (Philadelphia, PA). 2015;**35**(11):2364-2370

[23] Krawitz BD, Mo S, Geyman LS, Agemy SA, Scripsema NK, Garcia PM, et al. Acircularity index and axis ratio of the foveal avascular zone in diabetic eyes and healthy controls measured by optical coherence tomography angiography. Vision Research. 2017;**139**:177-186

[24] Zahid S, Dolz-Marco R, Freund KB, Balaratnasingam C, Dansingani K, Gilani F, et al. Fractal dimensional analysis of optical coherence tomography angiography in eyes with diabetic retinopathy. Investigative Ophthalmology & Visual Science. 2016;**57**(11):4940-4947

[25] Samara WA, Shahlaee A, Adam MK, Khan MA, Chiang A, Maguire JI, et al. Quantification of diabetic macular ischemia using optical coherence tomography angiography and its relationship with visual acuity. Ophthalmology. 2017;**124**(2):235-244

[26] Pedinielli A, Bonnin S, Sanharawi ME, Mané V, Erginay A, Couturier A, et al. Three different optical coherence tomography angiography measurement methods for assessing capillary density changes in diabetic retinopathy. Ophthalmic Surgery, Lasers & Imaging Retina. 2017;**48**(5):378-384

[27] de Carlo TE, Romano A, Waheed NK, Duker JS. A review of optical coherence tomography angiography (OCTA).

International Journal of Retina And Vitreous. 2015;**1**:5

[28] Simonett JM, Scarinci F, Picconi F, Giorno P, De Geronimo D, Di Renzo A, et al. Early microvascular retinal changes in optical coherence tomography angiography in patients with Type 1 diabetes mellitus. Acta Ophthalmologica. 2017;**95**(8):e751-e7e5

[29] Cao D, Yang D, Huang Z, Zeng Y, Wang J, Hu Y, et al. Optical coherence tomography angiography discerns preclinical diabetic retinopathy in eyes of patients with type 2 diabetes without clinical diabetic retinopathy. Acta Diabetologica. 2018;**55**(5):469-477

[30] Zeng Y, Cao D, Yu H, Yang D, Zhuang X, Hu Y, et al. Early retinal neurovascular impairment in patients with diabetes without clinically detectable retinopathy. The British Journal of Ophthalmology. 2019;**103**(12):1747-1752

[31] Dimitrova G, Chihara E, Takahashi H, Amano H, Okazaki K. Quantitative retinal optical coherence tomography angiography in patients with diabetes without diabetic retinopathy. Investigative Ophthalmology & Visual Science. 2017;**58**(1):190-196

[32] Yasin Alibhai A, Moult EM, Shahzad R, Rebhun CB, Moreira-Neto C, McGowan M, et al. Quantifying microvascular changes using OCT angiography in diabetic eyes without clinical evidence of retinopathy. Ophthalmology Retina. 2018;**2**(5):418-427

[33] Sun Z, Tang F, Wong R, Lok J, Szeto SKH, Chan JCK, et al. OCT angiography metrics predict progression of diabetic retinopathy and development of diabetic macular edema: A prospective study. Ophthalmology. 2019;**126**(12):1675-1684

[34] Lee H, Lee M, Chung H, Kim HC. Quantification of retinal vessel tortuosity in diabetic retinopathy using optical coherence tomography angiography. Retina (Philadelphia, PA). 2018;**38**(5):976-985

[35] Tang FY, Ng DS, Lam A, Luk F, Wong R, Chan C, et al. Determinants of quantitative optical coherence tomography angiography metrics in patients with diabetes. Scientific Reports. 2017;**7**(1):2575

[36] Kim AY, Chu Z, Shahidzadeh A, Wang RK, Puliafito CA, Kashani AH. Quantifying microvascular density and morphology in diabetic retinopathy using spectral-domain optical coherence tomography angiography. Investigative Ophthalmology & Visual Science. 2016;**57**(9):OCT362-OCT370

[37] Nesper PL, Roberts PK, Onishi AC, Chai H, Liu L, Jampol LM, et al. Quantifying microvascular Abnormalities with increasing severity of diabetic retinopathy using optical coherence tomography angiography. Investigative Ophthalmology & Visual Science. 2017;**58**(6):BIO307-BBIO15

[38] Tang FY, Chan EO, Sun Z, Wong R, Lok J, Szeto S, et al. Clinically relevant factors associated with quantitative optical coherence tomography angiography metrics in deep capillary plexus in patients with diabetes. Eye and Vision (London, England). 2020;7:7

[39] Sandhu HS, Elmogy M, Taher Sharafeldeen A, Elsharkawy M, El-Adawy N, Eltanboly A, et al. Automated diagnosis of diabetic retinopathy using clinical biomarkers, optical coherence tomography,

and optical coherence tomography angiography. American Journal of Ophthalmology. 2020;**216**:201-206

[40] Yu DY, Cringle SJ, Su EN, Yu PK, Jerums G, Cooper ME. Pathogenesis and intervention strategies in diabetic retinopathy. Clinical & Experimental Ophthalmology. 2001;**29**(3):164-166

[41] Toto L, D'Aloisio R, Di Nicola M, Di Martino G, Di Staso S, Ciancaglini M, et al. Qualitative and quantitative assessment of vascular changes in diabetic macular edema after dexamethasone implant using optical coherence tomography angiography. International Journal of Molecular Sciences. 2017;**18**(6):1-12

[42] Spaide RF, Fujimoto JG, Waheed NK. Image artifacts in optical coherence tomography angiography. Retina (Philadelphia, PA). 2015;**35**(11):2163-2180

[43] Coscas G, Lupidi M, Coscas F. Optical coherence tomography angiography in diabetic Maculopathy. Developments in Ophthalmology. 2017;**60**:38-49

[44] Zheng F, Zhang Q, Shi Y, Russell JF, Motulsky EH, Banta JT, et al. Age-dependent changes in the macular Choriocapillaris of Normal eyes imaged with Swept-source optical coherence tomography angiography. American Journal of Ophthalmology. 2019;**200**:110-122

[45] Dai Y, Zhou H, Chu Z, Zhang Q, Chao JR, Rezaei KA, et al. Microvascular changes in the choriocapillaris of diabetic patients without retinopathy investigated by swept-source OCT angiography. Investigative Ophthalmology & Visual Science. 2020;**61**(3):50

[46] Lopez Galvez M, Di Lauro S, Crespo MS. OCT angiografia y complicaciones retinianas de la diabetes. In: Gomez Ulla F, Ruiz Moreno JM, Arias-Barquet L, editors. Angiografía Por Tomografía De Coherencia Óptica (OCTA). 1. Spain: Sociedad Española de Oftalmologia (SEO); 2021. p. 632

Chapter 13

Analysis and Modeling of Polygonality in Retinal Tissue Based on Voronoi Diagram and Delaunay Tessellations

Nazario Bautista-Elivar and Ricardo Cruz-Castillo

Abstract

Several important properties of biological systems are directly related and even determined by the spatial distribution of their constituent elements. Those elements interact with each other and tend to use space in an optimal way, regarding their specific function and environmental constraints. A detailed methodology, based on Voronoi polygons and Delaunay triangles method employed to extract information on the spatial distribution of cells, is presented. On the other hand, diabetic retinopathy (DR) is defined as microvascular pathology. However, some data have suggested that the retinal photoreceptor (RPs) might be important in the pathogenesis of this ocular disease. In this study, the organization of the PRs in control and diabetic-induced rats was compared, using multiphoton microscopy. The PR mosaic was imaged at different locations in non-stained retinas. Thus, this work investigated the pathological changes in the cellular structures of the retina in the early stages of diabetes in laboratory animals. Of the different proposed tools that are highly reliable to be tested with human retinas, the metrics mean averaged distance and the mean square deviation of the angles are found ($P < 0.05$).

Keywords: multiphoton microscopy, diabetic retinopathy, Voronoi tessellations, computational geometry, bioinformatics

1. Introduction

Several biological/physical systems involve two-dimensional spatial arrangements with elements such as molecules, or cellular tissue, and the profiling in space has important repercussions to biological and physical investigations. The analysis of biological tissues often requires quantitative measurements to explore cell organization, in order to understand, identify, and monitor changes during pathology development and healing processes.

Measurements of cellular organization might not be always able to distinguish healthy and diseased tissues from each other [1]. It has also been revealed that the existing density measurements in cells present multiple restrictions [2–7]. In particular, some studies have reported that the density of retinal cones is not an appropriate parameter to identify pathological states in early stages of retina diseases [8, 9].

Maps of cellular distribution have to be considered linked to morphogenesis, mechanical structural stabilities and functional state of a given healthy tissue. Finding the connection that links form to disorder and is based on distance networks partition constructed from the position of cells when defined as mathematical nodes generators of Voronoi tessellations, then they can be used to construct summary functions [10], see **Table 1**. For example, Sudbø and Marcelponil Reith developed 27 algorithms based on Voronoi diagrams to describe the architecture of tissues [11]. Chiu showed that the minimum angles and areas of Delaunay triangles are responsive parameters when it concerns cellular distributions [12]. Voronoi analysis has also been used to determine the packing arrangement of cones at different retinal storage bins displayed with adaptive optics (AO) and hexagonal packing was found [13, 14]. Other authors have proposed to measure the regularity of convex polygons by successive measurements of irregular polygonal reconfiguration until regularity [15].

However, side number, distance between cones, according to proportion, any measurements derivative from the least distance will cause statistics to fail to identify healthy tissues and pathological tissues, which yield identical statistical densities measured from the shortest distances [1]. Other serious constraints developed from the method of counting the number of Voronoi cell sides result

Retinal photoreceptor	Real image (healthy tissues)	Voronoi polygon	Delaunay triangulation
Sprague-Dawley male rat	 Multiphoton microscope	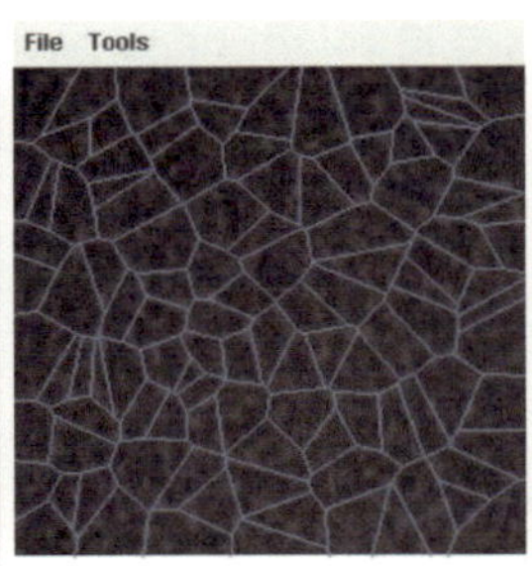	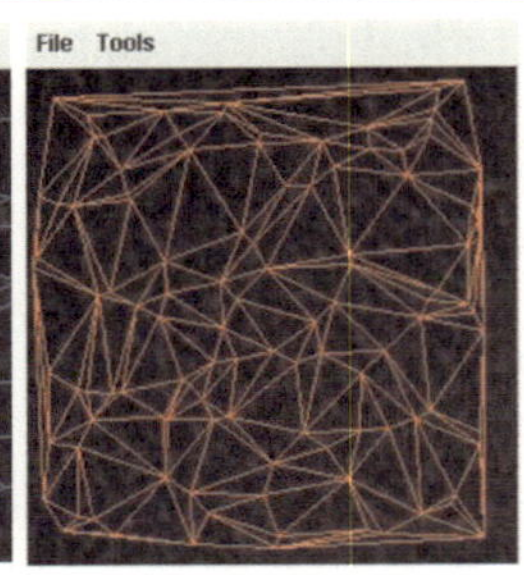
Human	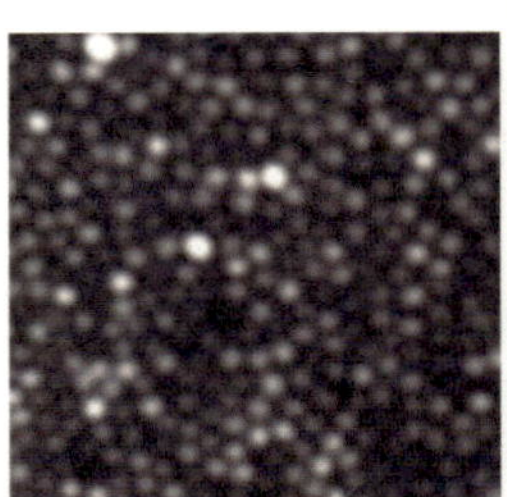 Adaptive optics scanning laser ophthalmoscope (AOSLO)	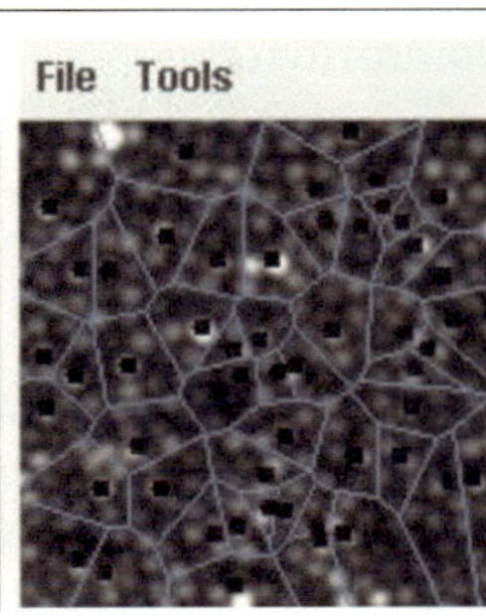	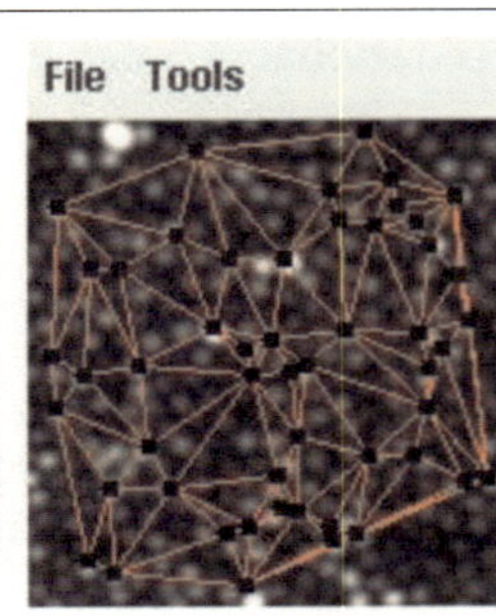

Table 1.
Voronoi polygons and Delaunay triangles in a retinal tissue.

from the fact that the number of cell sides will not change except for gross perturbations of the particle system. In addition, in Delaunay triangulation, no significant differences are observed by using Delaunay segments and Delaunay areas in tissues [16].

The general aim of this chapter is to establish an analysis for a comparison of the distribution of PRs in tissues with retinopathy diabetic, which is an important problem to mechanically understanding of the processes that lead to the experimental observations. This research presents only the model of the photoreceptor's spatial location (cones and sticks) considering photoreceptors small enough, in the suitable scale, to contemplate them as mathematical points. Then, Voronoi polygons and Delaunay triangles are formed by using these points. Therefore, Voronoi polygons do not represent the photoreceptor's shape. So, in this chapter, Voronoi polygons are not used to model biological cells nor their surrounding tissues.

This chapter is organized as follows: in Section 2, the description of several metrics using Voronoi polygon and Delaunay triangles and its integrated platform based on computational geometry, is given; in Section 3, multiphoton microscopy and image analysis is provided; in Section 4 we continue with a detailed description of retinal tissues, using Voronoi and Delaunay metrics described in Section 2; the Discussion is presented in Section 5, and finally the Conclusions are in Section 6.

2. Metrics/algorithm to computational biology

2.1 Description of metrics/algorithm

2.1.1 Internal distance

The internal distance d_i in a particular Voronoi cell, is the distance measured from the internal mathematical node (black dot, see **Figure 1**) of the Voronoi polygon to each neighboring point (blue dot, see **Figure 1**) which forms the polygon. This is an Ulam tree modified to measure distances, **Figure 1**.

2.1.2 Angular graph

The numbers ψ_i are the angles between the horizontal line which contains the internal mathematical node and the line which joins each neighboring point to the internal node, it is measured anticlockwise (Ulam tree modified to angles), **Figure 2**.

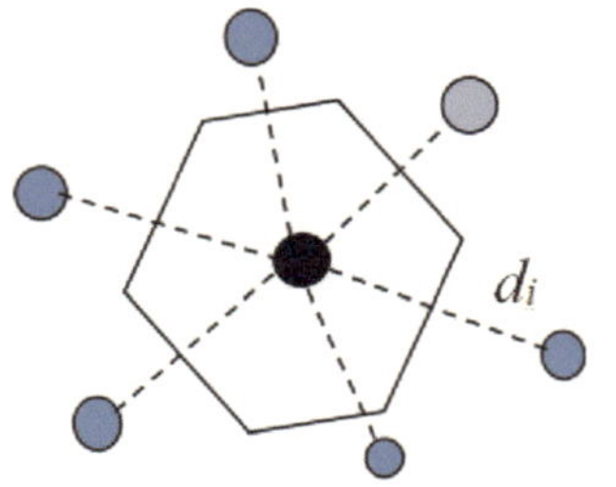

Figure 1.
Distance graph (Ulam tree modified) between neighbors in a 6-tides Voronoi polygon.

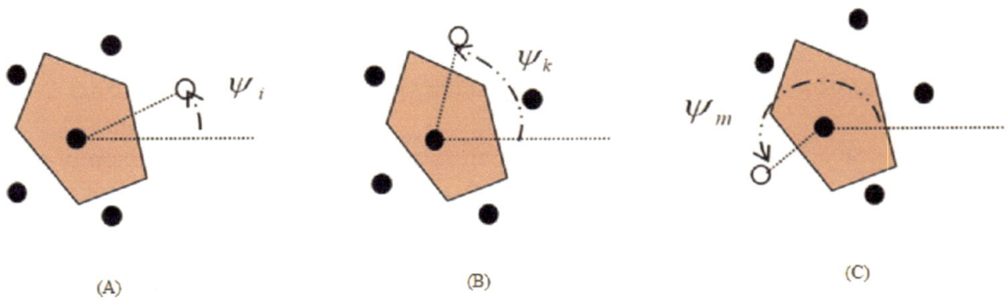

Figure 2.
Angle measurement between nearby points from a horizontal axis.

2.1.3 Internal angles of Delaunay triangles

These are the internal angles of any triangle in the Delaunay triangulation ω_i; the angles are measured in the positive direction (counterclockwise), **Figure 3**, using the following procedure:

i. First, measure the angle between two points containing the generating interior point of each cell.

ii. Arrange angles from least to greatest.

iii. Then measure the edge distances of the Delaunay triangulation containing the generating point.

iv. Finally, measure the angle between consecutive edges in which such a vertex is the generating point.

The sequence to measure the angle ω_i is in the following order: if you select first point 1 (vertex 1) then select point 2 (vertex 2), these points will form a starting line where the angle measurement starts, the point 3 (vertex 3) is where the angle measured ends. The selection and sequence of generating points will indicate the final angle obtained.

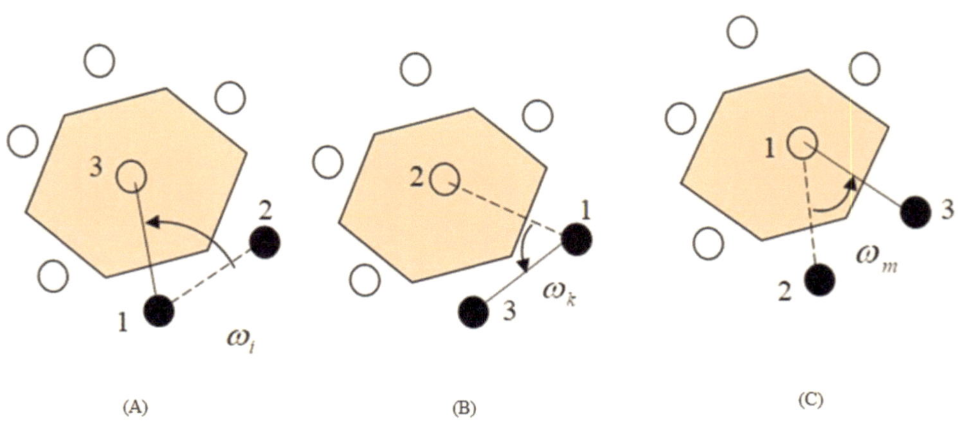

Figure 3.
Procedure to measure angles between three neighbors that form a Voronoi polygon and choosing one angle.

2.1.4 Mean distances average

This metric/algorithm determine the mean of average distances from the inner point in every Voronoi cell to its n neighbors and it is calculated by

$$\sum_{i=1}^{n} \frac{d_{\mathrm{i}}}{n^2} \tag{1}$$

where d_{i} is the internal distance defined above. It also represents a way to measure the cell size and it could be interpreted as a coefficient of expansion or contraction, **Figure 4**.

2.1.5 Polygonality index

This metric/algorithm generates the measure Ξ,

$$\Xi = \frac{1}{\sum_{i=1}^{n} |\chi_i - \beta| + 1} \tag{2}$$

where χ_i is the formed angle between consecutive neighbors for Delaunay triangle (irregular polygon, dotted arrow), β is the angle between consecutive vertex for a regular polygon (solid arrow), $\beta = 360\,\text{degree}/n$ and n is the number of neighbors of the Voronoi cell, **Figure 5**. The angle χ_i is invariant under any rotation movement. The measurement is performed counterclockwise.

If the value of Ξ is close to 1, then the Voronoi polygon is close to regularity, angles χ_i and β will have similar value. If Ξ is close to 0, then Voronoi polygon is irregular. The units of Ξ is the inverse in degrees.

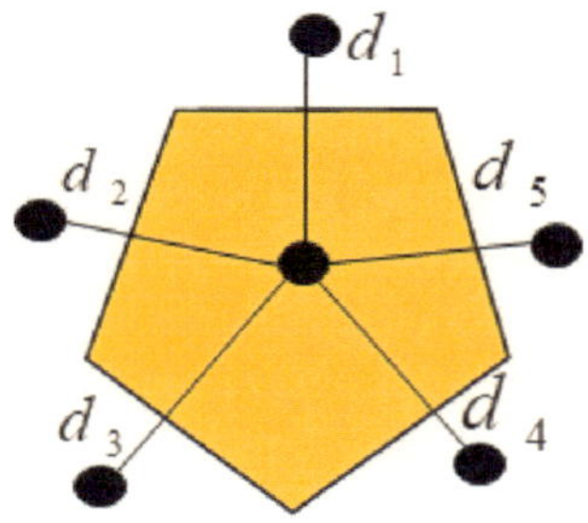

Figure 4.
Modified Ulam tree graph to measure distances in Voronoi cell.

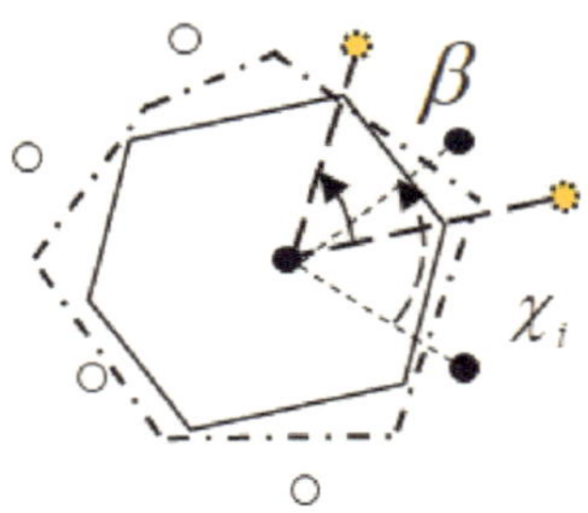

Figure 5.
The solid line is a regular polygon, the irregular polygon is represented by the dotted line, and the neighbors are the black circle. The internal black dot is a mathematical node.

2.1.6 Mean-square deviation of angles

This metrics/algorithms evaluate ε,

$$\varepsilon = \sqrt{\sum_{i=1}^{n} (\chi_i - \beta)^2} \tag{3}$$

the root square of mean deviation from the angles χ_i, with respect to angle $\beta = 360\,\text{degree}/n$ where n is the number of neighbors of the Voronoi cell for each Voronoi polygon. The magnitudes χ_i, β, and n are defined above (**Figure 5**). The metric ε is invariant under any rotation movement.

2.1.7 Variation index angle of differences

This metric algorithm gets δ ,

$$\delta = \frac{1}{\sqrt{\sum_{i=1}^{n} (\chi_i - \beta)^2 + 1}} \tag{4}$$

where χ_i and $\beta = 360\,\text{degree}/n$ are defined as above (**Figure 5**). If the value of δ is close to 1, then the Voronoi polygon is close to regularity, if δ is close to 0, then Voronoi polygon is irregular.

2.2 Software description

In view of the foregoing, we suggest development of an integrated platform based on computational geometry for bioinformatics and computational biology for analyzing spatial cellular organization which in turn use both Voronoi tessellation and Delaunay triangulation, for the purpose to measure the distance, internal angles, radius of circumscribed circle, amid nearby points mean distances average, angular polygonality, polygonality index, mean-square deviation of angles, and variation index angle of differences. The platform holds two options, either being performed by a user or operating with an automatic formulation. This software allows to create Voronoi polygons and Delaunay triangles from a set of *XY* coordinates, or generated by selecting in an imported image. It locates *XY* coordinates, using an auxiliary window S, **Figure 6**.

2.2.1 Voronoi frequency

This function displays graphics of frequency with respect to the number of sides in Voronoi mosaic with a data reading window, wider enough to avoid loss of data of polygons compared to other platforms [17].

2.2.2 Circumscribed circle

These metrics/algorithms are able to find the magnitude of the circumradius, the coordinates of the center of the circumcircle, and the coordinates of the vertices formed in each Delaunay triangle. *R* is the radius of the circle circumscribing a Delaunay triangle, some examples (a) and (b), **Figure 7**.

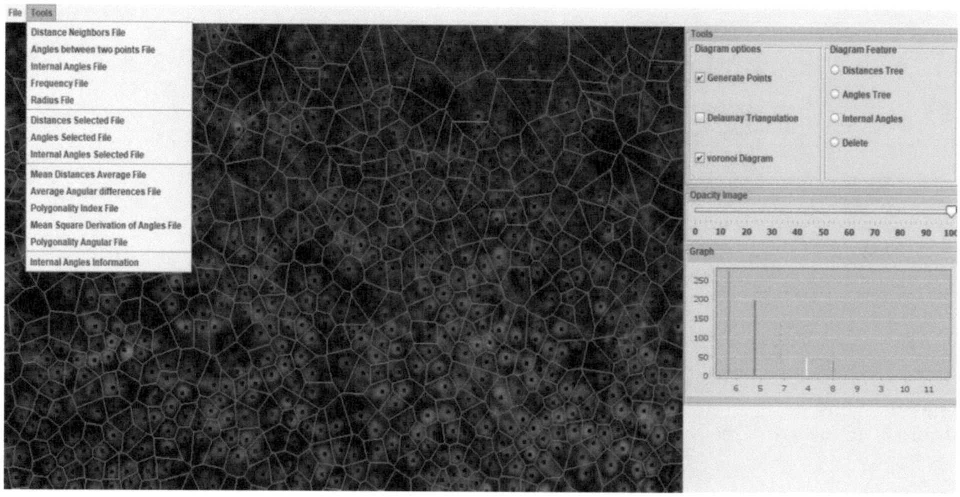

Figure 6.
Platform based on computational geometry for Voronoi polygons and Delaunay triangles to biological structures.

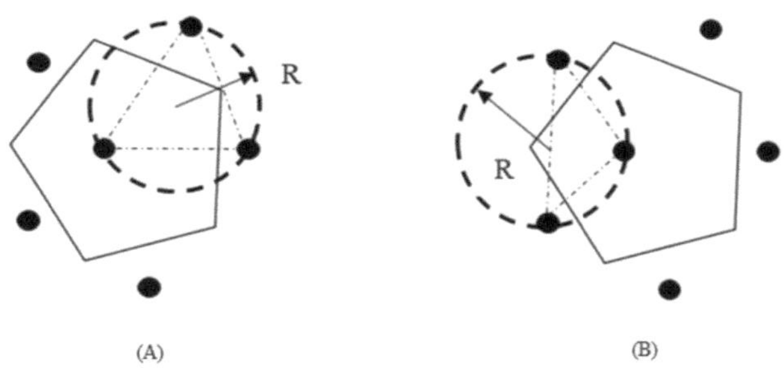

Figure 7.
Circumcircle and circumradius for each Delanuay triangle in a Voronoi polygon.

2.2.3 Distances selected

These metrics/algorithms are able to get the distance d_k between each pair of points selected by the user. First select the icon distances, located in Diagram Feature screen, after that choose a point of the polygon, by the icon select points, then select again the icon select point for another interest point, finally activate the icon selected file distances from Tools menu to get the data file with its coordinates and the distance that separates them. You might select different pairs of points to find out their distances in a single file, activating the icon selected for several couple points, for example (A), (B), (C), **Figure 8**.

2.2.4 Angles selected

These metrics/algorithms generate a file formed from each pair of points selected by the user. The angle v is relative to the horizontal axis and it works as the rangefinder. First, activate the *angles tree* icon (**Figure 6**), and then you can select different points for the same file using the select point button, to generate the Angles Selected file, **Figure 9**.

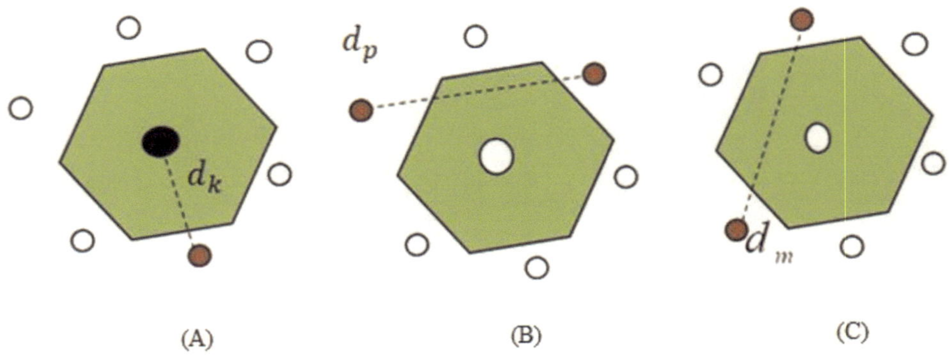

Figure 8.
Selection of distances to be chosen by the user in a Voronoi polygon.

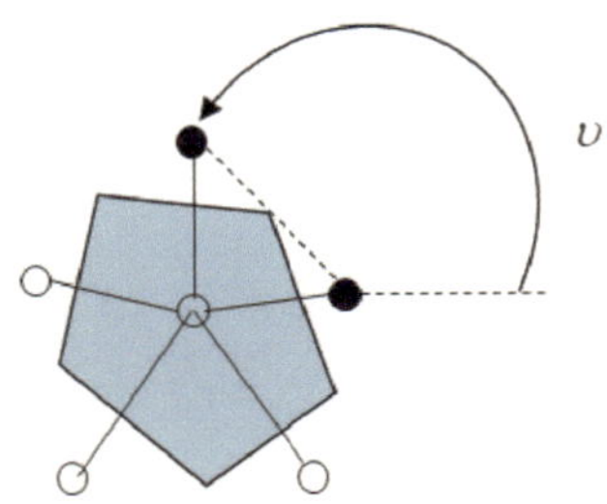

Figure 9.
Selection of angles between neighbors to be chosen by the user in a Voronoi polygon.

Internal angles selected. This metric algorithm generates a file for the angles $\gamma_i$of each Delaunay triangle selected by the user. First, activate radio button internal angles (**Figure 6**), then select points radio button to form the Delaunay triangle, selecting three points. The select order of each point defines the angle to be measured. First, if the black point is selected, then you can choose the white point. These two points form a line from which we start measuring the angle and ends at the line formed between the third point, the striped circle, forming an angle which is measured from for example, tree forms to obtain several internal angles in a Delaunay triangle, γ_k, γ_p, γ_i, **Figure 10**, (A),(B) and (C), respectively.

For example, for four tides polygon, if the option 2 is selected, the angle γ_i is shown in **Figure 11**.

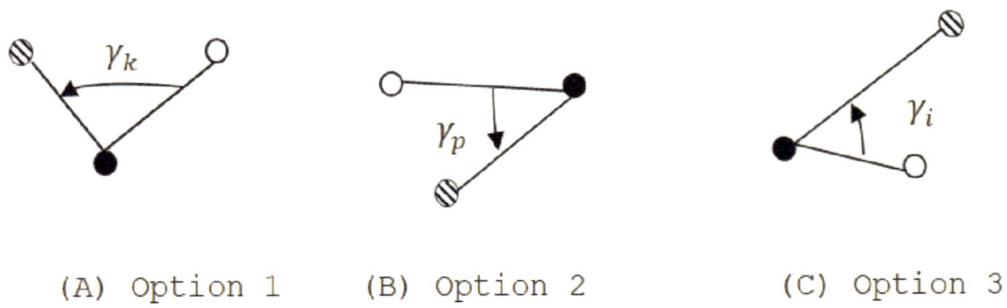

Figure 10.
Options to select nearby points to get an angle between them in a Voronoi mosaic.

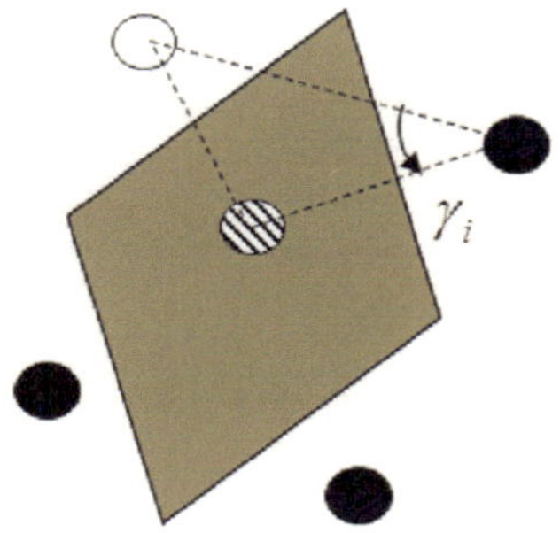

Figure 11.
Delaunay triangle, an angle selected between neighbors with option 2, ***Figure 10****.*

3. Multiphoton microscopy, image acquisition and processing

A multiphoton microscope was used to obtain images of the retinal mosaic in 16 healthy (C) mice and sixteen mice with diabetic retinopathy (DR). The multiphoton microscope combines a fs-laser system (760 nm), a scanning unit, a Z-motor, and a detector (photon-counting) within an inverted microscope. The whole system was computer-controlled. Nonlinear microscopy images were acquired using two imaging modalities: regular *XY* images and fast 2-photon imaging tomography, **Figure 12**.

Eight Sprague-Dawley male rats, weighing 200 g were administered intraperitoneal via with 55 mg/kg from *streptozotocin* diluted in citrate buffer were housed in a temperature-and humidity-controlled room maintained on a 12-hour light/dark cycle (lights on: 07:00–19:00 hours) and had free access to food and water. Retinas were evaluated after 6 weeks from diabetic-induced.

The retinal mosaic was estimated for each subject (both eyes), at 270, 810, 1350 and 1890 μm of eccentricities from the optic nerve along the nasal, temporal, dorsal and ventral of both eyes. The photoreceptors arrangement was analyzed using Voronoi polygon and Delaunay triangulation analysis; estimations were done by using a sampling window S of 90 × 90 μm image sections, **Figure 13**.

Through the Voronoi partition, some contours of the tessellations should be modified if other points outside the analysis window S (90 × 90 μm) were acquired.

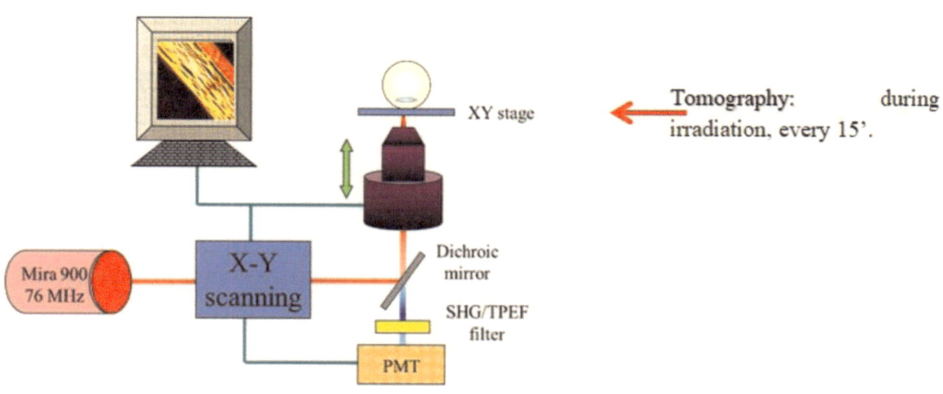

Figure 12.
Setup for scanning with a multiphoton microscope.

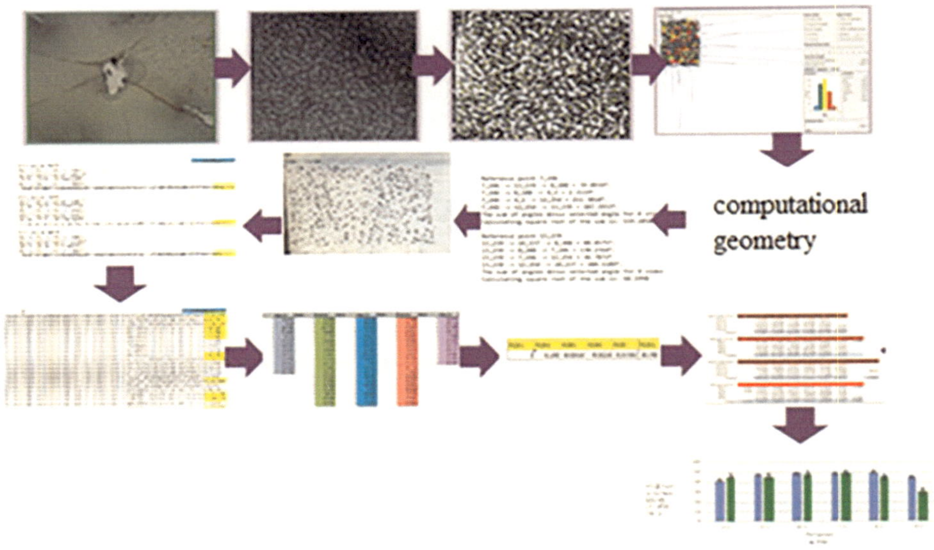

Figure 13.
Data processing diagram in retinal tissues for healthy photoreceptors and with DR, starting from raw data and applying image processing and segmentation, feature extraction and classification, and finally polygonality measurements.

These points are associated to the outline regions which are closer to the analysis window than to the considered point. The points which belong to such contour regions are considered to be at the border. All the marginal points are not noted in the subsequent calculations, because they cause statistical noise.

4. Retinal tissues analysis

We use some metric/algorithms of Section 2.1 to analyze and model the polygonality in retinal tissues, especially with DR.

4.1 Mean-square deviation of angles

Using the metric of mean-square deviation of angles ε (Eq. (3)), to know the angular distributions of photoreceptors in the rodent retina in order to identify healthy tissues (C) from tissues with pathology (R). The results are shown in **Figure 14**.

Results obtained during this analysis reported that at an eccentricity of 270 μm, there is a greater angular variation than 6 degrees in 4-sided polygons in tissues with pathology (R) with respect to its counterpart of healthy tissues (C). At an eccentricity of 810 μm a greater angular variation is observed in polygons of 10 and 9 sides, in addition to polygons of 6 and 7 degrees, respectively, in tissues with pathology (R). At an eccentricity of 1350 μm, an angular variation is presented up to 12 degrees in polygons of nine sides in tissues with pathology (R). At an eccentricity of 1890 μm, again the 9-sided polygons present an angular variation of 9 degrees in tissues with pathology (R). Likewise, we identify that as the eccentricity increases; the training of a greater number of sides of polygons is increasing in tissues with pathology which does not present healthy tissues (not presented here).

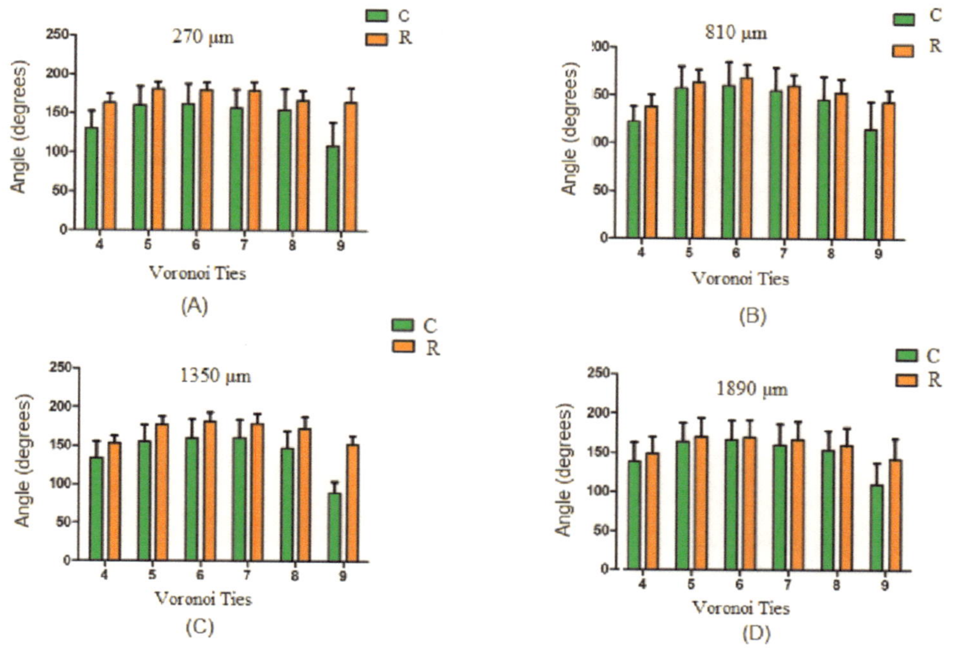

Figure 14.
Distribution of angular variation as eccentricity in retinal tissues, both healthy tissues (C) and diabetic retinopathy tissues (R): (A) 270 µm, (B) 810 µm, (C) 1350 µm, (D) 1890 µm.

Voronoi ties	*P*-value*		
	270 µm	1350 µm	1890 µm
5	0.006	0.002	0.022
6	0.025	0.0066	0.0204
7	0.001	0.018	0.0078
*Two-tailed.			

Table 2.
P-*value* to 5, 6, and 7 Voronoi ties.*

Is observed that if the angular variation is minor to 6.15 degrees, the value *P* is minor to 0.05. It is identified, then that to 810 and 1890 µm the angles of the polygons are minor to 30 degrees. For photography retinal, it is observed that to major eccentricity, the spacing of the photoreceptors is major, **Table 2**.

4.2 Detection of modal spacing

Using the metrics/algorithm of radius in a circumscribed circle for estimating photoreceptor spacing based on the circumradius of Delaunay triangle, as a metric that allows knowing how is the density/separation of photoreceptors in retinal healthy tissues and with diabetic retinopathy. This metric is an alternative form at the Yellott's ring [18]. The circumradius provides an estimation of the modal spacing in the retinal image of the photoreceptors. The distributions of density grouped by circumradius interval are: (a) 1.12–2.24 µm, (b) 2.244–3.36 µm, (c) 3.364–4.48 µm, (d)

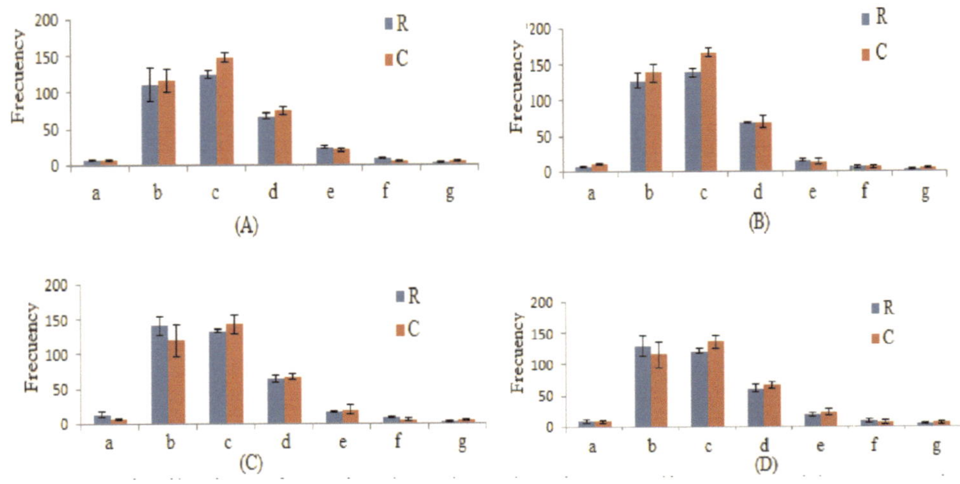

Figure 15.
Distribution of spacing based on the circumradius grouped by eccentricity in retinal tissues: (A) 270 μm, (B) 810 μm, (C) 1350 μm, (D) 1890 μm.

4.485–5.601 μm, (e) 5.605–6.721 μm, (f) 6.725–7.842 μm, (g) 7.846–9.62 μm. The results are shown in **Figure 15**.

To distribute the density by spacing of photoreceptors, we have proposed a standard criterion for arbitrary intervals of circumradius: 1.12–2.24 μm, 2.244–3.36 μm, 3.364–4.48 μm, 4.485–5.601 μm, 5.605–6.721 μm, 6.725–7.842 μm, and 7.846–9.62 μm. By using these intervals with the metrics/algorithms of circumscribed circle to obtain each circumradius, our results allow us to observe that the two dominant distributions of grouped density of photoreceptors are at intervals between 3.364–4.48 μm and 2.244–3.36 μm.

With these results, it has been observed that the percentage of circumradius in the range of 2.244–3.36 μm increases in tissues with DR as eccentricity increases. These results show a density of separating healthy photoreceptors to 810 μm of eccentricity with circumradius in the range of 3.364–4.48 μm (42.51%) and in the range of 2.244–3.36 μm (37.68%), **Table 3**.

It has been also identified that in cellular damaged tissues with DR the training of circumradius to greater eccentricity and also with a larger radius increases, with

Retinal tissue	Range 3.364–4.48 μm	Range 2.24–3.36 μm	Eccentricity (μm)
R	38.75%	30%	270
C	41.59%	33.61%	270
R	37.42%	32.63%	810
C	42.51%	37.68%	810
R	34.35%	35.11%	1350
C	37.05%	36.04%	1350
R	33.24%	37.56%	1890
C	36.93%	38.69%	1890

Table 3.
Percent density by eccentricity intervals.

Tissue	270 μm	810 μm	1350 μm	1890 μm
C	59.35 %	57.73 %	57.3 %	55.85%
R	55.68 %	56.9%	51.88 %	51.84%

Table 4.
Percentage of circumradius in the interval [3.364–5.601] μm.

respect to the control tissue, this is because they increase the spaces between photoreceptors that stop emitting fluorescence. It is also appreciated that the clustered density decreases in the photoreceptors of tissues with diabetic retinopathy, between the intervals of 2.244–3.36 μm and in 3.364–4.48 μm, as eccentricity.

However, in the interval [3.364–5.601] μm, that represents 55.8% of circumradius, they have a higher percentage behavior in control tissues than in tissues with DR, **Table 4**. Therefore, this shows that frequency of circumradius decreases in tissues with DR.

4.3 Mean distances average

To measure distances between neighbors that form each Voronoi cell is employed the metric/algorithm of mean distances average (Eq. (1)), as a measure for expansion or contraction of the polygon of Voronoi. The results are shown in **Figure 16**. This is a modification to the metric Ulam tree in each polygon. A measurement of spacing (or contraction) between neighbors is explained in terms of a bi-dimensional space with reference to the populations on flat surfaces. This metric allows us to measure the space between neighboring cells, as a result of leakage in photoreceptors.

In **Figure 16**, it can be seen that for the 5, 6 and 7-sided polygons, they have a similar spacing. In the same way it is observed that for polygons of four, eight and nine sides have a particular behavior of distance separating, the distances between diabetic cells increases, in relation to the healthy cells, because the distances between the cells increase because of the diabetic retinopathy.

Figure 16 depicts the mean averaged distance (Eq. (1)), as a function of the number of sides of Voronoi polygons for both control and pathological retinas. Since it

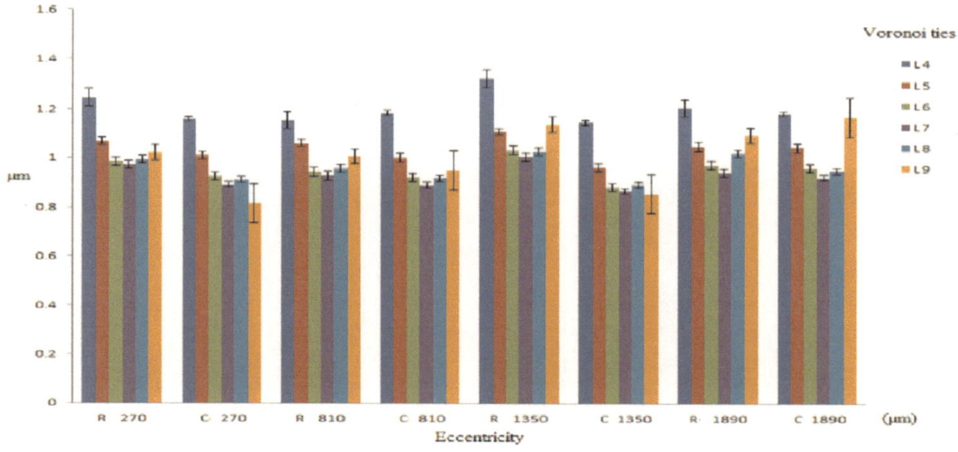

Figure 16.
Distribution of cellular spacing in healthy tissue and with diabetic retinopathy according to the eccentricity measured from the optic nerve.

has been just showed that the polygon frequency distribution does not change with retinal eccentricity (**Figure 20**), the data have been also averaged across all locations for better comparisons. Differences between both groups of retinas were statistically significant (paired t-test, $P < 0.05$).

Using the Ulam tree modified for distances, it is possible to characterize the environment of each cell and in a more general way, to study cellular interactions. This metric/algorithm appears to be useful for analyzing the effects of the cell surrounding on a given cellular function and vice-versa.

A topic as suitable to determinate of the average type of the spatial occupation, following isoperimetric inequality [19], see Eq. (5),

$$L(X)^2 - 4\mu A(X)^2 \geq 0 \qquad (5)$$

Where $A(X)$ is the area and $L(X)^2$ is the perimeter for a convex set.

4.4 Angular polygonality

With this metric/algorithm $\sum_{i=1}^{N_k} \frac{|\chi_i - \beta|}{n}$ is quantified that the Voronoi polygons of five, six, seven, and eight sides in healthy tissues and with diabetic retinopathy maintain a maximum range of angular values between 110 and 130 degrees measured from an arbitrary horizontal axis, defining an angular cluster of radio 10 degrees. It is shown that the Voronoi polygons of five, six, seven, and eight sides are sensitives.

However, the polygons of Voronoi in healthy tissues and with diabetic retinopathy of 3, 4, 9, 10, 11 and 12 sides are very irregular angularly, and the range of angular variation is from 60 to 180 degrees, defining an angular cluster radius of 60 degrees, **Figure 17**.

Other topics as suitable to capture regularity in convex Voronoi polygons is to measure how well they fit in a regular polygon or a regular polygon fits in them. This proposal has the characteristics to providing a way of fitting with convex polygons in

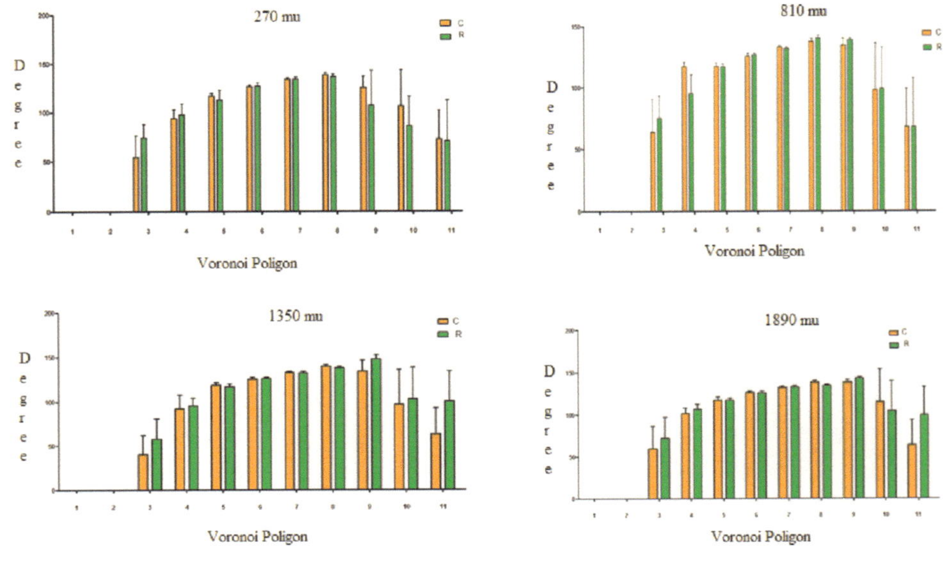

Figure 17.
Distribution of the angular polygonality relative to the side number in the Voronoi polygon.

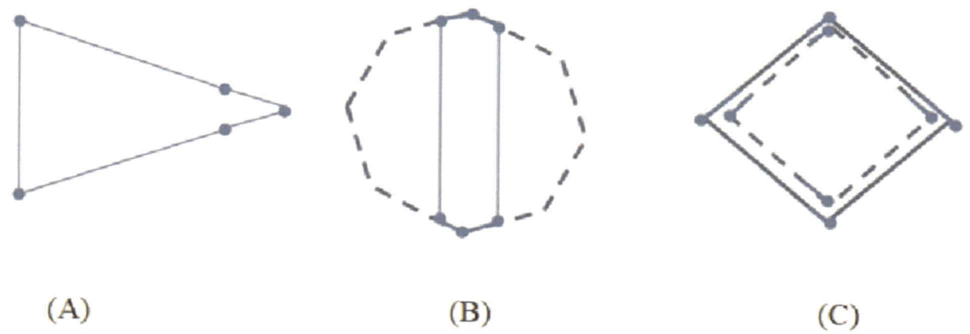

Figure 18.
In (A), a pentagon that almost looks like an equilateral triangle, (B) hexagon that almost looks like an octagon, (C) square that almost looks like a rhombus shape.

which they are very similar to regular polygons with a different number of edges [20], see **Figure 18**.

The procedure consists in transforming the given irregular polygon into a regular one, while measuring the amount of deformation required in such a process. The measurement of the angle variation gives a first parameter to consider in the final measurement of the regularity of Voronoi polygon. Using the Ulam tree modified to distances and the Ulam tree modified to angles gives a measure of the amount of deformation produced. Combining both procedures will be obtaining a measure of the regularity of the Voronoi tessellations on retinal tissues.

4.5 Frequency of Voronoi polygon

In order to quantify the distribution of polygons according to the eccentricity, frequency graphs were generated. In these it is observed that five and six sides polygons predominate, in healthy retinal tissues (C) and with diabetic retinopathy (R). In healthy tissues, with eccentricities of 270 and 810 μm, the frequency of polygons of five and six sides is greater, with respect to pathological tissues. However, with eccentricities of 1350 and 1890 μm, predominate 5-sided polygons, in tissues with diabetic retinopathy, **Figure 19**.

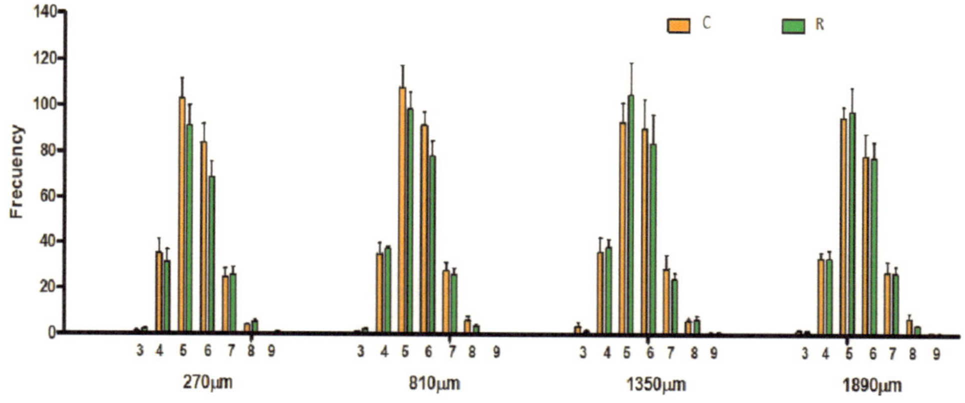

Figure 19.
Distribution of frequencies in Voronoi polygons by eccentricity in healthy retinal tissues (C) and with diabetic retinopathy (R).

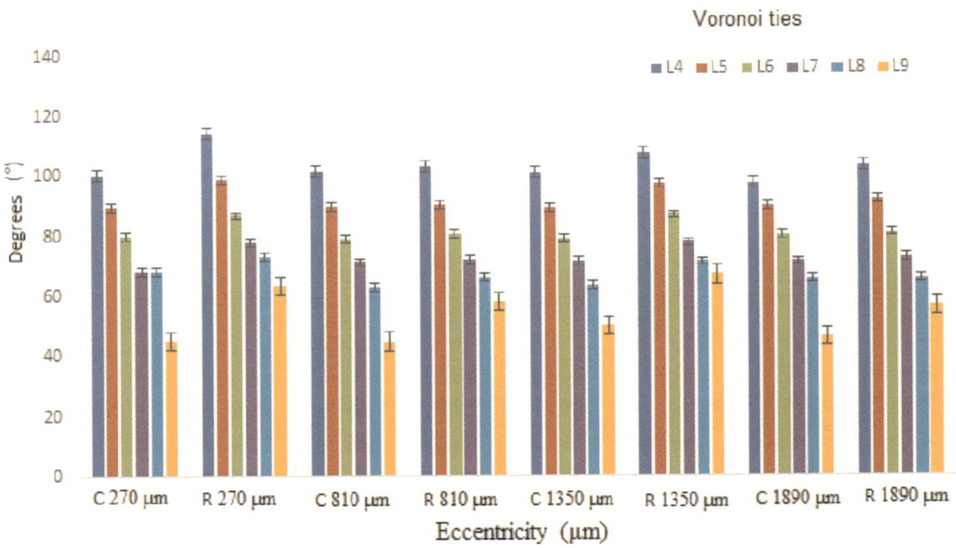

Figure 20.
Distribution of maximum angles χ_i relative to the side number (4,5,6, ...) in the Voronoi polygon.

We found that the spatial sampling of the images with S window, even using resizing of the recorded images of 90 × 90 µm, has a significant impact on the performance of the metric/algorithms, but also that an excessive upsizing does not substantially improve the measurements. We observed that the percentage of Voronoi polygon is the parameter in which is most affected by errors in photoreceptors detection, and for this reason the combined measurements of more parameters could be a better choice in order to characterize different retinal regions and the different subjects' retinas.

4.6 Minimum and maximum angles

Control (C) and diabetic retinopathy (R) tissues were characterized based on measuring the maximum angles χ_i and minimum angles χ_i of the Delaunay triangles in Voronoi polygons (**Figure 5**). Greater sensitivity is identified when quantifying maximum angles than minimum angles; see **Figure 20** and **Table 5**.

5. Discussion

Soliman et al. [21], using AO fundus camera to acquired images of parafoveal cones, from patients with type II diabetes mellitus with or without retinopathy, captured the cone mosaic at 0 and 2 degrees eccentricities along the horizontal and vertical meridians. The density of the parafoveal cones was calculated within 100 × 100-µm squares located at 500-µm from the foveal center along the orthogonal meridians. They found that the cone density was significantly lower in the moderate non-proliferative diabetic retinopathy (NPDR) and severe PDR/proliferative DR groups compared to the Control, No DR, and mild NPDR groups. Also, they found that the mean percentage of cones with hexagonal Voronoi tiles in the Control and No DR groups was 44.8% and 45.6%, respectively. In the DR groups, the percentage of cones with hexagonal Voronoi tiles ranged between 43.4% and 40.0%. They therefore

Voronoi ties	Control	Diabetic retinopathy	(±) Angular difference	*P*-value*
Maximum angles χ_i, 270 µm				
5	89.46	98.40	8.94	0.0208
6	79.75	86.66	6.91	0.0258
7	68.05	77.77	9.72	0.006
Maximum angles χ_i, 810 µm				
5	89.47	90.06	*0.59*	0.092
6	78.70	80.46	*1.76*	0.0596
7	71.09	71.90	*0.81*	0.0787
Maximum angles χ_i, 1350 µm				
5	88.79	97.11	8.32	0.0204
6	78.78	86.64	7.86	0.0198
7	71.30	77.45	6.15	0.0478
Maximum angles χ_i, 1890 µm				
5	89.63	91.51	1.88	0.06312
6	79.79	80.56	0.77	0.08258
7	71.13	72.25	1.12	0.07114

**Two-tailed.*

Table 5.
Value-P for maximum angles in 5, 6 and 7 Voronoi ties.

conclude that decreased cone density may be linked to the prior use of anti-VEGF therapy in these patients. Since VEGF is known to have a neuroprotective effect on photoreceptors, anti-VEGF agents may potentially have a deleterious effect on photoreceptors. Other progress against the wet form of the disease has come through the use of drugs that target vascular endothelial growth factor, or VEGF, a substance in the body that promotes the growth of new blood vessels. It has also been found that, cone photoreceptor counts in the control group reported in this study fall within the range reported in previous studies, high inter subject variability of cone density may also play a significant role [22].

Likewise, Li and Roorda showed that the percentage of hexagonal Voronois tended to decrease between 0.25 and 5 degrees from the fovea; a study on a post-mortem human retina showed that the cones were more hexagonally arranged near the edge of the fovea (between 0.20 and 0.25 degrees eccentricity) than in the foveal center [7, 23, 24]. According to the current study and previous work from others [25, 26] a model of the parafoveal mosaic by a lattice with continuous hexagonal regularity cannot be considered completely adequate to describe the cone mosaic arrangement in a healthy eye. In addition, in an AO retinal image of the photoreceptor mosaic, deviations from hexagonal order can be attributed to some phenomena, such as point defects and linear cracks. 'Point defects' of the cone lattice occur within otherwise intact mosaic areas and may be represented by smaller cones (S cones), cones with no wave guiding properties or isolated rods (it is plausible that rods cannot be always distinguished by point defects). Other phenomena that can contribute to change the hexagonal order are represented by local variance of the cone shape and the compression along the vertical meridian as a consequence of the expansion along the horizontal meridian of the photoreceptor mosaic [7, 24, 27–29].

Lombardo [30] identified several possible limitations based on the preferred packing arrangement of the cone mosaic: resolution of AO system, study size, and the presence of several sources of confounding orbias. Firstly, the resolution of the rtx1 camera is insufficient to assess the density of extremely tightly packed cones at the center of the fovea. Whether or not this loss of parafoveal cones reflects similar changes at the foveal center remains unclear. To date, the association of photoreceptor loss and vision loss in patients with DR remains obscure. Secondly, small sample size is another limitation of this prospective observational cohort study. This variability could be attributed to several factors, including the lack of a standardized approach to cone counting and differences in image processing software, AO systems, sampling window size, and foveal reference point location.

Methodology based on the optical coherence tomography (OCT) allows it to quantify retinal thickness in diabetic retinopathy. A total of 136 patients in different stages of diabetic retinopathy were examined with OCT [31]. In the controls, retinal thickness was 153 ± 15 μm in the fovea, 249 ± 19 μm in the temporal parafoveal region, and 268 ± 20 μm in the nasal parafoveal region. In diabetic patients, retinal thickness was increased to 307 ± 136 μm in the fovea, 337 ± 88 μm in the temporal retina, and 353 ± 95 μm in the nasal retina, respectively. The differences between diabetics and controls were highly significant ($P < 0.001$). There was an intermediate correlation between retinal thickness and visual acuity, particularly in patients without macular ischemia. Sensitivity of detecting clinically significant macular edema by measuring foveal retinal thickness was 89% and specificity was 96%. Apparent correlation between the increase and decreased visual acuity in the retina thickness, can be explained by the results of an increase in the thickness will be related to the increase in time axonal loss. In diabetic retinopathy, retinal spaces can take place between the inner and outer plexiform layer, outer limiting membrane or the outer plexiform layer. These results demonstrate the retinal tissue integrity, as a measure of the retention axon connection, and as an index of visual function. The strength of the correlation between the retention structure and visual function as expected decreases in the eccentricity increases from the center of the fovea.

There is disagreement in the literature concerning the effects of age on PR packing density. Curcio et al. [32] found a nonsignificant change in the number of cone photoreceptors with age. However, they reported that the range of peak density variation at older ages was narrower, overlapping the lower end of the cone density from younger subjects.

As mentioned above, there are mixed results of histology on age-related changes in PR packing. It is clear that nonhuman primates undergo changes in the central retina with age [33, 34]. Ordy et al. [35] studied the visual acuity and foveal PR density in the retina of aged rhesus monkeys, finding that the foveal photoreceptor density decreased significantly in the oldest age group of macaque monkeys compared with the middle age group. Other properties of the photoreceptors have been found to change with age, in addition to the cone packing density. Gartner and Henkind [36] reported loss of photoreceptor nuclei. Keunen et al. [37] and Kilbride et al. [38] found that the cone pigment density decreased as a function of age. Elsner et al. [39] showed that young healthy people typically have steep foveal peaks in photopigment density, but older people have shallower distributions.

Our approach emphasizes the local density of the PR rather than the total area. Thus, we found that a significant decrease in photoreceptor packing density occurred primarily, at distances less than 1890 μm from the center of the fovea.

Changes in the central fovea are also evident from the analysis of foveal shape by Gorrand and Delori [40], who found that the curvature of the foveola increases with increasing age. Elsner et al. [39], Bone et al. [41], and Chang et al. [42] found changes in the distribution of macular pigment with age, but Delori [43] did not. Since macular pigment is deposited preferentially in the photoreceptor axons and inner plexiform layers of the retina. Similarly a loss of PR could cause an increased curvature. An alternative possibility is that central cones spread outward, and the foveal curvature increases due to this spread, but again, the mechanism would be more complex and not easily tested by PR packing measurements alone.

However, despite the seeming transparency of DR pathogenesis and the progress in its treatment observed in recent years, a number of issues remain that warrant further study [44–46]. One of them is the temporal sequence of pathological changes in DR development [47, 48]. Studies in rodents have highlighted that biomarkers of inflammation, such as leukostasis, overexpression of adhesion molecules in retinal vascular endothelial cells and leukocytes, vascular permeability alteration, and aggravated production of nitric oxide, prostaglandins, cytokines, and other inflammatory mediators appears in the retina during 1–6 months of diabetes crisis [49].

Most developed therapies for DR, have primarily focused on the terminal stage of this disease, and as thus, failed to address the early potentially reversible stage of this disease. In addition, most of these therapies have been associated with severe sight threatening side effects [44]. With that, understanding of the temporal sequence and stages of pathological disturbances of DR development is of great prognostic and scientific value, as it might contribute to improvements to current methods or even the development of new methods of diagnosis and treatment of such a serious complication of diabetes.

6. Conclusions

The general aim of this chapter was to establish an analysis for a comparison of retinal tissues with retinopathy diabetic and healthy tissues, which is an important problem to mechanically understanding of the processes that lead to the experimental observations.

In retinal tissues, metrics as quantification of Voronoi polygons and Delaunay triangles, are not sensitive to register changes in cellular organization, because in the first geometry, the number of dominant polygons are both six and five sides in both cases, and in the second geometry are presented the same amount of triangles Delaunay, as it has been reported by many authors [2–7]. Similarly, Kaccie and Roorda [50] showed that Voronoi regions gradually increase in size at higher eccentricities.

In this chapter, we focused here on the photoreceptor degeneration in an animal model of retinal degenerative disease, retinopathy diabetic, in which we investigate how pathology affects mosaic organization. We analyzed 128 retinal tissues here, eventually we found abnormality in retinal tissues. This spacing rule is enough to simulate the geometry of mosaics, suggesting that interactions between the mosaic cells satisfy tessellation formations of healthy tissues and pathological damaged tissues. Once generated, cells migrate to their layer, and a simple rule controlling the spacing between cells of the same type suffices to control mosaic formation [51, 52]. This ensures uniform coverage of the retina by each type of cell, regarding the mechanisms that control the genesis of the different retinal cells.

From the Voronoi analyses, the parameter of Eq. (1), was also obtained. This has been reported to be very sensitive to changes in photoreceptors spacing [11]. Independently of the number of sides of the Voronoi polygons, the PR spacing increased in the samples with DR, what represents an expansion in cellular spacing.

Based on the results obtained, the metric that are suggested to detect morphological changes in retinal tissues with DR is the metric of the mean averaged distance (Eq. (1), **Figure 17**) and the mean square deviation of the angles (Eq. (3), **Table 2**), in both cases P value <0.05.

In this study, among the tools presented that are highly reliable and ready to be tested with human retinas are the mean averaged distance (Eq. (1)) and the mean square deviation of the angles (Eq. (3)), which have a high sensitivity to detect changes in DR tissues, by using retinal images obtained with a fundus camera or AOSLO. We consider that the tools mentioned (Eqs. (1) and (2)) are reliable enough to perform clinical level tests.

A much more effective developmental design, consistent with the experimental observations so far available, is that cell genesis and cell positioning are determined separately, which requires a combination of experimental and theoretical tools. Although we learn from comparing real data to obtain patterns, a mathematical model is needed to investigate the contribution from many retinal processes. The understanding of the distribution of cone density and spacing as a function of retinal eccentricity in the same eye and between fellow eyes of the same subject could be of great clinical utility when monitoring a subject longitudinally over time or when comparing controls with presumptive pathologic cases.

Several studies of diabetic retinopathy have focused especially on the retinal vasculature, but recent studies suggest that the neural retina also is involved. Oxidative stress and local inflammatory changes have been shown to play important roles in the pathogenesis of this retinopathy, but the source of reactive oxygen species has been less clear. Du et al. [53] accumulating evidence suggests that photoreceptor cells play a previously unappreciated role in the development of early stages of diabetic retinopathy, but the mechanism by which this occurs is not clear. The oxidative stress in retinas of diabetic mice emanates from neural photoreceptor cells, and elimination of these cells in diabetes inhibits both the oxidative stress and inflammatory changes shown to cause the vascular lesions of diabetic retinopathy. These studies suggest a mechanism by which neural cells can initiate the vascular injury characteristic of diabetic retinopathy.

Finally, we show in this chapter provides new insight into the mechanisms loss of cells observed of mice retinas, and could be used to rescue inner retinal neurons from secondary degeneration, enlarging the time window in which receptor transplants or substitution may be for the benefit of subjects suffering retinal degenerative diseases.

Conflict of interest

The authors declare that the research was conducted in the absence of any commercial or financial relationships that could be construed as a potential conflict of interest.

Author details

Nazario Bautista-Elivar[1*] and Ricardo Cruz-Castillo[2]

1 Electrical and Electronic Engineering Department, National Technological of Mexico/Technological Institute of Pachuca, Mexico

2 Academic Area of Mathematics and Physics, Institute of Basic Sciences and Engineering, Autonomous University of Hidalgo State, Mexico

*Address all correspondence to: nazario.be@pachuca.tecnm.mx

References

[1] da Fontoura Costa L, Rocha F, Lima SMA. Characterizing polygonality in biological structures. Physical Review E. 2006;**73**:011913-10-011913-11

[2] Song H, Chui TYP, Zhong Z, Elsner AE, Burns SA. Variation of cone photoreceptor retinal eccentricity with packing density and age. Investigative Ophthalmology & Visual Science. 2011; **52**:7376-7384

[3] Li KY, Tiruveedhula P, Roorda A. Intersubject foveal photoreceptor variability of cone density in relation to eye length. Investigative Ophthalmology & Visual Science. 2010;**51**:6858-6867

[4] Lombardo M, Serrao S, Ducoli P, Lombardo G. Variations in the image optical quality of the eye and the sampling limit of resolution of the cone mosaic in axial length with young adults. Journal of Cataract and Refractive Surgery. 2012;**38**:1147-1155

[5] Garrioch R, Langlo C, Dubis AM, Cooper RF, Dubra A, Carroll J. Repeatability on in vivo cone spacing and density measurements. Optometry and Vision Science. 2012;**89**: 632-643

[6] Hirsch J, Miller WH. Does resolution limit cone positional disorder? Journal of the Optical Society of America. 1992;**4**: 1481-1492

[7] Curcio CA, Sloan KR. Packing human cone photoreceptors of geometry with eccentricity variation and evidence of the local anisotropy. Visual Neuroscience. 1992;**9**:169-180

[8] Godara P, Siebe C, Rha J, Michaelides M, Carroll J. Assessing the photoreceptor mosaic over drusen using adaptive optics and SD-OCT. Ophthalmic Surgery, Lasers & Imaging. 2010;**41**:S104-S108

[9] Godara P, Wagner-Schuman M, Rha J, Connor TB Jr, Stepien KE, Carroll J. Imaging the photoreceptor mosaic with adaptive optics: Beyond counting cones. Advances in Experimental Medicine and Biology. 2012;**723**:451-458

[10] Okabe BA, B. and Sugihara, K. Spatial Tessellations: Concepts and Applications of Voronoi diagrams. New York: Wiley; 1992

[11] Sudbø J, Marcelponil Reith R. New algorithms based on the Voronoi diagram applied in a pilot study on normal mucosa and carcinomas. Analytical Cellular Pathology. 2000;**21**: 71-86

[12] Chiu SN. Spatial point pattern analysis by using Voronoi diagrams and Delanuay tessellations, a comparative study. The Biochemical Journal. 2003;**45**: 367-376

[13] Headington K, Choi SS, Nickla D, Doble N. Single cell imaging of the chick retina with adaptive optics. Current Eye Research. 2011;**36**(10):947-957

[14] Kisilak ML, Bunghardt K, Hunter JJ, Irving EL, Campbell MC. Longitudinal in vivo imaging of cones in the alert chicken. Optometry and Vision Science. 2012;**89**(5):644-651

[15] Pinelis I. A characterization of the convexity of polygons in terms of cyclic center angles. Journal of Geometry. 2007;**87**(1):106-119

[16] Rossi C, Strettoi E, Galli-Resta L. The spatial order of horizontal cells is not

affected by massive alterations in the organization of other retinal cells. The Journal of Neuroscience. 2003;**23**(30): 9924-9928

[17] Khiripe N, Khantuwan W, Jungck JR. Ka-me: A Voronoi image analyzer. Bioinformatics. 2012;**28**(13):1802-1804

[18] Cooper RF, Langlo CS, Dubra A, Carroll J. Automatic detection of modal spacing (Yellott's ring) in adaptive optics scanning light ophthalmoscope image. Ophthalmic & Physiological Optics. 2013;**33**(4):540-549

[19] Marcelpoil., R. and Usson, Y. Methods for the study of cellular sociology: Voronoi diagrams and parametrization of spatial relationships. Journal of Theoretical Biology. 1992;**154**: 359-369

[20] Chalmeta R, Hurtado F, Sacristan V, Saumell M. Measuring regularity of convex polygons. Computer-Aided Desing. 2013;**45**:93-104

[21] Soliman MK, Sadiq MA, Agarwal A, Sarwar S, Hassan M, Hanout M, et al. High-resolution imaging of parafoveal cones in different stages of diabetic retinopathy using adaptive optics fundus camera. PLoS One. 2016;**11**:1-13

[22] Curcio CA, Sloan KR, Kalina RE, Hendrickson AE. Human photoreceptor topography. Journal of Comparative Neurology. 1990;**292**(4):497-523

[23] Li KY, Roorda A. Automated identification of cone photoreceptors in adaptive optics retinal images. Journal of the Optical Society of America. A. 2007; **24**:1358-1363

[24] Wojtas DH, Wu B, Ahnelt PK, Bones PJ, Millane RP. Automated analysis of differential interference contrast microscopy images of the foveal cone mosaic. Journal of the Optical Society of America. A. 2008;**25**: 1181-1189

[25] da Fontoura CL, Oliveira Bonci DM, Saito CA, de Farias Rocha FA, de Lima Silveira LC, Ventura DF. Voronoi analysis uncovers relationship between mosaics of normally placed and displaced amacrine cells in the thraira retina. Neuroinformatics. 2005;**5**:59-77

[26] Hendrickson AE, Youdelis C. The morphological development of the human fovea. Ophthalmology. 1984;**91**: 603-612

[27] Chui TYP, Song H, Burns S. Adaptive-optics imaging of human cone photoreceptor distribution. Journal of the Optical Society of America. A. 2008; **25**:3021-3029

[28] Williams DR. Topography of the foveal cone mosaic in the living human eye. Vision Research. 1988;**28**:433-454

[29] Pum D, Ahnelt PK, Grasl M. Iso-orientation areas in the foveal cone mosaic. Visual Neuroscience. 1990;**5**: 511-523

[30] Lombardo M, Serrao S, Ducoli P, Lombardo G. Eccentricity dependent changes of density, spacing and packing arrangement of parafoveal cones. Ophthalmic & Physiological Optics. 2013;**33**:516-526

[31] Goebel W, Kretzchmar-Gross T. Retinal thickness in diabetic retinopathy: A study using optical coherence tomography (OCT). Retina. 2002;**22**: 759-767

[32] Curcio CA, Millican CL, Allen KA, Kalina RE. Aging of the human photoreceptor mosaic: Evidence for selective vulnerability of rods in central

retina. Investigative Ophthalmology & Visual Science. 1993;**34**:3278-3296

[33] Francis PJ, Appukuttan B, Simmons E. Rhesus monkeys and humans share common susceptibility genes for age-related macular disease. Human Molecular Genetics. 2008;**17**: 2673-2680

[34] Ulshafer RJ, Engel HM, Dawson WW, Allen CB, Kessler MJ. Macular degeneration in a community of rhesus monkeys: Ultrastructural observations. Retina. 1987;**7**:198-203

[35] Ordy JM, Brizzee KR, Hansche J. Visual-acuity and foveal cone density in the retina of the aged rhesus-monkey. Neurobiology of Aging. 1980;**1**:133-140

[36] Gartner S, Henkind P. Aging and degeneration of the human macula. 1. Outer nuclear layer and photoreceptors. The British Journal of Ophthalmology. 1981;**65**:23-28

[37] Keunen JEE, Norren DV, Meel GJV. Density of foveal cone pigments at older age. Investigative Ophthalmology & Visual Science. 1987;**28**:985-991

[38] Kilbride PE, Hutman LP, Fishman M, Read JS. Foveal cone pigment density difference in the aging human eye. Vision Research. 1986;**26**: 321-325

[39] Elsner AE, Burns SA, Beausencourt E, Weiter JJ. Foveal cone photopigment distribution: Small alterations associated with macular pigment distribution. Investigative Ophthalmology & Visual Science. 1998; **39**:2394-2404

[40] Gorrand JM, Delori FC. Reflectance and curvature of the inner limiting membrane at the foveola. Journal of the Optical Society of America. A. 1999;**16**: 1229-1237

[41] Bone R, Landrum J, Fernandez L, Tarsis S. Analysis of the macular pigment by HPLC: Retinal distribution and age study. Investigative Ophthalmology & Visual Science. 1988;**29**:843-849

[42] Chang Y, Lee FL, Chen SJ, Chen SF. Optical measurement of human retinal macular pigment and its spatial distribution with age. Medical Physics. 2002;**29**:2621-2628

[43] Delori FC. Autofluorescence method to measure macular pigment optical densities fluorometry and autofluorescence imaging. Archives of Biochemistry and Biophysics. 2004;**430**: 156-162

[44] Stitt AW, Lois N, Medina RJ, Adamson P, Curtis TM. Advances in our understanding of diabetic retinopathy. Clinical Science (London, England). 2013;**125**:1-17

[45] El Rami H, Barham R, Sun JK, Silva PS. Evidence-based treatment of diabetic retinopathy. Seminars in Ophthalmology. 2017;**32**:67-74

[46] Rajalakshmi R, Prathiba V, Mohan V. Does tight control of systemic factors help in the management of diabetic retinopathy? Indian Journal of Ophthalmology. 2016;**64**:62-68

[47] Schorr SG, Hammes HP, Müller UA, Abholz HH, Landgraf R, Bertram B. The prevention and treatment of retinal complications in diabetes. Deutsches Ärzteblatt International. 2016;**113**: 816-823

[48] Lechner J, O'Leary OE, Stitt AW. The pathology associated with diabetic retinopathy. Vision Research. 2017;**139**: 7-14

[49] Chen M, Stitt A. Animal models of diabetic retinopathy. In: Chan CC, editor. Animal Models of Ophthalmic Diseases. Cham: Springer International Publishing; 2016. pp. 67-83

[50] Li KY, Roorda A. Automated identification of cone photoreceptors in adaptive retinal images. Journal of the Optical Society of America. A. 2007;**24**:5

[51] Galli-Resta L, Resta G, Tan S-S, Reese B. Mosaics of Islet-1 expressing amacrine cells assembled by short range cellular interactions. The Journal of Neuroscience. 1997;**17**:7831-7838

[52] Galli-Resta L. Assembling the vertebrate retina: Global patterning from short-range cellular interactions. Neurology Report. 2001;**12**:A103-A106

[53] Yunpeng D, Veenstra A, Palczewski K, Kerna TS. Photoreceptor cells are major contributors to diabetes-induced oxidative stress and local inflammation in the retina. Proceedings of the National Academy of Sciences of the United States of America. 2013;**41**: 16586-16591